Chinese Traditional Herbal Medicine
Vol 1. Diagnosis and Treatment

Michael Tierra, L.Ac., OMD, A.H.G.
and Lesley Tierra, L.Ac., A.H.G.

LOTUS
PRESS

DISCLAIMER

This book is a reference work, not intended to diagnose, prescribe or treat. The information contained herein is in no way to be considered as a substitute for consultation with a qualified health-care professional.

First Edition 1998
Printed in the United States of America

ISBN 978-0-9149-5531-3
Library of Congress Catalogue Number 98-66146

DEDICATION

To Dr. Miriam Lee, a courageous pioneer of Traditional Chinese Medicine in California. Suffering legal harassment in the early years, she most generously and openly shared her wisdom and skill with a whole generation of Western practitioners, who revere her with great honor and respect.

ACKNOWLEDGMENTS

Dr. Naixin Hu, TCM Doctor and former professor of herbal medicine at the Traditional Chinese Medical College in Shanghai, for critically reviewing and contributing many valuable suggestions.

Thomas Garan, who helped in compiling and editing many portions of the text.

Bill Schoenbart, TCM practitioner, who was able to bring his deep understanding of Traditional Chinese Medicine and his skill as an editor to this book.

Ewan Klein, TCM practitioner in Scotland, who helped review the manuscript.

Marjorie Wolfe who helped with the editing and collating of the text and thus developed her computer skills.

Baba Hari Das, Yogi and Healer for his inspiration and transmission of yogic pranayamas.

CONTENTS

FOREWORD

Chinese Herbal Medicine, one of the most precious resources from my mother country, is finally beginning to achieve the recognition it deserves in the Western world. Today we see how not only acupuncturists, but a wide range of health care practitioners, including medical doctors, herbalists, chiropractors, nutritionists, and midwives, are increasingly using Chinese herbs for their patients. Acupuncture has been well known for some time as an independent health care method, but people are just now beginning to understand more clearly that acupuncture and herbal medicine are the two parts of a complete system of healing, called Traditional Chinese Medicine (TCM).

The organization of training in Chinese medical universities can give some insight into the scope and depth of TCM, and the balance between the different parts of TCM. Each province in China has one government sponsored University of TCM. The largest in Beijing has a staff of several thousand, maintains a large hospital, and runs more than a dozen independent research institutes.

There are usually three departments: Materia Medica, Acupuncture and Herbal Medicine. The Materia Medica department is concerned with pharmacological and botanical descriptions ofthe herbal medicines, plant collection, storage and preparation. Graduates get four years of training, and occupy positions similar to pharmacists here. They also carry out scientific research to ensure safety and efficacy of the herbal materials. They do not prescribe. Students in the acupuncture department study for 5 years, with the same basic medical theory as herbal doctors, but with more attention on needling and less on herbs. Their training is similar in format to graduates of American acupuncture schools, but one to two years longer. The department of herbal medicine is by far the largest university department, typically occupying approximately 60% of the classroom space, compared to 25% for materia medica, and perhaps only about 15% for acupuncture. This is quite the reverse in the West where acupuncture has thus far defined the public and legal recognition of TCM.

It is my one sadness that Chinese herbalism has not yet achieved its own independent prominence, as befits its stature in China. Only recently with the separate certification by the National Commission for the Certification of Acupuncturists (NCCA) has there been a separate testing and certification procedure for the certification of Chinese herbalists. While not officially recognized in all states, it nevertheless easily and facilely establishes the possibility for the recognition of a professional class of herbalists in America, albeit Chinese herbalists. It is up to the new generation of herbalists to form these laws. TCM students of the herbal medicine department major in herbal medicine, minor in acupuncture, and, after graduation, prescribe herbal medicines to their patients. Unlike in the West--where there is huge schism between traditional medicine and conventional Western allopathic medicine--TCM doctors occupy positions equal in stature to the Western style family doctors. They practice side by side as equals in all Chinese hospitals under the combined Western/TCM system throughout China. What a great benefit to our Western patients if there was greater acceptance, respect and dialogue between Western and Traditional doctors. If more Western doctors could learn to embrace the well established efficacy of TCM, there would be much less abuse of extreme therapeutic procedures and the unnecessary use of conventional Western drugs for conditions that herbs or acupuncture could better treat. After all, Chinese herbs excel at nourishing and detoxifying the body at a deep and fundamental level, and supported in this way the body has a much greater capacity to heal itself; can anyone deny this truism? Western medicine, in contradistinction, is powerful and heroic, and able to maintain life in times of severe crisis or dysfunction. Yet it is difficult to name a single prescription pharmaceutical which can nourish the lungs,the kidney, the heart or the Spirit in order to prevent the onset of crisis.

From my years of teaching herbal medicine to Europeans studying at the Chengdu University of TCM (Sichuan province), and my more recent experiences treating Westerners at Chrysalis Natural Medicine Center in Wilmington, Delaware, I have become acutely aware of the problems confronting Western students of Chinese Herbal Medicine. Even for the Chinese student, it is a formidable task, requiring 5 years of medical school, with 6-8 hours a day of study, six days a week. Their training covers TCM medical theory, pharmacology, acupuncture, internal medicine, diagnostics, and prescription formulation. Students must be able to read, comprehend, and recite passages from the ancient textbooks (many written in our Classical language), and know the properties and uses of over 1,000 herbal medicines and hundreds of formulas. Recently standards have been increased, with several years of postgraduate study, including study of Western medicine, necessary to become a doctor. How much more difficult it must be for the Westerner, who does not have direct access to the literature, the herbal medicine university, or the teaching hospital.

Chinese Medicine has faced many challenges over the centuries, from political opposition in the past to the recent opposition of those claiming that it has no basis in science. Yet it has met and overcome all of those challenges, and is now flourishing allover the world, in large part due to the efforts of the many pioneers who have strived, at great cost and effort to themselves, to bring the knowledge of the healing powers of Chinese herbs to the aid of those who are suffering and sick. I consider my close friends and colleagues Michael Tierra and Lesley Tierra to be two of those pioneers. Michael, after distinguishing himself more than thirty years ago in the field of Western herbalism, was among the small group of visionaries who recognized the importance of Chinese herbalism at that time, and along with his wife, Lesley, were among the handful who have steadfastly pursued the arduous task of mastering the essence of that knowledge. Their new work, written in their characteristicly clear and lucid style, will bring a wealth of traditional knowledge to all those fortunate enough to realize its significance.

Naixin Hu, OMD
L.Ac Co-director of Chrysalis Natural Medicine Center
Former Acupuncturist to the Royal Family of Egypt

INTRODUCTION

The inspiration for this book grew out of a need for an accessible and comprehensive introductory text which would combine all the most salient aspects of Traditional Chinese Herbalism, such as the history, theory, diagnosis, Materia Medica, formulary, dietary guidelines and treatment protocols. After years of teaching Chinese Herbalism through the East West correspondence course and the American School of Herbalism, it became obvious that there was a need for a single volume that includes all the information needed by a new student.

The basis of Chinese medical theory is rooted in Confucian, Taoist and Buddhist philosophy. The perspective is always one of activating and supplementing the body's innate healing capacity to restore biological balance and harmony. From there, it extends to assume universal value and meaning beyond cultural and philosophical sectarianism. The theories and principles of Traditional Chinese Medicine (TCM) are being successfully applied to the use of Western drug therapy, vitamins, minerals and other supplements. Chinese physiology, as described in this book from a TCM perspective, has been fully validated in our own research to reflect the most profound and significant aspects of Western physiology. The difference is simply that the orientation of TCM is more functional, referring to in-depth physiological interactions, while Western scientific physiology is more mechanically specific.

For example, when reading the description of the meaning of the Kidneys in the chapter describing the TCM definition of the Organs, it can be seen that besides the actual function of the anatomical kidneys, the TCM Kidneys include the adrenal glands and the entire endocrine system. Another great Organ constellation of TCM is the Spleen. The Western spleen is a blood and lymphatic organ while the TCM Spleen, by interpreting its designations, refers to the pancreas as well as the most fundamental aspects of cellular metabolism.

So why is this important, one may ask? Why are such seemingly imprecise descriptions of two well known physiological organs, expressed in obtuse TCM jargon, useful to the Western physiologist-researcher or to the most fundamental understanding of medical practice throughout the world? To resort to the well known cliché, "the proof is in the pudding." If by applying the principles of TCM we are able to utilize therapies, treatments and herbs to safely and effectively benefit the endocrine glands or strengthen cellular metabolism, two mechanisms which have profound significance in terms of maintaining health, optimal longevity, and successful treatment of what are regarded as incurable conditions, this would be a definite enhancement of all systems of medical practice. Economically it is of tremendous advantage since the practice of TCM, unlike contemporary Western medicine, is remarkably low-tech. Biochemists and pharmaceutical companies, if they were liberated from current economic demands and constraints, could investigate the traditional indications of Chinese herbs to understand deep complex physiological responses and processes. These qualities make a particular herb, such as Astragalus membranaceus (Huang Qi), beneficial for the immune system and cellular metabolism), or Rehmannia glutinosa (Sheng Di Huang or Shu Di Huang) a safer and less crippling alternative treatment strategy to the use of cortisone.

The most important aspect of traditional Chinese herbal medicine that will probably take most people more than a lifetime is the art of diagnosis. It is one thing to present all the various aspects of it in a text, but altogether another to be capable of evaluating the information derived from an assessment of symptoms to arrive at a successful therapeutic result. This can only come from experience and practical hands-on guidance from an experienced practitioner.

To learn Chinese medicine one must be guided, at least in the beginning years, to focus on narrowing down centuries of accumulated knowledge to what is essential for beginning practice. Eventually one must learn nearly 400 herbs in the Materia Medica and at least 50 to 100 formulas with possible variations.

Today we see attempts, including in our own books, *Planetary Herbology* and *The Herbs of Life,* to expand the practice of Chinese Herbalism to include herbs and healing modalities from around the world and several healing disciplines. While doing this, it must be remembered that Chinese Herbalism, while capable at least theoretically of such expansion, is a circular system where theory, energetics, diagnosis and practice are all interdependent. An energetic system such as Chinese Herbalism is complete in itself because it attempts to describe dynamic living relationships between all aspects of human existence.

Despite the necessity to achieve precision, diagnosis, as important as it is, becomes only a prelude or hypothetical strategy for treatment. Just as all herbalism is fundamentally empirical, the success of a diagnosis is always tested in the result of treatment. From that perspective, Yin or Yang Deficiency, for instance, has no further meaning than if through the use of appropriate Yin or Yang tonics we are able to achieve a successful result. For this reason, Chinese herbalism can seem ambiguous and confusing because, with the centuries of accumulated information, it virtually has an infinite number of strategies that can be applied to diagnosis and treatment.

The practice of Chinese Herbalism is like a detective mystery where diagnosis becomes the gathering of evidence. Differential diagnosis means that no single piece of evidence necessarily tells all. One interprets a particular TCM condition based on the primary complaint, after which it is confirmed through the process of assessing the various patterns, conditions and pulse and tongue signs. For this, the most important tool is our discretionary powers of observation and evaluation. There is a considerable level of subjective evaluation, but there must always be enough objective evidence in order to initiate an effective treatment.

Another vision that led to writing this book was to describe the holistic aspect of TCM through the integration of complementary healing modalities, including diet, exercise, lifestyle and meditation. Too often we have seen patients who have received acupuncture and/or herbal treatment with poor results because the diet or some other lifestyle factor was not appropriately modified. The ancient approach of TCM further included emotional and spiritual aspects of living, Barefoot Doctor techniques such as moxibustion, dermal hammer, scraping and cupping and therapeutic exercises, like Tai Chi and Qi Gong. While it is not within the scope of this book to be exhaustive in all these aspects, we feel that we present enough of these accessory healing modalities to provide an integrated therapeutic model for including these therapies along with the specific indicated herbal formulas for each of the disease pattern syndromes.

Like the writing of any such book, this has been a particularly laborious process which we sincerely hope will meet with appreciation by students and practitioners who desire to learn one of the most inspired natural healing systems on earth.

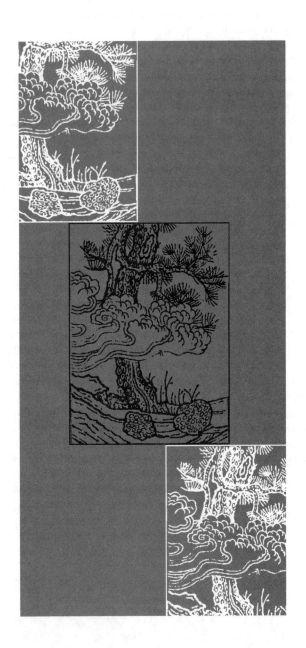

ONE

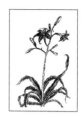

HISTORY OF CHINESE HERBALISM

As with all traditional cultures, the knowledge of the therapeutic properties of plants and other natural substances is empirical. This means that the knowledge of their properties and uses was and still is primarily based upon trial and error. At first the experience of the uses of herbs was passed down orally. Later, the accumulated knowledge of their therapeutic effects was written.

The earliest recorded Chinese herbal was the *Shen Nong Pen T'sao Jing* or Emperor Shen Nong's Classic Herbal. Shen Nong, the God-Farmer, was one of three legendary kings of ancient Chinese history. He was also known as Di Huang, King of the Earth, while the other two were Tian Huang, the King of Heaven, and Ren Huang, the King of Humans.

Before Shen Nong, Chinese society was based on hunting and gathering. Legend states that to encourage greater social stability and continuity, Shen Nong was the first to teach farming and agriculture to the Chinese people. In addition, he was also the first to bestow upon them the knowledge of medicinal herbs. The legend goes on to state that because of his compassion for the sick, each day he would go into the fields and forests and poison himself a hundred times by tasting various plants and substances, each time finding a natural antidote. The result of Shen Nong's discoveries was the knowledge of the healing properties of plants, which were first recorded in the *Shen Nong Pen T'sao*, meaning Shen Nong's Herbal.

Out of myth and legend, Chinese herbalism evolved, and every official herbal has since been titled Pen T'sao in honor of Shen Nong's contribution. The first *Shen Nong Pen T'sao* published in 200 BC was lost, but subsequent references inform us that it contained 365 herbs. These were subdivided as follows: 120 emperor herbs of high, food grade quality which are non-toxic and can be taken in large quantities to maintain health over a long period of time; 120 minister herbs, some mildly toxic and some not, that have stronger therapeutic action to heal diseases; and 125 servant herbs that have specific actions to treat disease and eliminate Stagnation. Most of those in the last group are toxic and are not intended to be used daily over a prolonged period of weeks and months.

Hua Tuo (100-208 AD) is regarded as one of the greatest acupuncturists and surgeons of Chinese medical history. He is famous for the discovery and use of a special set of accessory points along the spine which are called "Hua-Tuo" points. He was also a highly skilled herbalist.

There is a famous story that describes the psychological aspect of healing that was part of his practice. It involved a famous governor who, having been sick for a prolonged period, bestowed generous gifts on his renowned physician, Hua Tuo, in expectation of herbal treatment. The governor eventually became increasingly frustrated and angry because, despite his lavish endowments, Hua Tuo did not give any medicine to relieve his malady. In fact, he would taunt and scoff at the governor. This eventually resulted in the necessity of Hua Tuo having to flee the district for his life to escape the governor's wrath. Fortunately, the governor was unable to apprehend the exiled Hua Tuo. His anger, however, rose to such a pitch of intensity that he vomited dark bile and blood, after which he completely recovered.

Between 220 and 589 AD, China was once again wracked by civil wars. As a result, the *Shen Nong Pen T'sao Jing* was threatened by abuse and neglect. During this time Buddhism was promulgated throughout the Northern and Southern Dynasties of China. Northern Chinese society was strongly influenced by the cultures of the steppe and the Sino-Tibetan frontier region, tended to lack strong central direction, and was warlike and illiterate. In contrast, the Southern Dynasty situated around the Yangtse basin was aristocratic and sophisticated. Famous Buddhist caves with giant carvings were created as natural sanctuaries, and the emperor came to be regarded as the living Buddha. There was a wide dissemination of knowledge between distant cultures as Chinese monks such as Faxian ventured into India during the 5th century, and Indian monks of the 6th century disseminated Indian culture throughout China. Because of commercial trading, there were also influences to and from Japan, Korea and far-off Arab lands.

During this time alchemy was further developed. Taoism, medicine and alchemy being closely linked, the Taoist quest for longevity begun in earlier times persisted with research and experimentation in the consumption of cinnabar that unfortunately led to a plethora of characteristic symptoms of mercury toxicity prevalent at this time.

With the interest in alchemy came the development of pharmaceutical science and the creation of a number of books, including

Tao Hong Jing's (456-536) compilation of the *Pen T'sao Jing Ji Zhu* (Commentaries on the Herbal Classic), based on the *Shen Nong Pen T'sao Jing*. In that book 730 herbs were described and classified in six categories: 1) stones and metals (minerals), 2) grasses and trees, 3) insects and animals, 4) herbs, fruits and vegetables, 5 grains, 6) named but unused. This has become the most influential and oldest herbal still intact to be found in the Tun Huang District northwest of Kansu Province.

Because of frequent wars, medicine developed to the extent that the first Chinese text on surgery was written during this time. Another contribution of the Chinese Middle Ages was the establishment of the first formal Chinese medical school, created in 443 by the Emperor's physician Qin Chengzu. Before this time medical knowledge was exclusively passed down from master to pupil.

During the 2nd century, Wang Shuhe compiled all previously known knowledge of the pulse in his famous *Maijing* (Pulse Classic). This in turn led to the introduction of pulse diagnosis into Arabic medicine.

The Tang Dynasty (618-907) is regarded as the greatest dynasty in Chinese history because of the many contributions to art, medicine and the sciences made during that period. The *Tang Xin Pen T'sao* (Tang Materia Medica), the official materia medica of the Tang Dynasty, was China's first illustrated herbal and contained 844 entries. Besides officially sanctioned herbals, many works by independent citizens were also generated during the Tang, including the *Yue Xing Pen T'sao* (The Book of Herb Properties) by Zhen Quan. It was when Zhen Quan was 120 years old that Emperor Tai Zong (629-649) visited him and the aged herbalist bestowed his herbal upon the Emperor.

Sun Simiao (581-682), regarded as the King of Doctors, was perhaps the most popular figure in Chinese medicine. Having steeped himself in the three pillars of Chinese wisdom based on Confucianism, Taoism and Buddhism, Sun, being of fragile health, decided to dedicate his life to the study and practice of medicine.

Sun refused tempting offers of wealth and prestige from various emperors of the time to live the life of a humble country doctor. As a result Sun Simiao is revered as a great humanitarian. His practice and knowledge are known only through two works, *Qianjin Yaofang* (Prescriptions of the Thousand Ounces of Gold) and *Qianjin Yifang* (Supplement). Because Sun regarded human life as precious, the term gold reflects his regard for human life.

Sun regarded the integration of acupuncture, moxibustion and the use of drugs as a complete system of medicine. Relying solely on the

Four Methods of Diagnosis (observation, listening, interrogating and palpation), Sun considered that pulse should only be studied after listening to the patient, observing the tone of voice and complexion. He also strongly advocated prevention and pre-diagnosis to be superior than the treatment of disease. The ideal physician, Sun Simiao's interest and influence extended to his incorporation of the principles of the Shang Han Lun, proper harvesting of medicinal plants, the causes of disease and his enthusiastic advocation of maternal and infant care.

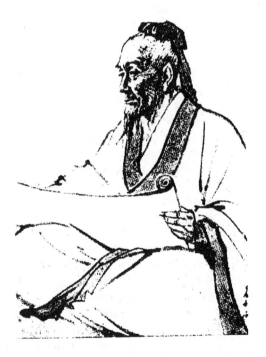

Sun Simiao

In *Qian Jin Shi Zhi*, Sun said: "In the old days, herbalists collected herbs themselves at the right time and in the right place, and they processed the herbs properly. That is why they were able to cure nine out of ten of their patients. Nowadays, doctors only know how to prescribe. Most of the herbs they are using were not collected and processed properly so they can only cure five or six out of ten of their patients." More than any of his particular contributions, the exalted personage of integrity, compassion and benevolence of Sun Simiao remains as a shining influence and ideal for the future practice of medicine.

During the Song dynasty (960-1279), the first herbal that was officially published was the *Kai Bao Pen T'sao* (Kai Bao was the name of the emperor of that time) in 973. It was later revised and enlarged by the Taoist, Liu Han, and others and published as *Kai Bao Zhong Ding Pen T'sao* (Revised Kai Bao Herbal).

In 1552, during the later Ming Dynasty (1368-1644), another one of the greatest Chinese herbalists, Li Shi Zhen (1518-1593) began work on the monumental *Pen T'sao Kan Mu* (Herbal with Commentary). Li dedicated his life to travel throughout the distant reaches of the empire to consult directly with people in many places regarding local remedies. He further consulted 277 herbals as references, as well as the classics, histories and many other books — a total of approximately 440 in all. After 27 years and three revisions, the *Pen T'sao Kan Mu* was completed in 1578. The book lists 1892 drugs, 376 described for the first time, with 1160 drawings. It also lists more than 11,000 prescriptions.

Li's compilation of the *Pen T'sao Kan Mu* represented an attempt to correct the errors of his predecessors regarding the names and descriptions of medical substances. He also carefully noted the time and methods of harvest and the preparation and use of drugs. He derided as foolish the belief that the Ling Zhi mushroom (Reishi or Ganoderma lucidum), could prevent death. Besides his monumental Materia Medica, Li Shi Zhen was also the author of the *Binhu Maixue* (A Study of the Pulse) and *Qijing Bamai Kao* (An Examination of the Eight Extra Meridians). During his lifetime he was also regarded as a great physician who set forth the hitherto unique concept of the brain as the location of the principal vital influence, i.e., mental awareness. Li relied heavily on the classics, the *Huangdi Neijing* and the *Shang Han Lun,* yet maintained a fresh critical stance whenever he personally observed in practice situations and conditions that were at variance with tradition. Among his many contributions to pathology was his observation of cholelithiasis as a disease distinct from mere hypochondriac or epigastric pain. He also promoted the use of ice to bring down fever and the technique of disinfection which involved soaking patient's clothes in a steam bath to protect family members from contamination. To protect patients from epidemic disease, Li advocated the burning of Atractylodes lancea (Cang Zhu) as a fumigant.

As with Sun Simiao and other great Chinese physicians, Li attributed greater significance to prevention than cure, following the approach of the *Neijing*, which states: "To cure disease is like waiting until one is thirsty before digging a well, or to fabricate weapons after the war has commenced." Thus the *Pen T'sao Kang Mu* lists more than 500 remedies to maintain and strengthen the body, with over 50 of these created by Li Shi Zhen himself. He described the use and preparation of a wide variety of preparations, including ointments, pills and powders, and recommended the preparation of various medicinal broths with herbs, including wheat, rice, chestnut, radish, garlic, ginger and vital organs and parts of various animals.

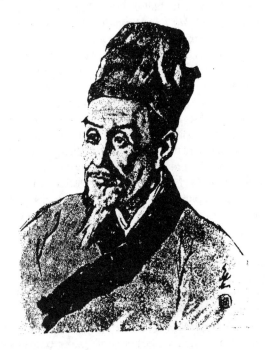

Li Shi Zhen

Li Shi Zhen was a great pharmacognocist, pharmacologist, physician, zoologist, botanist and mineralogist and made a profound and lasting contribution to humanity as well as the Chinese people in particular. Like Sun Simiao, he was also a great humanitarian with high Confucian-inspired medical ethics, promoting all to the care and welfare of their fellow humanity. The most popular image we have of him is observing the flower of the Datura.

During the Qing dynasty, beginning in 1644 to the first Opium war in 1839-42, more than 20 herbals were published. These included the *Pen T'sao Kan Mu Shi Yi* (Herbs Not Listed in the Pen T'sao Cao Kang Mu). During this period European influence gradually spread into China. The *Huangdi Neijing* (Yellow Emperor's Classic of Internal Medicine) became recognized as the bible of Chinese medicine, with wide interest from commentators extending from the 17th to the 19th century. The fame and reputation of the *Shang Han Lun* as well as the companion book, *Chin Kuei Yao Lueh* (Prescriptions from the Golden Chamber), both by Chan Chung Ching, also grew during this period. One of the most important evolutions that occurred during this period was the treatment of diseases caused by Heat, in contrast to the Shang Han Lun (Cold induced diseases). While the notion of Heat as a Pathogenic Influence was first formulated by Liu Wansu, it became more firmly established as a Pathogenic Influence during the 17th century, when Wou Youxin postulated and observed the effect of epidemic pestilence and plague as Heat diseases entering through the mouth and nose.

From 1842-44 various treaties, missionaries and foreign doctors established hospitals, treaty ports and the translation of Western medical works. Chinese doctors began to be educated in Western medicine and were even sent abroad to study. Along with Western medicine, the practice of Chinese medicine, based on time honored tradition, continued throughout the period from 1840 to 1911. The physician Zhu Peiwen, author of *Huayang Zangxiang Yuezuan* (1892), conceptualized a comparative understanding of the Organs based on Chinese and Western concepts. He decided that there were both advantages and disadvantages to Chinese and Western approaches.

From 1911 to 1949, with the establishment of the People's Republic, the nationalist government under Sun Yat-sen declared in 1924 that China must grasp the initiative and not remain backward. Since Sun Yat-sen received Western-style medical training, he probably was a strong advocate of establishing Western medicine as the primary medical approach. There were considerable benefits in improved public hygiene, especially in urban areas, with clear running water and the establishment of a central bureau to help combat epidemics. In rural China, however, Traditional Chinese Medicine continued to be practiced, with training continuing to be based on student apprenticeship.

It was the vision of Mao Zedong, who declared Traditional Chinese Medicine a national treasure, that we must strive to explore it fully and raise it to a higher level. As a result, Traditional Chinese Medicine represents an attempt to rationalize Chinese Medicine with Western scientific medicine, by initiating state sponsored research of herbs and treatments and downplaying the role of Taoist-Buddhist psycho-spiritual practices. With the introduction of TCM in the West, there is currently a renewed interest in the value of a psycho-spiritual orientation to the treatment of disease, which is the original basis of Chinese Medicine.

TWO

THE THEORY OF YIN AND YANG

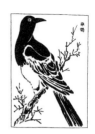

The practice of Traditional Chinese Medicine seeks to understand and evaluate the state of balance or imbalance of a person using the bipolar principle of Yin and Yang. Yin is the expression of the receptive or passive polarity, while Yang is an expression of the aggressive or active polarity. In terms of Chinese herbalism, Yin embodies the qualities of cold, damp, immobility and substance, while Yang embodies the qualities of warmth, dryness, movement and ephemerality. Yin is like a vessel that receives the energy or Qi of life, while Yang is that which warms, enlivens and circulates.

Following the paradigm of Yin and Yang, all herbs and foods as well as physiological symptoms are classified as Hot or Cold, Dry or Damp, External-acute or Internal-chronic, heavy or light. Also included are various pscho-physiological qualities such as aggressive or timid, happy or sad, and so forth. Rather than limiting diagnosis to specifically named pathologies, the symptoms and signs of imbalance in terms of the various Yin-Yang diagnostic parameters are truly wholistic and specifically interconnect with the use of herbs, foods, exercise and lifestyle to restore balance and health.

Even beyond this, Yin-Yang is the foundation of Traditional Chinese Medicine. Like the grandest and noblest music of life, the physician's goal, at least from one perspective, is to assist the patient in perceiving and experiencing the underlying harmony and unity through all diverse moods and complexities. In this, it is not unlike one of the great monuments of classical keyboard music, Bach's *Goldberg Variations*, where with repeated hearing, we gradually perceive more of the unity of divine energy or Qi. This is represented by the beginning theme as it evolves, transforms and dances through the moods and complexities of the 30 variations, only to return in the end to the simplicity and purity of the original theme. This great music, like our life, seems to exist as a compelling challenge from some unknown source. We are able to witness the myriad diversity of things, through the various signs and symptoms of TCM, to reconnect with our inner and outer nature and to help reestablish our experience of unity and wholeness.

Is this not also in harmony with the inner meaning of healing, which is "to make whole", to perceive those finely woven strands of themes and melodies that weave in and out of each life, along with their many contrasting moods, as a variation or phase of the greater whole? It is sad to consider that perhaps many of us may never reach the point in our lifetime were we can perceive the essential purity of existence in this way, as we become entranced with the eternal Yin-Yang dance where action continually engenders reaction. Disease becomes, then, the ultimate challenge to make our peace, within and without, to finally return to an awareness of what is of essential importance throughout. It is out of the perception of that greater unity that the wise physician invokes all three kingdoms of nature; in the process selecting those particular foods and herbs from the vegetable kingdom, minerals from the mineral kingdom and parts from the animal kingdom as a gesture of healing reintegration.

All life is a dance, as we continuously posture and reposition ourselves with all the elements of our lives, our ancestry and parentage, our food, our personal relationships, our work, and the climate we live - all the unique stresses and stimuli that sometimes propel us forward while at other times seem to cause us to bog down. It is the play of light and dark and of all the dual expressions of Yin and Yang dancing through the elements of physical manifestation.

From the beginning to the end we have universal life energy or Qi connecting and animating all phenomena. Then what need is there to presume a personal divine hand in it? The occasional sounding of a compassionate note in the harmonies of one variation or a caring glance from a friend or healer should be enough to intuit the presence of the divine as a positive motivating spirit underlying the music of life.

Even if there were no other practical value associated with the study of Traditional Chinese Medicine other than its ability to train the senses to perceive the expression of Qi or vital energy throughout all of nature, this alone would make it a worthwhile endeavor. However, there are the practical rewards of being able to enlist the healing forces of nature for the benefit of ourselves and others that deeply adds to our experience.

Taoism, the religious philosophy from which TCM emanates, believes that Qi is equivalent to the Great Spirit of creation. And so, the closeness of the Great Spirit to our very essence is reflected in the fact that Qi also connotes 'breath' in Chinese, which in turn is similar to the Yogic definition of 'Prana' or 'life breath'. Beyond this, according to the Hindus, lies the supreme 'Atman' made visible through the eternal dance of Shiva and his consort, Shakti. This would also agree with the old testament, where it is stated that no man has ever seen God or that the Supreme Name of God is unutterable. How could anything so all pervasive and unlimited be adequately conceived in the limited minds of humans, except through intuition? To diverge even further, the Moslems invoke God by the two syllable formula "Al-lah". Here one primal syllable is simply the reverse of the other, reflecting the supreme as the two poles of duality similar to the Chinese concept of Yin-Yang. Yin and Yang is an expression of the natural law of homeostasis. As simply and eloquently stated by T.Y. Pang:[1] " The virtue of Yin is in tranquillity while that of Yang is action. Yang gives life, Yin fosters it; Yang creates, Yin grows; Yang kills, Yin preserves; Yang generates energy, Yin makes form. Yin and Yang are relative and are related. There is Yang within Yin and Yin within Yang."

Yin represents the negative or receptive pole, while Yang is the positive. (The terms negative and positive are not qualitative terms but a simple description of one of the most fundamental laws of the universe.) The Chinese character for Yin literally means the cold, dark, or Northern side of the mountain, while the character for Yang is the sunny, or Southern, side. The ancient Chinese learned to apply the concepts of Yin and Yang to all aspects of natural phenomena, eventually developing the philosophies that became Taoism.

The Taoist priests who developed the principles of herbal medicine based on Yin-Yang theory extended them to the classification of foods, herbs, activities and diagnosis. The ideal was (and still is) to achieve a balance between the outer Yin-Yang influences of diet, activity, environment and seasons and the inner influences of one's constitution.

The balance of Yin and Yang, however elusive it may be to achieve, represents ideal health. Imbalance remains the simplest definition of sickness and disease. Qi is the dynamic energy that is constantly transformed from negative to positive and vice versa as it flows between these two poles.

BACKGROUND

The "Oracle of Changes", known as the *I-Ching*, dates back to around 700 B.C., and is the earliest attempt to graphically represent the various cycles and transformations of Yin into Yang and vice versa. The *I-Ching* utilizes a combination of broken Yin lines and unbroken Yang lines. The addition of a third line in various positions forms eight trigrams. Juxtaposition of these trigrams in various permutations creates the 64 hexagrams that are the basis for the entire book. The significance of the various permutations of broken and unbroken lines graphically represents the various cycles of Yin-Yang transformation. What is most impressive about the study of the *I-Ching* is the insight that Yin-Yang is not static, but a dance of transformation and change. When this process ceases, chaos and death result.

In Western physiology the closest approximation we have to the concept of Yin-Yang is the principle of homeostasis. However, the concept of Yin-Yang explaining the integration and relationship of all natural phenomena in a practical way is unique to Traditional Chinese Medicine.

Many think of traditional Chinese society as fundamentally orderly. Certainly when one considers the many remapping changes that Western European nations have undergone over the last 2000 years, we might agree. On the other hand, as Chinese culture has been able to evolve even through Mongol invasions and even greater devastation wreaked by European influences, the enduring philosophies of Yin-Yang and the Five Elements stand as a testimony to their cohesiveness.

Even in popular Western literature, Chinese heroes and villains behave with great protocol and decorum and follow very specific paths to achieve their goals. This tendency is due to the pervasive influence of Yin-Yang philosophy and Confucianism, which teaches that everything and everyone has its appropriate role, opportunity, time and place.

These great Chinese philosophies evolved in reaction to the early period of total unrest and chaos called the Warring States (476-220 BC). This time was similar to, but even more chaotic than, the Middle Ages of European feudalism. In any case, there arose a profound need for order and a philosophy that would support the establishment of that order.

Political influences not withstanding, Chinese philosophy and medicine are fundamentally holistic, with their roots in nature and empiricism. The Yin-Yang and Five Element doctrines emanated from the so-called Naturalist School, primarily expounded upon by Zou Yan (350-270 BC), and forms the theoretical basis of Traditional Chinese Medicine.

THEORY

Qi and the Yin-Yang theory are the unifying theoretical basis of Traditional Chinese Medicine (TCM) and connect the individual with all aspects of being. The principles are not always easy to apply to the state of a given individual, but the theory in itself represents an essential thought process for gaining an understanding and intuitive feeling for all natural phenomena. To even begin considering things in terms of Yin and Yang is a profound healing idea regardless of the conclusions.

Yang includes the outgoing masculine or motivating force as well as the body's capacity to generate and maintain warmth. It can be equated with hyper-metabolic qualities which affect all organic processes, including warmth, libido, appetite, digestion and assimilation. Its normal manifestation is comparable to our concept of zest for life.

Yin is receptive, fluidic, cooling and equated with hypo-metabolic qualities and conditions. Physiologically it represents innate capacity or substance, including blood and all other fluids in the body. These nourish, nurture and moisten all aspects of the body including the organs and tissues.

There are four major aspects of the Yin-Yang relationship: opposition, interdependence, mutual consumption, and inter-transformation. They are described as follows:

1) **Opposition**: Yin and Yang are opposite states of expression contained in all of life. For example, Heaven is Yang while Earth is Yin, rising is Yang and descending is Yin, outward is Yang and inward is Yin, light is Yang and dark is Yin, activity is Yang and rest is Yin.

In the body, signs that are hot, restless, dry, hard and fast are Yang, such as fever, restless sleep, dry eyes or throat, hard lumps and talking fast. Signs that are cold, quiet, wet, soft and slow are Yin, such as chills, lack of desire to talk, loose stools, soft lumps and walking or talking slowly.

However, Yin and Yang are not absolutes, but relative, as there is a seed of Yang within Yin and vice versa. They are in a dynamic and constantly changing relationship with one another, a flowing balance of many opposite forces. A summary of these opposite forces is as follows:

Qualities:	Yang	Yin
	Heaven	Earth
	sun	moon
	immaterial	material
	generation	growth
	energy	form
	creation	materialization
	activity	rest
Tendency	develop, expand	condense, contract
Position	outward	inward
Structure	time	space
Direction	ascending; right	descending; left

Compass	east, south	west, north
Color	bright	dark
Temperature	hot	cold
Weight	light	heavy
Catalyst	fire	water
Light	light	dark
Construction	exterior	interior
Work	physical	psychological
Attitude	extrovert	introvert
Biological	animal	vegetable
Energy	aggressive	receptive
Nerves	sympathetic	parasympathetic
Tastes	spicy-sweet	sour-bitter-salty
Season	summer	winter

2) **Interdependence**: While opposite qualities of each other, Yin and Yang are also interdependent; one cannot exist without the other. Everything contains these opposite forces which are both mutually exclusive and dependent on one another.

For instance, if the stomach and intestines do not move, food and drink can't be digested or absorbed. Yin (Blood) depends on Yang (Qi) to circulate it throughout the body, while the organs that produce Qi are dependent on Blood to nourish them. Thus, structure (Yin) is dependent on function (Yang) and vice versa. Without structure, the function would not perform while, without function, the structure would lack movement and ability to perform.

The qualities of interdependence of Yin and Yang can be seen in the following theorems:

Theorems of Yin and Yang
1. Infinity divides itself into Yin and Yang.
2. Yin and Yang result from the infinite movement of the Universe.
3. Although they are opposite ends of a continuum, Yin and Yang are complementary and form a unity.
4. Yang contains the seed of Yin and Yin contains the seed of Yang.
5. Yin is centripetal and Yang is centrifugal; together they produce all energy and phenomena.
6. Yin attracts Yang and Yang attracts Yin.
7. Yin repels Yin and Yang repels Yang.

18

8. The force of attraction and repulsion between any two phenomena is proportional to the difference between their Yin-Yang constitution.
9. All things are ephemeral and constantly changing their Yin-Yang constitution.
10. Nothing is neutral; either Yin or Yang is dominant.
11. Nothing is solely Yin or Yang; everything involves polarity.
12. Yin and Yang are relative: large Yin attracts small Yin and large Yang attracts small Yang.
13. At the extreme of manifestation, Yin turns into Yang and Yang turns into Yin.
14. All physical forms are Yin at the center and Yang on the surface.

3) **Inter-transformation**: As stated before, Yin and Yang are dynamic states which actually transform into each other. At their extremes, Yin can change into Yang, and Yang can change into Yin. We are familiar with this in the daily cycles of our lives as night turns into day and then day turns into night; winter eventually turns into summer while summer moves into winter; and birth eventually turns into death.

This waxing and waning of Yin into Yang and vice versa is not random, but only occurs when the condition is ripe for it, when a certain stage of development has been reached. This is experienced in the body when we work without cessation (Yang), ultimately ending up exhausted and depleted (Yin).

In pathological terms, an excess of Cold can change into Heat and vice versa. For instance, a cold may begin with chills and progress to severe fever and even pneumonia. Frostbite can result in a burning inflammation. Heat changing to Cold occurs as a result of an acute inflammatory symptom that weakens the vital force and degenerates to a more chronic, Cold condition. Further, during the course of an extreme fever with restlessness, irritability and a strong pulse (Yang), the patient suddenly becomes listless, the temperature lowers, the face turns pale and the pulse becomes very weak (Yin). In many hot tropical countries, food is heavily spiced with chili peppers. This results in excessive perspiration which makes one feel cooler.

Deficiencies and Excesses can also cause manifestation of their opposites. A Deficiency of Spleen energy can result in an Excess of Dampness, while a Kidney or Liver Yin Deficiency can lead to an Excess of Liver Yang (hypertension).

This thinking also extends to the use of Yin or Yang foods and herbs. Too much Yang sweet flavor will cause Yin exhaustion. Overuse of tonic herbs can have the paradoxical opposite effect of causing exhaustion and stagnation. In excess, extremely hot spices can over-stimulate and exhaust the Qi.

Recognizing that Yin and Yang are mutually transformative is an important way of helping us refrain from overdoing anything that could ultimately upset our balance and health. A summary of the inter-transformation of Yin and Yang is stated in the following Laws:

Laws Governing Yin and Yang
1. All things are the differentiated apparatus of One Infinity.
2. Everything changes.
3. All antagonisms are complementary.
4. No two things are identical.
5. Every condition has its opposite.
6. Extremes always produce their opposite.
7. Whatever begins has an end.

4) **Mutual Consumption:** The dynamic balance of Yin and Yang is maintained by a continuous adjustment of each of their relative levels. In the waxing and waning of the seasons, when winter is ending Yin begins to decrease while Yang increases; when day comes to an end, Yang decreases while Yin increases with the development of night. Thus, while continuously balancing one another, they also consume each other. When one increases the other must decrease: when Yin increases, Yang is consumed, and when Yang increases, Yin is consumed.

In the body this is seen in four possible states of imbalance: Excess of Yin, Excess of Yang, Deficiency of Yin and Deficiency of Yang. Thus, when Yin is in Excess (Cold Dampness, for instance), it consumes the Yang (the warming fires get dampened and put out). Likewise, when Yang becomes Excess (Heat and activity), Yin is consumed and becomes Deficient (exhaustion and weakness).

Further, when Yin is Deficient, it causes Yang to appear greater than it is, while when Yang is Deficient, it causes Yin to appear greater than it is. This gives rise to the terms "false Yin" and "false Yang" as neither is a case of true Yin or Yang Excess, but an apparent state of Excess occurring only because the other is Deficient.

Empty ("*xu*") and full ("*shi*") are further terms used to describe Deficiency and Excess. Because it is important to see the difference between these four states, the following is a more detailed description of their pathological imbalances.

Full Yin imbalances bring about symptoms of excessive fluid retention and lethargy. People experiencing full Yin, or an Excess of Yin, tend to retain water, may be more plump or swollen and have symptoms of Dampness, and yet may have adequate energy. Spicy, warm-natured herbs, such as ginger and cinnamon, and diuretics, such as Fu Ling mushrooms, can help promote the elimination of excess water in such cases.

Empty Yin diseases are strumous (Deficient), involving emaciation and weakness with wasting Heat symptoms, termed "false Yang". Such individuals are nutritionally depleted to the point that they begin to manifest false Heat symptoms, but in the context of Deficiency rather than Excess. For instance, an individual who is emaciated, runs on nervous energy, talks fast but peters out quickly, sleeps poorly, and has little stamina and low resistance is experiencing Empty Yin, or Yin Deficiency.

Quite often, these people show a greater than average resistance to antibiotic therapy, which makes their infections particularly troublesome to treat. They require more neutral or cool-natured tonics, either alone or in judicious combination with heat-clearing herbs, for effective treatment. In this case you want to tonify the Yin with appropriate Yin tonics, such as ophiopogon root, asparagus root, marshmallow root and rehmannia root. Milder Qi tonics with Yin nourishing properties can also be used, such as polygonatum (Solomon's seal root).

Full Yang symptoms represent a significant degree of Heat, such as high fever, restlessness, red complexion, loud voice, aggressive actions, strong odors, yellow discharges, rapid pulse and hypertension. Heat clearing herbs that detoxify, drain Fire and Heat and promote bowel movements are most useful here. These can include the Ayurvedic formula called "Triphala", red clover blossoms, cascara bark, rhubarb root, lonicera blossoms or chrysanthemum flowers, to name a few.

Empty Yang is a type of Yang Deficiency accompanied by symptoms of lethargy, coldness, edema, poor digestion and lack of libido. Here there is a lack of Heat and activity to perform adequate functions in the body. Foods and herbs that tonify Yang and Qi are needed here, such as more red meat, root vegetables like carrots, and herbs such as ginseng, astragalus, Dang Gui (which, although it is a Blood tonic, has warming, circulation-enhancing properties), ginger, cinnamon, fenugreek, cuscuta, psoralea, morinda and eucommia.

Excess Yang and Deficient Yin are both associated with too much heat, irritability and other Yang symptoms. However, in each of these cases, the symptoms arise from two entirely different imbalances, so the two syndromes are not the same. With Excess Yang there are true Heat signs, but with Deficient Yin, there is an underlying weakness with superficial Heat signs.

Similarly, a Deficiency of Yang has similar symptoms to an Excess of Yin, but because each originates from a different point of either Excess or Deficiency, they also are not the same. A Deficiency of Yang causes Coldness and hypo-functioning of the Organs with the result of tiredness, lethargy and edema occurring, since there is little Heat and activity to give energy or transform Fluids. An Excess of Yin, on the other hand, results in significant Dampness in the body, from copious discharges to a full rounded body.

YIN AND YANG IN CHINESE ANATOMY AND PHYSIOLOGY

All parts of the body have a Yin-Yang relationship to each other. Here is a general classification:

YANG	YIN
external (skin)	internal (Organs)
upper body	lower body
posterior-lateral	anterior-medial
back	front
functional-transportive	structural-transformative
Qi	Blood and body fluids
defensive Qi	nutritional Qi
six Yang organs	six Yin organs

The six Yin Organs of transformation are considered the most important in Chinese medical theory. They are the Heart, Spleen, Lungs, Kidneys, Liver and Pericardium. The six Yang Organs of transportation are hollow and serve a more external function as transport for food and waste. They are the Small Intestine, Triple Warmer, Stomach, Large Intestine, Bladder and Gall Bladder.

A balance of Yin and Yang function is essential for the proper functioning of all organs. In Traditional Chinese Medicine the Yin-Yang theory is applied to the state of individual Organ functions, such as the " Yin of the Kidney" (referring to that aspect of Kidney function that relates to Fluid balance and urine), or the "Yang of the Kidney" (relating to the function of the adrenal glands). Because the Kidneys are central to the entire theory of Chinese Medicine, they are considered the "storehouse of Qi" and the "root of Yin and Yang" for the whole body. This means that through the complex action of adrenal medulla and cortical hormones the Kidneys are able to regulate the organic functions of the entire body.

Thus, the Kidneys are fundamental to the basic inherited constitution of the individual as a whole and the storehouse of "Inherited Qi" or "Ancestral Qi." Herbs that tonify Kidney Yin are demulcent diuretics, such as asparagus root and rehmannia glutinosa, while herbs that tonify Kidney Yang have warming diuretic properties, such as juniper, dogwood berries and cinnamon.

The Lungs need to maintain a proper balance of moisture (Yin) and dryness (Yang). They also need Yang strength for inhalation and the Yin potential for release and exhalation. Therefore, there are specific treatments for the "Yang of the Lungs" or the "Yin of the Lungs." Herbs that increase the Yang of the Lungs are Qi tonics such as ginseng, codonopsis and astragalus, and herbs that are warming and stimulating, such as anise seed, elecampane and angelica. Herbs that increase the Yin of the lungs are cooling, demulcent herbs, such as comfrey and marshmallow roots.

The Heart also needs a proper balance of Yin (Blood and Fluids) and Yang (neurological impulse) to function correctly. The Yang function of the Heart refers to the impulse, arterial and venous pressure, while the Yin function is related to the quality and amount of blood present. Many Heart problems are caused by exhaustion of Heart Qi, a Yang phenomenon improved by herbs such as ginseng. Other conditions are related to a lack of Heart Yin and Blood, a Yin phenomenon that is treated with herbs such as Dang Gui and biota seeds. The Pericardium, sometimes called the "Heart Protector," is the sixth Yin Organ and for all practical purposes serves as an extension of the TCM Heart.

Stagnant conditions of Yin Fluid and Blood may be caused by an excess of both Yang and Yin. This results in impaired Organ function that can be improved through the use of diuretic and blood-moving (emmenagogue) herbs, such as hawthorn berries and/or motherwort herb. Problems can also stem from an imbalance known as "Heart Fire", a general condition of hyper-function of the Heart and circulation usually associated with an acidic condition of the Blood. Alterative herbs such as coptis, golden seal, and oregon grape root are appropriate.

As the Liver tends to require more Yin (Blood and Fluids) for proper function, it is most frequently threatened by an Excess Yang syndrome associated with hypertension, depression and anger. Thus, beneficial herbs for the Liver might be cooling herbs, such as dandelion root, herbs to tonify Blood and Yin, such as Chinese lycium berries, or herbs to relieve Wind or spasms, such as lobelia or cramp bark. A category of warm-natured herbs useful for regulating and smoothing Liver Qi are carminative herbs, such as fennel seed, cyperus and citrus peel. These herbs actually help stimulate the production and secretion of enzymes by the Liver to aid digestion.

The Spleen-Pancreas, on the other hand, has a basically Yang function responsible for a variety of actions associated with digestion and assimilation of food and fluids. Therefore, the most frequent problem of the Spleen-Pancreas is "lack of Spleen Yang," a condition associated with edema, damp swelling, poor digestion, hypoglycemia, fatigue and tiredness. Herbs that tonify Qi, such as ginseng, codonopsis and astragalus, as well as diuretics, such as atractylodes, the mushroom Poria cocos and Western gravel root, are all good Spleen-strengthening herbs.

Yin and Yang in Relationship to Seasons, Diet and Activities

Yin and Yang is a way of describing the relative states of balance or imbalance between the individual and any or all external factors affecting his or her existence. Based on these principles, it is important to adjust diet and herbs according to seasonal and individual lifestyle differences so that they can be truly healing. During the cold seasons, it may be more appropriate to eat foods of a more substantial, Yang-warming nature, such as cooked whole grains with a little animal protein, and cooked rather than raw vegetables and fruit. On the other hand, during the hotter seasons one might use more seasonal raw fruits and vegetables.

Because children have a much higher metabolism than adults, they can usually tolerate more Yin-cooling fruits. Similarly, a woman who is pregnant might require less Yang-heating foods and more Yin-cooling substances at different stages of her pregnancy, due to a higher Yang metabolism during that time. In all cases, whole grains are the "staff of life" and represent a balance of all parts of the life cycle of a plant and of Yin and Yang energies. Therefore, they should constitute the central pillar of our "daily bread." Above all, we must learn to adjust our diet and health program so that it is in harmony and balance with all external and internal emotional changes we might be experiencing.

Since Yin and Yang are mutually related, there is always a tendency for the body to compensate an Excess of one with an apparent Deficiency of the other. We can see this clearly in the progression of daily and seasonal cycles. Daytime is Yang and night is Yin. Individuals lacking in Yin-strength will experience more symptoms in the evening, the time of Yin.

Similarly, winter is Yin and summer is Yang. This means that our bodies must adjust to the change of the coming season over the course of Spring or Fall. As the Yin of Winter changes during the Spring to the Yang of Summer, or the Yang of Summer changes back in the Fall to the Yin of Winter, we are particularly vulnerable to the excesses of the previous season. These may manifest as allergies and other upper respiratory diseases as well as a variety of gastrointestinal problems.

Our body adjusts to outer Yin or Yang seasonal influences by complementary relationships within the body. When it is cold outside, our body counterbalances the outer cold with a greater concentration of inner warmth. Conversely, when it is hot outside our body counterbalances with a greater concentration of internal coolness. In this way homeostasis is maintained.

We see how this works particularly in terms of how our digestion and eating habits change throughout the seasons. During the Summer, our inner gastric fires are weaker, and we should eat lighter foods and resist the temptation to overindulge in excessively cold Yin foods that can further suppress our digestive fires. Most people notice that as the heat of summer progresses, digestion becomes more sensitive, and there is an increased tendency towards gastrointestinal diseases, dysentery, heat stroke and other conditions described as "Summer Heat", which can include all of the above plus feverish symptoms.

In the Winter, despite the outer cold, our digestion becomes capable of handling larger quantities of heavier, calorie-rich foods. This is like stoking the fires of a wood-burning stove to ward off the outer cold. If we continue to eat raw, cool natured, Yin-type foods and do not supply our body with sufficient proteinaceous, higher-calorie foods, our body will tend at first to burn off its own excess reserves. For those who have too much excess to begin with, this is good, but those who have already consumed their excess run into problems as the body starts to chip away at vital nutrient stores in order to maintain sufficient strength to withstand the outer Cold-Damp influences. It is something like burning your house down to keep warm. This is one cause of Yin Deficiency.

Food and activity are natural means of creating a balance with our external environment. It is not easy to describe, because each person's needs differ according to our pre-existing Yin-Yang constitution, balance and activities. Potential dietary imbalances, especially an excess of calorie-rich foods, can be balanced with greater levels of activity and exercise. A diet with fewer calories and less protein can be balanced by a reduction in physical activity. The key in all cases is balance.

Foods that are more appropriate for Spring and Summer are vegetables, seasonal fruits, lighter grains, beans and legumes and a small amount of dairy. Foods that are more appropriate for Fall and Winter seasons include squashes, root vegetables, heavier grains such as brown rice, mochi (pounded sweet rice), beans and animal protein (such as fish). Cooked foods are more appropriate in the Winter while a somewhat greater quantity of raw fruits and vegetables can be eaten in the Summer.

Since food is considered the best tonic, tonic herbs for empty conditions are best taken cooked in soups or sweet rice congee porridge (see Chapter 13 for specific instructions and recipes). In most other cases, tonics are best taken before meals to prepare the body for effective absorption. Cleansing herbs are better taken after meals, to promote thorough elimination.

YIN AND YANG IN HERBAL HEALING

Chinese medicine is based on the systematic application of Yin-Yang principles to diagnosis and treatment. Every symptom and every herbal treatment can be evaluated in terms of Yin and Yang. All pathologies, herbs and foods are classified accordingly. There are four basic treatment choices:

1. To tonify Yang
2. To tonify Yin
3. To eliminate excess Yang
4. To eliminate excess Yin

Herbs, too, are classified according to Yin-Yang characteristics, as they have the potential to either raise the organic metabolic function of an organ process that may be too weak or low, or lower one that is too high and congested. Thus, like foods, herbs are classified according to their basic energetics: their relative hot-warm-neutral-cool-cold characteristics. Based on these classifications, they are given to individuals to balance Excessive or Deficient states.

Herbs can also play a role in helping to maintain balance through the seasons. Generally, we take herbs that are warming and tonifying during the Winter and cooler-natured herbs that nourish Yin-essence during the Summer. Herbs that are good to include with food during the Winter include Chinese ginseng, astragalus root, Dang Gui, angelica, cinnamon bark, garlic and ginger. Beneficial herbs that are good during the Summer include ophiopogon root, rehmannia root, American ginseng and asparagus root. Chrysanthemum flower tea is particularly good to drink throughout the Summer and Fall because it is cooling and has slight Yin tonic properties. Chamomile tea is also appropriate during this time of year. During the summer months, American ginseng is a better choice than Chinese ginseng because it is more lubricating and cooling.

Pathologies of Yin and Yang

Pathologies of Yin and Yang involve their four basic states: Deficient Yin, Deficient Yang, Excess Yin and Excess Yang. They are described in detail in the Chapter, Patterns of Disharmony.

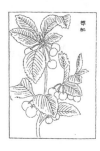

THREE

THE FIVE ELEMENTS

Next to the Yin-Yang doctrine, the Five Elements, or Five Phases (Wu Xing), is the second most important principle of Traditional Chinese Medicine. Five Element Theory recognizes that qualities and things can simply be what they are without necessarily being the opposite of something else. As such, it provides an alternative to the dualistic approach of the Yin-Yang doctrine.

The Five Elements 五行 were first described around 3000 years ago in the Yellow Emperor's Classic of Internal Medicine (*Huangdi Neijing*) as follows: "Heaven has four seasons and five elements to allow cultivation, growth, harvesting and storing. It produces cold, heat, drought, humidity and wind. Man has five vital organs that transform the five influences to engender happiness, anger, vexation, sadness and fear." It probably originated around 4000 to 5000 years ago.

The Chinese Five Elements, described as Wood, Fire, Earth, Metal and Water, represent interactive phases or processes that are fundamental to humankind and nature. Originally the Five Elements were probably a further subdivision of Yin-Yang aspects, extending into four subdivisions with Earth in the center. Eventually, Earth, with its own set of relationships, began to be thought of as one of the five.

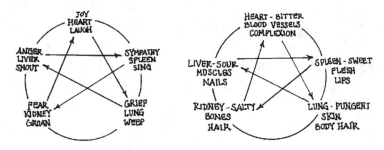

The Five Elements describe the dynamic functional relationship between all aspects of nature as well as the energetic relationship between

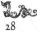

the twelve internal Organs and other physiological processes. It goes further to describe the interaction of all parts of an individual, including both internal physiological and psychological processes, with external factors such as season, climate, foods and other variables. In this way it shows us how an imbalance in one phase or Organ process can influence an imbalance in all other phases. It is inclusive of the Yin-Yang concept but goes a step further by subdividing the energies according to their influence on particular Organs.

Implicit in each of these systems is the perspective of life as a process of constant flow, interaction and change. All phenomena, including herbs and foods, are contained within the Chinese Five Element cycle, allowing a balance of creative engendering and control. This system, therefore, is another way to describe the vision of health as balance and of disease as a manifestation of imbalance.

The Five Element concept evolved out of an ancient people who lived closely with the earth and followed the cycles of nature. Today, with artificial lighting and heating, foods imported from all around the world and jet travel, many of us have forgotten the once powerful influence of the seasons upon our daily lives. Ancient sages, however, perceived the cycles of seasonal change, the cycles of each day and the progression from birth, infancy, puberty, adolescence, adulthood to old age as a predictable and orderly process that exists through all aspects of life.

As a result the Five Elements are an expression of those natural cycles, beginning with the seasons and extending out to explain the principles of transformation and change throughout all of nature and human psycho-physiological processes. The following table outlines the primary correspondences of the Five Elements:

	WOOD	FIRE	EARTH	METAL	WATER
Planet	Jupiter	Mars	Saturn	Venus	Mercury
Direction	East	South	Center	West	North
Color	Green	Red	Yellow	White	Black
Season	Spring	Summer	Indian Summer	Autumn	Winter
Injurious Climate	Wind	Heat	Moisture	Dryness	Cold
Yin Organ	Liver	Heart	Spleen-Pancreas	Lungs	Kidneys-Endocrine
Yang Organ	Gall Bladder	Small Intestine	Stomach	Large Intestine	Bladder
Power	Birth	Growth	Transformation	Harvest	Storage
Sense	Sight	Speech	Taste	Smell	Hearing
Body Part	Muscles/Ligaments	Blood Vessels	Flesh	Skin	Bones
External Manifestation	Nails	Complexion	Lips	Body Hair	Head Hair

Body Orifice	Eyes	Tongue	Mouth	Nose	Ears, anus, Urinary organs
Bodily Secretion	Tears	Sweat	Lymph	Mucous	Saliva
Bodily Sound	Crying	Laughter	Singing	Sobbing	Groaning
Spiritual Quality	Ethereal Soul/*Hun*	Spirit/*Shen*	Thought/*YI*	Corporal Soul/*PO*	Will/*Zhi*
Emotion	Anger	Joy/Levity	Worry	Grief	Paranoia
Dynamic	Spiritual	Visionary	Intellectual	Vitality	Will
Controls	Spleen	Lungs	Kidneys	Liver	Heart
Activity	Seeing	Walking	Sitting	Reclining	Standing
Grains	Wheat	Corn	Millet	Rice	Beans
Vegetable	Leek	Shallot	Hollyhock	Scallions	Leaf of Bean Plant
Animal	Chicken	Lamb	Cow	Horse	Pig
Fruits	Plum	Apricot	Date	Peach	Chestnut
Benefits when eaten	Sweet	Sour	Salty	Bitter	Spicy
Injures when overeaten	Spicy	Salty	Sweet	Sour	Bitter

Each of the Five Elements has a dynamic inter-relationship with the others. These relationships are incorporated into two cycles: the **Shen cycle** and the **Ko cycle**. The Shen cycle moves clockwise and is the engendering or creative movement. Thus, Fire creates an ash that engenders Earth; Earth creates or engenders Metal; Metal turns into a liquid when it melts to engender fluidity; Water nourishes the growth of the plant kingdom so it engenders Wood; and finally, Wood feeds Fire when it burns. This engendering cycle is described as a parent-child relationship where Fire is the parent of Earth, Earth the parent of Metal, and so forth. Therefore a parent is responsible for nurturing its child, or the following Element.

The Ko cycle is sometimes called the controlling cycle. By this definition, Wood controls Earth by pushing through soil during its growth, Earth controls Water by damming it, Water controls Fire by putting it out, Fire controls Metal by melting it and Metal controls Wood by breaking it. The controlling cycle reflects the role of the grandparents as protectors of custom and tradition in traditional Chinese society, and their control over the behavior of the grandchildren. Thus, Wood is the grandparent of the grandchild-Earth, Earth is the grandparent of the grandchild-Water, and so forth. As such, the grandparent controls, or keeps in check, its grandchild Organ.

Within each phase there are closely related Yin and Yang Organs that follow the Husband-Wife Law. This states that to help one is to benefit the other, and that to harm one is to harm the other. Thus, the Stomach is the husband of the Spleen-Pancreas; the Colon is the husband of the Lungs; the Kidneys are the wife of the Bladder, the Liver is the wife of the Gall Bladder and the Small Intestine is the husband of the Heart. Thus, treating the husband-Stomach assists the process of assimilation represented by the wife-Spleen-Pancreas; to treat the wife-Kidneys helps the husband-Bladder, and so forth. On the other hand, a depletion of the wife-Lung can cause a depletion of the husband-Large Intestine and similarly for the other Elements.

Each of the Five Elements embodies a particular energy, or Power, as follows: Wood embodies birth, ideation, creativity, expression; Fire: impulse, consciousness, spirit, mental processes; Earth: centeredness, nourishment, thought processing; Metal: elimination, letting go, regulation and conduction of energy throughout the body; Water: will power, essential power, inherited constitution, fluidity. All these qualities can appear active when the Organ is in balance, or over-stimulated or suppressed if the Organ is correspondingly Excess or Deficient.

For example, an imbalance in Wood can cause an Excess or Deficiency in one's creativity and expressiveness with resultant feelings of frustration that give rise to anger, moodiness and depression. An individual with an Excess in Wood will tend to have a shouting, angry tone of voice even in normal speech, while a person Deficient in Wood may be very timid and repressed with little tendency towards self-expression.

An imbalance in Fire is represented by an inappropriately happy or over-indulgent partying mood which would be an Excess, or a marked lack of happy feelings, which would be a Deficiency. Fire corresponds to the Heart, and since the Heart also rules the Mind, conscience and speech, one with an imbalance of Fire and Heart Qi may exhibit a variety of psychological problems which affect one's ability to relate to the external world, such as neurosis or schizophrenia.

An Earth imbalance is represented by problems in assimilation of either food, drink or, on a more subtle level, ideas and concepts. There may be a lack of centeredness and grounding, a tendency to look to others for personal support, a yellowish pallor and an overly sweet manner of expression with perhaps a singsong voice or total absence of vocal inflection.

An imbalance in Metal may cause a general blockage of energy flow, giving rise to stiffness, rigidity, or an inability to let go of past occurrences. The individual may have a whining or sobbing sound to their voice, a whitish pallor, a tendency towards mucus, physical weakness, lung problems, sinus congestion and/or cough.

A Water imbalance will be associated with inherited weaknesses, lack of will power, lack of power or strength, aching feelings in the lower back or joints and a tendency towards fatigue, dark coloration and a low, groaning or gravely sound to the voice.

It is possible to become skilled at identifying a person's Five Element imbalance by observing how they walk, their taste and color preferences, the tone of voice, personality types and so on. For example, patients who worry about money, express negative attitudes of insufficiency and inadequacy, need to sit and cannot stand long, have a light low groaning tone in their everyday voice and a darkish pallor, especially under the eyes, are recognized as being a Deficient Kidney-Adrenal type. In other words, who we are and how we act, as well as our physical-mental-emotional imbalances, reveals our predominant constitutional Element.

Although this aids in identification of the underlying constitution, often the Five Element understanding alone does not provide enough information to effectively treat acute colds, flu, skin conditions or digestive disorders. When we look closely to find Five Element correspondences, we usually find that all Five Element indications are present in everyone, and thus the key is in recognizing the primary imbalance. While Five Element analysis offers a more constitutional or underlying cause of disease, other TCM systems such as Eight Principles or Symptom-Sign diagnosis afford a more direct strategy for treatment. Five Element imbalances tend to remain even after the presenting complaint is resolved, because we all exhibit a predominance or deficiency of one Element or another.

Thus, instead of a treatment protocol, the Five Element system is like a "user's guide" to the specific needs and requirements of the individual body. By learning to recognize our tendencies and limitations within the Five Element system, we are better able to understand them and utilize their various aspects to create greater harmony and well-being in our lives. If there is one dominant principle of Chinese Medicine and Five Elements, it is to keep the energy flowing with as much integrity, grace, compassion and awareness as we can. It is to this end that acupuncture, diet and herbal medicine are ultimately intended.

Following is a description of the characteristics of each of the Five Elements.

WOOD

In the Five Element system we begin with Wood because that is where the new energy first arises. As a young sapling is eager to burst forth in the Spring to realize the opportunities of the new light, the Wood person displays a similar need for expansiveness and growth.

Motivation, daring and planning are the Positive qualities of the Wood person, while control over those individuals and circumstances that may impede their ambitions are the negative ones. Confronted with obstacles, the Wood person experiences extreme frustration, anger and possibly depression. The key personality characteristics of the Wood person are controlling, planning and organizing. Comparing each of the personality traits of the Elements, Fire generates enthusiasm, Earth grace and leisure, Metal detachment and letting go, Water apprehension and fear, and Wood planning and organizing.

1) **Yin Organ: Liver**
The Liver is like a "general" or "planner" in charge of formulating strategies to serve the purpose and goals of the body-mind. Physiologically it has the most complex functions. It is responsible for detoxifying, filtering, nourishing, restoring and storing blood. In doing this, the Liver chemically counteracts foreign toxins that enter the blood and eliminates these through the bile, along with the waste of broken down blood cells.

These toxins are either endogenous or exogenous. Exogenous, or external, toxins occur from environmental pollutants, additives, preservatives and hydrogenated oils in foods, impure water and air, and other toxins. Endogenous, or internal, toxins are created as a hormonal or neuro-transmitter response to external stimuli. This includes the secretion of adrenaline in response to fear and anger, the secretion of sexual hormones and, in general, the ability to switch between the mobilizing functions of the sympathetic nervous system and the nourishing and maintaining functions of the parasympathetic nervous system.

These secretions, manufactured and sent into the blood from diverse areas of the body, serve as a command for various physiological processes to occur. These include regulating and transforming glycogen stored in the liver to maintain normal blood sugar levels, stimulating digestive and sexual secretions and a wide range of other more subtle hormonal responses.

When the body-mind response is no longer required because the original need for the mobilizing hormonal secretion has passed, the hormonal secretions need to be canceled. A healthy Liver neutralizes hormonal secretions which are no longer needed. If the Liver is backed up with other vital tasks, such as filtering and eliminating complex exogenous toxins, the hormones continue to circulate in the blood and become endogenous toxins. Unfortunately, if the system becomes overloaded beyond capacity with both endogenous and exogenous toxins, like a frustrated commander or general, the Liver gives a chemical 'file it' command for them to be stored in various cells throughout the body awaiting future detoxification and elimination. This can put a burden on the body, especially the various tissues and cells that must accommodate the presence of the various toxins.

If they are allowed to remain, however, they are capable of causing cysts and tumors in the area where they are located. In women this may include various fatty tissues such as those found in the breasts (near the Liver) and female reproductive organs. They can also be lodged in other organs and glands in the body which themselves may have been the site of extraordinary stress, such as the lungs (from smoking), the gastrointestinal tract, the pancreas or the Liver itself. Certain glands and organs, such as the female ovaries or male prostate, can also become the Liver's dumping ground for metabolic waste and toxins.

The capacity to overcome addictions, let go and relax is the result of a healthy Liver. Because of its ability to regulate the sympathetic and parasympathetic nervous systems, the Liver governs the entire nervous system. From all of this we understand how TCM considers the Liver's ability to regulate Qi of paramount importance. Both the Liver and its Yang counterpart, the Gall Bladder, control proper neuro-muscular tension throughout the body-mind. This includes the ligaments and tendons responsible for neuro-muscular coordination.

Because the Liver is involved with the storage of the Blood, it is responsible for maintaining a wide range of other physiological functions and systems. These range from sexual potency, regularity of the monthly menses of women, the condition of the fingernails and toenails, and the eyes. In addition, it regulates various psycho-spiritual processes including our creativity, drives and ambitions.

The Liver is involved in a wide variety of complaints, ranging from hepatitis, cirrhosis, gallstones, diabetes, hypoglycemia, female menstrual cycle issues, problems associated with menopause, infertility, leukorrhea, herpes simplex, hypertension and depression, to name a few. It is remarkable that, for the many conditions that modern Western medicine employs suppressing drugs and tranquilizers and an increasing variety of chemical mood regulators (most of which have Liver toxicity as a prominent side effect), the ancient Chinese created herbal formulas to regulate the many complex Liver functions involved as the underlying cause for these conditions.

2) Yang Organ: Gall Bladder

In the government of the body-mind, the Gall Bladder is the official of pure and proper judgment. It is responsible for our ability to make decisions and to manifest the courage necessary to execute them. Just as in folk parlance we associate the phrase "a lot of gall' with the gall bladder, an inability to formulate decisions or a lack of courage is psychospiritually a sign of Gall Bladder imbalance.

As the Yang Organ counterpart of the Liver, the Gall bladder is directly responsible for the discharge of bile, which in turn greatly facilitates the digestion of fats and oils. Diverse conditions ranging from gall bladder issues to problems with the ligaments and tendons and tension headaches can indicate Gall Bladder imbalances.

3) Season: Spring

Spring, the season for Wood, signals the new growth of plants. This is an ideal time to consume wild edible greens such as dandelion leaves, chickweed, watercress, malva and lamb's quarters leaves, all of which impart the energy of Spring to the Liver and aid in its blood-detoxifying and Qi regulating functions.

4) Climate: Wind

Diseases and conditions aggravated by Wind reflect a Wood imbalance. In Chinese medicine, Wind refers to those pathological conditions that tend to proliferate and spread such as colds, influenza, allergies and various skin diseases, all of which are considered External Wind. It also exists as Internal Wind, manifesting in diseases that involve muscular coordination and tension such as migraine headaches, tremors and epilepsy.

5) Direction: East

The direction for Wood relates the injurious effects of the East Wind on diseases caused by an imbalance of the Wood element.

6) Time of Day: 11 P.M. - 3 A.M.

For each of the Five Elements and their associated Yin and Yang Organs, there is a time of day that is optimum for the function of its corresponding Organ. For the Gall Bladder it is between 11 P.M. and 1 A.M., while for the Liver it is between 1 A.M. and 3 A.M.

This means that a significant portion of the complex functions of detoxification, regulation and nourishment involved with the Wood Element are accomplished during 11 P.M. - 3 A.M., the normal sleep hours. By so doing, imbalances characteristically created from an overabundance of physical and mental activity during the day are processed and put to rest in the evening. To accomplish this, during sleep and Liver time a large amount of the body's blood is stored in the Liver. This poses a problem for many who work at night or regularly go to bed late, as then the Gall Bladder and Liver are unable to adequately perform their vital functions, ultimately resulting in an imbalance in these organs.

7) Color: Green

Green is the color associated with Spring. When we detect a greenish pallor on the skin, it is associated with a possible imbalance of the Wood Element.

8) Flavor: Sour

The Flavors are a direct sensory experience of the chemical constituents of therapeutic substances such as herbs. As such, they serve a similar purpose for the traditional herbalist as chemical constituents do for the biochemist and pharmacist. In TCM, there are many instances where the flavors assigned to an herb are more a reflection of their therapeutic properties and effects than their actual tastes.

The sour taste is associated with fermented foods and substances that tend to be high in enzymes useful for digestion. It also has a mouth-puckering, astringent or contracting quality that is used to help retain fluids, stop hemorrhage and leakages, and contract and restore tissue that has lost its tone.

9) Sound: Shouting

Stagnant Liver Qi is associated with anger and frustration. The individual has a need to assert control over many situations, which causes them to develop a shouting angry tone of voice even in normal conversation.

10) Smell: Rancid

Individuals who have a Wood Element imbalance may have a sour or rancid body odor.

11) Body Orifice: Eyes

The Liver nourishes and supplies essential nutrients to the eyes. One of these is beta carotene, abundantly present in Chinese Lycii berries

(Gou Qi Zi) which tonify the Blood of the Liver. Red or dry eyes and excessive tearing or a lack of tearing all indicate Liver imbalances.

12) **Body Part: Muscles and Ligaments**
Lack of either mental or physical flexibility can indicate a Wood imbalance. The Liver and Gall Bladder must appropriately retain and secrete bile into the Small Intestine, making them the model for all restraining and contracting functions. If this process becomes imbalanced or exaggerated as a result of psychological or metabolic imbalance, it mirrors this contracted state to other tissues such as the muscles and ligaments, whose job is also involved with contracting and releasing.

13) **External Manifestation: Nails**
Problems associated with the nails of the hands and feet are an indication of Wood imbalance. This includes any conditions of brittleness, yellowness, striations, paleness or fungal degeneration.

14) **Emotion: Anger**
Anger arises out of fear (which precedes it as part of the Water Element). When plans and expectations are blocked, the result is anger. As with all the emotions corresponding to each of the Five Elements, either an Excess or complete lack of the correlating emotion can be indicative of Wood imbalance. However, what most aggravates the Wood personality is being blocked or unable to manifest their dreams, and anger is the result.

An Excess Liver manifests as an aggressive overbearing temperament with a shouting voice. Using the Shen cycle of the Five Element system, Liver-anger is aggravated from fear and paranoia, the emotion of the Water Element. Following the Ko cycle, Liver anger is controlled with grief and sadness, the emotion of Metal. From this we see how Five Element psychotherapy can employ supporting or counterbalancing emotions to move blocked emotional patterns and attitudes and effect positive mental changes. This is advantageously employed in a kind of traditional psychotherapy and counseling characteristic of shamanistic healing.

15) **Inner Resource: *Hun***
Chinese medical philosophy sees body, mind and spirit as integrated with each other, and each Organ has its unique psycho-spiritual potential. The Liver is the house of the *Hun* or Ethereal Soul. This is the aspect of the Soul that survives after death, returning to the world as pure spirit.

It is the Soul counterpart of *Shen*, the Spirit. The opening to the Liver and Hun, the eyes, are often termed the "window of the Soul".

Hun is rooted and nourished by Liver Yin and Blood. It is most active at night during sleep and helps determine the quality of sleep experienced. Hun pertains to mental and spiritual achievement and provides psychic abilities, intuition and inspiration. It is also responsible for balancing and harmonizing the Seven Emotions. Hun is also that quality of the psyche which gives us the capacity to plan our life and find a sense of direction and purpose.

Balanced Wood Type

The balanced Wood type tends to be creative, expressive and highly motivated. As such we might think of them as having an entrepreneurial temperament. They require an outlet to vent and express the unique aspects of their creative nature and temperament. Wood types are those individuals who are driven to excel in their focused endeavor. Like the young sapling first breaking through the earth with freshness and enthusiasm in Springtime, they thrive on opposition and resistance as they pursue their goals and ambitions. Acute diseases that are likely to occur with the Balanced Wood types involve Qi congestion and stagnation as it mainly affects the digestive tract: food stagnation, bloating, gas, indigestion and constipation.

Deficient Wood Type

The Deficient Wood type, still manifesting a tendency to outer drive, has an inner hollowness that causes them to fall short of their goals and ambitions. This brings with it a kind of brittle sensitivity that frequently dips into depressive states. While there is a desire for expression and creativity, they seem, for various reasons, unable to manifest their dreams. One of the problems with Deficient Wood types is infertility, for example,.

Peculiarly enough, both the Deficient and Excess Wood types still strive to manipulate and control their outer circumstances, sometimes with a tendency to aggression towards others. The difference is that, while the Excessive Wood type is more extroverted and overt in their method, the Deficient Wood type is more covert, but in their own way just as determined.

Deficient Wood types tend towards Qi, Blood and Fluid stagnation and Deficiency and should be treated with the appropriate herbal and dietary approaches. Women tend to have trouble with their menstrual cycles. Both men and women have a tendency to excessively push against their limitations and develop anxiety, insomnia and hypertension so that some degree of mild sedation and tranquilizing is also indicated.

Some herbal formulas that are used for Deficient Wood types include those that regulate Liver Qi, such as **Bupleurum and Peony Combination** (Xiao yao wan) and **Disperse Vital Energy in the Liver Powder** (Chai hu su gan san); those that sedate and nourish the Liver, such as **Zizyphus Combination** (Suan zao ren tang), and those that relieve depression, such as the above mentioned **Bupleurum and Peony Combination** (Xiao yao wan) and **Bupleurum, Dragon Bone and Oyster Shell Combination** (Chai hu long gu mu li tang). Herbs that nourish Blood and Yin include **Rehmannia Six Combination** (Liu wei di huang wan) and **Dang Gui Four Combination** (Si wu tang).

Excess Wood Types

Excess Wood epitomizes the extreme of Excess and stagnation syndromes. While stagnation and congestion are the primary characteristic imbalances of Wood, the Excess type is more archetypal. The personality of this type is the classic aggressive dominating personality whose voice even in normal speech sounds shouting.

These individuals are motivated to dominate any pursuit with which they are involved. As such they are the classic type A personality with all of the associated shortcomings as well as physical and psychological symptoms. Psychologically, these include irritability, aggression, hysteria and depression. Physiologically, Excess Wood types have problems with hypertension and other cardio-vascular complaints, chest tightness, abdominal bloating, gas, constipation, insomnia, nervous twitching, spasms and all problems associated with the Liver and Gall Bladder.

Therapeutically they are treated with a diet low in primary protein including dairy and meat, and tend to improve on a lighter vegetarian diet. As indicated, they should use herbs and formulas that promote elimination, including cholagogues (herbs that discharge bile) such as capillaris (Yin Chen Hao), coptis (Huang Lian), scutellaria (Huang Qin) and gardenia fruit (Zhi Zi); laxatives such as rhubarb root (Da Huang) and mirabilitum (Mang Xiao); herbs that relieve congestion such as green citrus (Qing Pi), bupleurum (Chai Hu) and cyperus (Xiang Fu); and herbs and minerals that calm and sedate such as Zizyphus spinosa (Suan Zao Ren), dragon bone (Long Gu) and oyster shell (Mu Li).

Formulas such as **Major Rhubarb Combination** (Da cheng qi tang) and **Minor Rhubarb Combination** (Xiao cheng qi tang) are indicated when there is constipation; for Liver and Gall Bladder toxicity problems use **Capillaris Combination** (Yin chen hao tang), **Coptis and Rhubarb Combination** (San huang xie xin tang), **Pueraria, Coptis and Scutellaria Combination** (Ge gen huang lian huang qin tang) or **Siler and Platycodon Combination** (Fang feng tung sheng san); and for stagnation and congestion consider **Bupleurum and Peony Combination** (Xiao yao wan) and **Disperse Vital Energy In The Liver Powder** (Chai hu su gan san).

FIRE

Fire represents light and warmth. Life is the capacity to moderate and contain the energy of the sun in plants and animals. It is the energy of Fire that is the very essence of Qi, and it imparts vitality, liveliness, joyousness and love to the universe and throughout all living beings.

To be without the essential spark of life is to be cold and alienated from everyone and everything. The energy of Fire is joy and gaiety. Laughter, the sound associated with the Fire Element, is an expression of our inner Fire energy, and like fire, it easily spreads and elicits a similar happy response from others. Our capacity to give and receive love is in proportion to the strength of the Fire Element, so that it governs our ability to communicate and relate to others.

1) Yin Organs: Heart and Pericardium
Fire is the only Element that has four corresponding organs. The Heart is a Yin Organ and is considered the supreme controller presiding over all aspects of psycho-physical activities throughout the body-mind. As in common folk knowledge, the Heart is not only responsible for circulation but includes all mental processes including our thoughts, aspirations and dreams, so that it is responsible for insight and enlightenment.

The other Yin Organ of Fire, the Pericardium, is actually the sac-like tissue that surrounds the physical heart. It is also known as Heart Protector or Circulation Sex. Despite its physicality, the Pericardium is a function rather than a specific Organ and, as such, is regarded as an extension of the Heart. The fact that it is sometimes called Circulation Sex reflects its importance as the Organ function governing relationships and sexuality.

2) Yang Organs: Small Intestine and Triple Warmer
The Small Intestine is the Yang Organ corresponding to the Heart, and it represents the Fire Element's potential for clarity. As the Chinese state, "the Small Intestine separates the pure from the impure," which is reflected in good digestion and assimilation as well as enhanced mental clarity.

The Triple Warmer, having no specific physicality or location, is even more of an Organ function than a specific Organ. It is divided into the Upper, Middle and Lower Warmers: the internal organs and area from the base of the sternum upwards is the Upper Warmer, from the base of the sternum down to the navel is the Middle Warmer and the area below the navel is considered the Lower Warmer. The Triple Warmer regulates warmth and water metabolism throughout all the internal systems and is the process by which the body-mind relates physically and mentally to all of its parts.

3) Season: Summer

Summer is a time when the sun is at its zenith and all living things flourish in the abundance of resources.

4) Climate: Hot

Either a strong preference for, or abhorrence of, hot weather is an indication of a Deficiency or Excess of Heat. According to TCM theory, all heat and warmth emanate from the Heart, so that hot weather can be injurious to the psycho-physical functions of the Heart-Mind. If there is Heart Deficiency, on the other hand, one is less able to tolerate cold weather.

5) Direction: South

This is the area that receives the greatest concentration of light and warmth from the sun. It is the exposure to the sunlight of the South that provides for maximum plant growth.

6) Time of Day: 11 A.M. - 3 P.M.

Based upon sun time, from 11 A.M. to 1 P.M. is Heart time and from 1 - 3 P.M. is Small intestine time. Then from 7 - 9 P.M. is the Pericardium time and finally from 9 - 11 P.M. is the Triple Warmer time.

7) Color: Red

Red, whether it is a flush on the complexion, a reddened area of inflammation or even a show of blood during hemorrhage, indicates Heat or Fire.

8) Flavor: Bitter

One of the paradoxes of the Five Element system is that while the Fire Element represents heat and warmth, it is assigned the bitter flavor, which is energetically cooling and detoxifying. The bitter flavor is a dominant quality in most medicinal herbs that are used for toxicity and inflammation. This is because the biochemical constituents of bitter tasting herbs include various alkaloids and bitter glycosides that have the potential to neutralize toxic wastes in the body as well as possessing antibacterial and antiviral properties. Herbs with a bitter flavor are also drying, so that in addition to their detoxifying effects they help resolve purulent and inflammatory discharges. Finally, digestive bitters, an alcoholic liqueur taken before or after meals, is traditionally used to aid digestion and to relieve gas and bloating.

9) Sound: Speech and Laughter

Laughter and speech are the sounds of the Fire Element. Individuals whose normal speech is punctuated with frequent laughter may indicate a Heart imbalance. Conversely, a noticeable absence of laughter reflects a Heart-Mind Deficiency. Similarly, an imbalance of Fire is also reflected in the individual who either talks too much or too little and/or when their speech manifests a great deal of excitement.

10) Smell: Scorched

Often it is possible to detect a noticeable scorched or burnt smell on an individual who has a Fire imbalance.

11) Body Orifice: Tongue

The Heart opens to the tongue. Talkativeness, lack of desire to talk, stuttering and aphasia all indicate Heart conditions.

12) Body Part: Pulse and Blood Vessels

The blood vessels are the way all parts of the body communicate with each other through the Heart. The condition of the blood vessels is strongly influenced by the activity of the Heart, which serves as a pump sending blood throughout the body. Conditions such as hardening of the arteries or increase of undesirable forms of cholesterol and lipids in the veins and arteries put more stress on the Heart, which can lead to heart disease.

13) External Manifestation: Complexion

The face is rich in blood vessels, which are controlled by the Heart; thus, its condition is reflected in the face through its color and luster. When the Heart functions well, Blood is plentiful and the face will be a normal red color with sheen and moisture. When Heart Blood is insufficient, the face will be pale and lusterless. If Heart Blood is stagnant, the face will be purple.

14) Emotion: Joy

Joy is the emotion of the Heart. For most of us, joy has a very positive connotation and certainly not what we would be inclined to consider as an imbalance. From another perspective, people who party and celebrate excessively, if for no other reason than overindulgence, are frequently prone to heart attacks. The Heart governs the blood vessels, and an overindulgence in the enjoyment of rich desserts causes fatty deposits in the arteries which can lead to heart attacks and strokes.

It is no accident that the Heart, the seat of the Mind and the emotions, is a universal symbol for love and affection. Further, bodily heat and warmth comes from the Heart, which, on a psychological level, extends into charisma and warmth for others.

15) Inner Resource: Spirit (*Shen*)

The Chinese Five Element Theory, together with most of the great religions, refer to the Heart as the seat of the Divine. Spirit is an essential diagnostic indication, the lack of which prevents healing of any disease. On the other hand, an abundance of Spirit is an inspiration and healing not only to one's self, but to all who encounter its influence.

Spirit is a lack of negativity. It manifests as boundless positive creative energy and compassion for others. Certainly this transcends the physical implications of the physical heart, which in the modern world has become a disposable organ and accepted candidate for organ transplant and replacement. The attainment of Spirit can come from inspiration, and is a potential with which one is either innately born or one acquires as a result of consciously maintaining a positive outlook, regardless of outer circumstances.

To some extent Spirit is at least partially inherited and partially acquired, but there is another more spiritual-physical aspect that is reflected in an inner harmony of body and mind and that might also have a material chemical component. Individuals who have experienced altered states of consciousness through the use of hallucinogenic substances under some circumstances seem to discover latent spiritual resources that they had not previously realized.

Yet, altered states of consciousness can be achieved without the aid of hallucinogenic substances through meditation, chanting, prayer and ritual irrespective of any religious affiliation. In our time, there is an increased tendency to seek out occasions that will heighten spiritual awareness — the awareness of ourselves and all existence as spirit. Considering that Heart disease is the number one cause of death in the Western world, does this not also reflect agreement with traditional beliefs that modern humankind is indeed starved for more Spirit in their lives?

Balanced Fire Type

Fire has to do with excitement, communication and relationship. A balanced Fire type communicates with a great deal of innate enthusiasm and interest. They have a naturally positive, happy and spirited way, even when confronted with what others might consider to be a negative experience. They are great talkers and their speech frequently tends to be too rapid. Having a more sensitive temperament, they seem to have a lively concern and involvement in whatever their interest may be.

They are easily excited by various circumstances and events and are capable of an extreme display of emotional enthusiasm. Because of this, it is not always easy to determine their deeper concerns, so that underneath their outer enthusiasm may be a lurking sadness or depression. Acute diseases, to which they are most prone, are inflammatory in nature, such as infections and inflammations.

Deficient Fire Type

Individuals who are lacking in Fire typically have "hypo" type symptoms such as hypothyroid, hypoglycemia and hypo-adrenals, although the latter two are applicable to Earth and Water Deficiencies as well. However, it is not uncommon for one to have multiple similar metabolic imbalances simultaneously.

The opposite of the Balanced Fire type, Deficient Fire individuals tend to be noncommunicative, reclusive, timid and shy in nature. While they tend to be uninterested in outer physical events, they have a decided introspective leaning with a marked interest in things that are more psycho-spiritually oriented. Deficient Fire individuals tend to feel colder, with a pale complexion that is more the absence of redness than the white color associated with Metal. They are more prone to chronic complaints associated with their low metabolism.

Dietarily, Deficient Fire types do well with all cooked foods, more red meat, especially lamb, and warm natured Qi, Blood and Yang tonics that include Dang Gui (Angelica sinensis), ginseng (Panax ginseng), codonopsis (Dang Shen), as well as internal Yang warming herbs such as cinnamon bark and ginger. Formulas that one might consider are **Vitality Combination** (Zhen wu tang), **Ginseng and Astragalus Combination** (Bu zhong yi qi tang) and **Aconite, Ginger and Licorice Combination** (Si ni tang).

Excess Fire Type

Excess Fire individuals display an exaggeration of most balanced Fire traits. They have a tendency to excessive and rapid talk, even to the point of irritation and obnoxiousness, with a penchant to interject their opinion regardless of the level of information or even the appropriateness of their remarks. Their degree of insensitivity to what is happening around them is manifested in their impetuousness and impatience as well as a quality of joviality and laughter that seems almost always present in their manner and vocal inflection. Because of their tendency to over-socialize and indulge themselves, Excess Fire types are prone to a variety of inflammatory as well as cardio-vascular diseases. These include arteriosclerosis, angina, heart disease and strokes.

Dietarily, Excess Fire Types require little or no animal protein, and should especially avoid high-fat flesh foods such as beef and lamb. They should limit their fat and oil intake and eat a larger proportion of fresh vegetables and fruits. They need herbs that are more detoxifying and eliminative with cholagogue (bile dispersing), laxative, diuretic and decongesting properties. They can use formulas that contain rhubarb root, mirabilitum, Chinese skullcap (Scutellaria baicalensis), coptis and gardenia fruit. Formulas that are useful for this type include **Coptis and Rhubarb Combination** (San huang xie xin tang), **Pueraria, Coptis and Scutellaria Combination** (Ge gen huang lian huang qin tang)and **Siler and Platycodon Combination** (Fang feng tung sheng san).

EARTH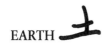

The Earth Element relates to processes involved with nourishing and supporting life. This includes digestion, assimilation and transportation of food and fluids and represents solidity and stability. This also encompasses personality and mental concepts such as grounding, focusing and centering as part of its manifestation in the individual person.

Originally Earth was in the center of Four Elements. This was because it supported all the other elements and their corresponding Organs. Eventually, it became part of the five with its own corresponding Organs and qualities. Notwithstanding, the Earth Element, which includes the Stomach and Spleen-Pancreas, is the source of acquired Qi from food and drink, and therefore has a unique role to play in supplying Qi to each of the Organs.

1) Yin Organ: Spleen-Pancreas

The Spleen-Pancreas transforms and transports food and fluids, deriving from them the essential factors that ultimately create Blood and Qi in the body. Thus, the Spleen includes as part of its functions the Pancreas (with its regulation of blood sugar and digestive enzymes). The basic indications for Earth imbalance include diseases associated with digestive imbalances and appetite, either too much or not enough. Concomitant with digestive weakness are mental symptoms of lack of focus and ungroundedness associated with pancreatic weakness and low blood sugar.

2) Yang Organ: Stomach

The Stomach is in charge of receiving ingested food and drink and then "ripening" and "rotting" it through its digestive process. It then sends the pure portion to the Spleen for its metabolic processes, and the impure part to the Small Intestine for further digestion. The Stomach "hates to be hot or dry and likes moisture", the opposite of the Spleen.

3) Season: Late Summer

Late summer is a time when all living things reach their stage of maximum maturity and fruition, and this time of year correlates to the Earth Element. However, because the Earth Element is neutral in relation to all other Elements, it also corresponds to the end of each season when each Element's energies returns to the Earth Element for replenishment.

4) Climate: Humidity (Dampness)

It is in warm tropical climates that diverse and abundant life thrives. Because Dampness is an External Pathogenic Influence that can injure Earth, overweight individuals who have problems with edema and Dampness may have an adverse reaction to damp and humid climates.

5) Direction: Center

Because the Earth Element is the source of Qi and Blood in the body and thus supports the activities of all the other Organs, it is considered to be the center. Thus, being off-centered reflects our being out of balance with Earth.

6) Time of Day: 7 - 11 A.M.

The biological time for the Stomach is from 7 - 9 A.M.; for the

46

Spleen it is from 9 -11 A.M. For this reason, the Chinese believe that this is the optimal time to receive quality nourishment.

7) Color: Yellow

Yellow is the color associated with Earth. Many people have trouble with this designation because a characteristic yellow pallor is associated in Western medicine with liver and gall bladder diseases such as hepatitis. From a TCM perspective, a yellow pallor may reflect a problem that began with the Liver and then later extended itself via the controlling, or Ko, cycle to invade or attack the Spleen (Earth Element). A pale yelow color indicates a Spleen imbalance due to Deficiency. A bright yellow in TCM signifies Damp Heat, and whether we are considering hepatitis from the perspective of Western medicine or Damp Heat from the perspective of TCM, the herbal treatment for both is essentially the same, employing the use of cholagogues and diuretics to clear Dampness.

8) Flavor: Sweet

The flavor for Earth is sweet. We crave sweet flavor not only because we have spoiled our palette but because the essential flavor associated with nourishment is sweet. A craving for sweet, therefore, reflects malnourishment. The stronger our craving, causing us to desire sugary excessively sweet foods, the greater our need for balanced nourishment from complex carbohydrates such as whole grains, beans, dairy and meat. Simple, refined sugar tends to stimulate our Earth Organs and launch them into an addictive reactive response that ultimately leaves us exhausted, depressed and asking for more.

In TCM, food is considered the first tonic. Sweet and/or acrid flavored tonic herbs, such as ginseng (Ren Shen), astragalus (Huang Qi), atractylodes (Bai Zhu), jujube dates (Da Zao), become superior tonics when cooked with foods such as soups and congees (porridge).

9) Sound: Singing

The Singing sound corresponds to the Earth Element. We frequently encounter individuals with a sing-song speech inflection. Not uncommonly they may also impress us with their "sweet" manner and sound. Considering that "sweet" diseases, such as hypoglycemia, are associated with Spleen-Earth imbalances, and that this disease is often associated with a kind of unfocused "spacy" or "dreamy" attitude, it is not uncommon that an exaggerated "sweetness" together with a sing-song vocal inflection is associated with Earth imbalances. Musically, the grounded sound of the drum corresponds to the Earth.

10) Smell: Fragrant

The smell associated with Earth is fragrant or sweet. While in many cases this can invoke the fragrance of blooming flowers and ripe fruit on the trees, the odor on a person with an Earth imbalance is a kind of cloying sweet fragrance.

11) Body Orifice: Mouth

Because food, drink and air first enter the mouth where the initial location of digestion occurs, the lips and mouth are traditional correspondences for the Earth element. The tissue of the GI tract extends itself to the mouth and gums, and the state of these bodily areas is indicative of the condition of the Stomach and Spleen.

12) Body Part: Flesh

Flesh is governed by Earth and includes muscles and fatty tissues. The areas where this is most likely to show up in excess are the buttocks, abdomen and thighs. When these parts of the body appear flabby and enlarged, it is a sign of Earth imbalance caused by weakness of the Spleen Qi in transforming and transporting Fluids. In Western medicine this corresponds to the abundance of swollen lymph nodes in these areas.

13) External Manifestation: Lips

The lips directly connect with the mouth, the orifice of the Earth Element, and so show the condition of the digestive Organs. Dry lips or inflamed gums indicate Stomach Heat, while swollen lips indicate Spleen Dampness.

14) Emotion: Pensiveness

Pensiveness, or over-thinking, includes both the negative aspect of worry and the seemingly less negative process of over-thinking. In some sense nostalgia, dwelling on the past, and sympathy, or over-concern for another, are also encompassed by the Earth Element. Any repeated or fixated process, be it physical or mental, can lead to stagnation of Qi through the Five Elements. Students who intensely study for an examination frequently experience chest discomfort, an indication of stagnant Qi, and digestive problems associated with bloating and gas.

On the other side, so many individuals with known problems associated with the Spleen and Pancreas, such as high or low blood sugar, complain of being unable to quiet their thoughts. Sometimes these have no particular emotion but are simply repetitive and obsessive.

Nostalgia and sympathy are two other thought processes which, if habitual and repetitive, indicate an imbalance of the Earth Element. In some sense an excess of either of these thought processes reflects some lack of contentedness with the present. With nostalgia, a sweet feeling, one may overly dwell on fond events of the past. To the extent that it causes one to escape or not be fully in the present, this becomes an imbalance. With sympathy, it is more difficult because most of us would like, and indeed need, to be more compassionate and sympathetic of others. This becomes a problem when our overly sympathetic feelings towards others become projections of our inner fears of inadequacy, and they can then interfere with the normal and customary flow of Qi.

There are individuals who simply are unable to say no to the expressed desires and needs of others. If, in overly attempting to satisfy the needs of others, we damage or incapacitate ourselves, such sympathetic response might be inappropriate. From the opposite perspective, an insatiable craving for sympathy indicates a deep emotional hunger and consequently, an Earth Deficiency.

15) Inner Resource: Thought (*Yi*)

Earth is responsible for thought, ideas and inspirations. Overthinking and worry, on the other hand, injures Earth energy. Individuals who are prone to excessive worry or are unable to control or stop their thoughts have a Spleen imbalance. Occupations that require little physical activity and a great deal of thought increase physical Damp stagnation that manifests as obesity, indicating Spleen Dampness.

As we digest and absorb food and drink, we also assimilate and absorb information and ideas. Therefore, it is not uncommon for individuals who are distracted and worried to have difficulty with digestion. Just as there must be a balance of diet and emotions for physical health, there must also be a balance of thought and activity.

Balanced Earth Type

Balanced Earth people present a balanced, strong physical appearance and an easy going, casual but compassionate manner. They tend to have an abundance of Qi and virility, good digestion, strong practical opinions, and an appreciation for pleasure as well as aesthetics in the form of art and music. They have a well established sense of "center" and Self, making them both practical and strongly self-motivated in all their endeavors.

Deficient Earth Type

A Deficient Earth person is frequently in need of sympathy and support from others. They tend to have low energy and weak digestion. The stool is generally loose and unformed with frequent, clear urine. Sexuality may be more for closeness and warmth rather than pleasure and lust. Lacking a strong inner drive, they require reassurance from others for many aspects of their life and are very guarded in taking on difficult projects that require prolonged effort. They may also have issues involving abnormal sweet cravings. They do best in warm sunny climates but may be less comfortable in either extreme cold or hot climates. Emotionally, they tend to be overly compassionate, identifying sometimes inappropriately and without any basis in fact with the discomfort of other individuals or creatures.

Diet should consist of mostly cooked foods high in whole grains, protein and some regular use of flesh foods. Vegetables should include potatoes, squash, cauliflower, carrots and broccoli. Herbs for the Deficient Earth type primarily include Qi and Blood building tonics such as astragalus root (Huang Qi), ginseng (Ren Shen) and codonopsis (Dang Shen). Formulas include **Major Four Herbs** (Si jun zi tang), **Major Six Herbs** (Liu jun zi tang) and **Eight Precious Herbs** (Ba zhen tang).

Excess Earth Type

An Excess Earth person exhibits excessive signs of Dampness and edema throughout the body. They may be overly opinionated with difficulty understanding another's point of view. Their digestion tends to be slow and congested with a tendency towards constipation or gas. They crave sweets but also appreciate hot, spicy foods which help to disperse stagnation. While they require more physical activity to maintain balance, they are generally slow moving and phlegmatic. Climatic humidity is a cause for much discomfort.

They are often individuals who state that at one time they had a great amount of physical energy but later in their life cycle, because of being weighed down by Damp accumulation, they easily tire and complain of a lack of physical stamina. They can be compassionate towards that which they understand but have difficulty in comprehension. Aesthetically they tend to appreciate those art forms that tend to stimulate and arouse strong emotions and passions.

Diet for the Excess Earth type should be low in animal protein, including all dairy. In contrast, it should be higher in whole grains, vegetable protein and leafy vegetables. Herbs should consist of reducing and eliminative herbs including laxatives such as rhubarb root (Da

Huang), cholagogues such as bupleurum (Chai Hu), coptis (Huang Lian) and gardenia fruit (Zhi Zi), and diuretic and Spleen Dampness removing herbs such as poria cocos (Fu Ling), alisma (Ze Xie) and pinellia (Ban Xia). Excess Earth also needs herbs that clear food congestion and promote digestion (Qi regulation). Herbs that remove food congestion include crataegus (Shan Zha) for digesting meat, Masa fermentata (Shen Qu) and Chicken gizzards (Ji Nei Jin), sprouted rice (Gu Ya) and sprouted barley (Mai Ya) for digesting grains. Carminative herbs that regulate Qi include cardamon (Sha Ren), saussurea (Mu Xiang) and tangerine peel (Chen Pi).

Laxative formulas include **Major and Minor Rhubarb Combinations** (Da cheng qi tang and Xiao cheng qi tang). Formulas that promote digestion include **Stomach Purging Decoction with Pinellia** (Ban xia xie xin tang) and **Citrus and Crataegus Formula** (Bao he wan). Formulas that remove Excess Dampness include **Poria Five Herb Combination** (Wu ling san), **Stomach Purging Decoction with Pinellia** (Ban xia xie xin tang) and **Hoelen and Areca Combination** (Wu pi yin).

METAL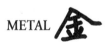

Today we think of Metal as a metaphor for dense material manifestation. With the dawn of the age of Metal being in close proximity to the time when the Five Element theory was evolving, ancient people undoubtedly had a much different idea concerning the metaphorical meaning of Metal than we do in our time. Their perspective of Metal included not only the utilitarian uses of iron and brass, but more precious metals such as silver and gold that were harder to mine. To ancient people, therefore, Metal signified a refined aspect of material manifestation.

Perhaps one of the most important metaphors associated with Metal is its correspondence with Autumn as a time of letting go and detachment. Thus, Metal is, in a sense, the most spiritual of all the Elements and involves transmutation from the base physical matter of Earth to its spiritual essence of Metal. It is from the refined essence of Water, Wood, Fire and Earth that the finest metals, such as gold, evolve. For this reason, the power of Metal is sometimes referred to as alchemical, the transmutation of base substances into gold.

There are many profound lessons to be learned about evolution as we meditate upon the significance of Metal. The connection of receiving cosmic spiritual energy is akin to the breath, for it is upon the essential rhythm of the breath that all physical activities depend. It is also from breath control, as found in the "inner" teachings of Yoga and Chinese Qi Gong, that the secret of quieting and focusing the mind is achieved and spiritual powers are made manifest. Thus, the Lungs are regarded as the home of the Corporeal Soul (*Po*). It is at this level that we experience our feelings from the most base sensations of pain and itching to emotional feelings of grief and sadness. It is through the experience of these uncomfortable feelings and sensations that we are prompted to learn to detach ourselves from the base material of the body to come in contact with the refined Metal essence of the Spirit.

Thus, the personality of Metal is one who is naturally detached and protected from negative outside influences (be it demons or viruses) and in touch with their spiritual essence. While Metal is present everywhere, to find or utilize its virtues requires effort and patience. With each calm, rhythmic breath cycle we take in positive cosmic energy of heaven and release negative tendencies and energies that are no longer needed for growth and survival.

People who have fallen out of rhythm with their breath by becoming off-centered tend to lose rhythm with the cycles of their higher needs, and they become vulnerable to outer negative spiritual and pathogenic influences. In this sense, upper respiratory allergies mystically represent some level by which we are out of rhythm with some factors of our external environment. One of the most frequently used methods for treating allergies is immunization, where Western medicine injects small quantities of allergens to protect us from outer viral diseases. Interestingly, homeopathy also utilizes the same reactive, allergenic substances but in submicro potencies to help attune us to those aspects of our outer environment which are the cause of our allergic reaction.

Asthma and emphysema are diseases where one literally loses one's breath. Certainly there are many causes including hereditary, environmental and dietary, that aggravate these terrible conditions, but one of the most important treatments for these conditions is the study and practice of pranayama (Yogic breath control) and/or Qi Gong (Chinese Taoist breathing practices). To overcome all obstacles in life, heal disease, manifest supernormal powers and strength, the object is ultimately for us to learn to get in harmony and regularity with our breath and ultimately, our lives.

1) Yin Organ: Lungs

Assigning the Lungs, which have to do with air and breath, to the Metal Element at first seems to present some difficulty. Air is the least solid element and yet it is this that is assigned to what may superficially be considered as the most dense of all the Five Elements. Only if we consider the importance of iron for the circulation of oxygen and food throughout the blood and into the cells of the body, as well as the processes of excretion governed by the Lung's Yang counterpart, the Large Intestines, are we able to understand how the ancient Chinese had such a profound understanding of complex physiological processes.

Minerals, dense though they may be, are vital catalysts for some of the most complex physical reactions in the animal and vegetable kingdoms. Thus, the Lungs are responsible for creating physical strength. They govern the Exterior and are responsible for preventing colds, flu, allergies, acute rheumatic and skin conditions through the Wei Qi. The Wei Qi in TCM is equivalent to the external immune system and is governed by the Lungs. Weakness, or Deficiency, of the Lungs is characterized by increased sensitivity and vulnerability to External diseases.

2) Yang Organ: Large Intestine
The Large Intestine represents the gross process of elimination on all levels. Without proper elimination, the body will become toxic and weak.

3) Season: Autumn
As stated previously, Autumn is the time of letting go as the energy retracts back into a state of Winter storage.

4) Climate: Dryness
Autumn is also the dry season. The primary complaints associated with both the Lungs and the Large Intestines are either excessive Dryness or Dampness in the form of mucus.

5) Direction: West
West represents the setting sun, the time of life to harvest, store and let go for the coming Winter.

6) Time of Day: 3 - 5 A.M.
This is the optimal time to perform Chinese Qi-Gong or Yogic pranayama or breath control exercises. Problems that regularly occur during this two-hour time period can indicate a Lung imbalance. Between 5 - 7 A.M. is the biological time for the Large Intestine and the optimal time for defecation.

7) Color: White
This the non-color of purity, detachment and withdrawal from

worldly affairs. A pale cast on the face can be an indication of either Blood Deficiency or Metal imbalance. Since the Lungs govern the circulation of Blood and Qi, there is a corresponding relationship between the two concepts.

8) Flavor: Spicy or Acrid

The spicy, or acrid, flavor indicates the presence of volatile oils that disperse outwards and downwards for elimination either through the perspiration or from the Urinary Bladder. Herbs such as cinnamon and ginger and foods such as onions and garlic are typically used to promote perspiration and treat colds and flu. Warm spicy herbs are also used to promote urination, especially when taken cool.

9) Sound: Sobbing or Crying

Since the corresponding emotion for Metal is grief and sadness, a sobbing tone of voice, even when there is no ostensible reason or awareness of sadness, is indicative of a Metal imbalance.

10) Smell: Rotten

It is during Autumn that dead leaves and decaying things assume a rotten odor. Similarly, the odor of mucus expelled from the lungs is typically a metallic, rotten smell.

11) Body Orifice: Nose

The nose is the outer opening of the Lungs. It also has an Elemental Yin-Yang relationship with the Large intestine. Both Lung imbalances and constipation can manifest as upper respiratory and sinus congestion.

12) Body Part: Skin

The Skin is considered the 'third' Lung because to maintain life, like the Lungs, it accomplishes a certain amount of respiration, absorption of nutrients (such as vitamin D) and elimination of waste through sweat. The pores must be capable of dilating to promote perspiration and elimination, and contraction to keep out External Pathogenic Influences. The energy that specifically accomplishes this emanates from the Lungs and is called the Wei Qi, or Defensive energy, and is an important aspect of the immune system in general. Many skin diseases are the result of constipation and can be treated by promoting bowel elimination.

13) External Manifestation: Body Hair

Any abnormal manifestations of the body hair, as opposed to head hair which is governed by the Kidneys, can indicate an imbalance of Metal.

14) Emotion: Grief

Grief and sadness are the emotions of letting go and releasing the past. While they are capable of plunging us into the depths of despair, they can also promote detachment from other worldly concerns and promote the possibility of greater self knowledge and strength. On the other hand, prolonged or intense grief can injure the Lungs, causing asthma, bronchitis or pneumonia.

15) Inner Resource: Corporeal Soul (*Po*)

The Lungs harbor the *Po*, or Corporeal Soul. As such, they represent the relation between our spiritual and physical being. It is through the rhythm of breath that we are able to coordinate our true inner needs and drives with the outer world. The breath also promotes the creation of Qi and activates the circulation of Qi and Blood throughout the entire body.

Balanced Metal Type

Metal represents the highest degree of adjustment, refinement and sensitivity. There is a sense of belonging and order, both in terms of the personal relationship with one's self as well as with the macrocosmic order of climate and outer relationship with events and others. A balanced Metal type is neither thrown off balance by outer atmospheric influences that might generate cold or allergic reactions, nor by emotional shock which can influence the rhythm of one's breath.

Consider how when one travels there is, for most at least, a period of bowel irregularity. With the balanced Metal type there is an even rhythm both in receiving on the subtle level of the psyche as well as the physical level of breath and, on the gross level of the large bowel, a letting go. In a word, the balanced Metal type is able to regulate their physical and emotional life with outer climate, circumstances and events.

Deficient Metal Type

The Deficient Metal type lacks the inner strength to withstand either atmospheric fluctuations, such as minor airborne irritants like dust or pollen for instance, or psycho-physical shocks that might precipitate an irregular breathing pattern, represented by such diseases as asthma and emphysema. We see them as being highly sensitive and emotionally vulnerable as well as having Deficient Wei Qi, or a weakened outer defensive immune system. This makes them highly susceptible to colds, flu, sinus congestion and allergies. They may have problems with bowel irregularity, not so much because of Excess congestion and stagnation, but from a lack of energy to effect a complete and regular bowel evacuation.

Psychologically these individuals require rhythmic evenness and regularity that will allow them to organize the various aspects of their psycho-physical lives, which is what Metal types are most inclined to want to achieve. Because of their inability to create such organization for themselves, they tend to fall victim to outer irregularities and mishaps.

Diet for Deficient Metal types should include regular servings of rice, the specific grain for strengthening the Lungs. If there is phlegm, dairy should be avoided (although boiling or precooking dairy will lessen its mucus forming propensity). Herbs for treating Metal Deficiency include Qi and Immune tonics such as astragalus root (Huang Qi), polygonatum (Huang Jing), ophiopogon root (Mai Men Dong), American ginseng (Xi Yang Shen) and pseudostellaria (Tai Zi Shen). Formulas to consider are **Jade Screen Immune Tonic** (Yu ping feng san) and **Ophiopogon Combination** (Mai men dong tang).

Excess Metal Type

Excess Metal is physically manifested as congestion, characterized by the tendency towards either yellow or Hot Phlegm, or white or Cold Phlegm. Here one characteristically is reacted upon once again by outer airborne influences or inner emotional responses to release and discharge that which has accumulated. By harmonizing with the Autumnal aspect of this event, which is to shed or let go of that which is no longer needed, the Excess Metal type is easily able to restore balance and normal circulation. Fasting and withdrawal from worldly concerns is most appropriate for Excess Metal, since what is to be eliminated is that which has been taken on as a result of the Excess of Earth.

Excess Metal commonly involves Phlegm congestion and allergies. Herbs used to treat asthma and allergies include ephedra (Ma Huang) and xanthium (Cang Er Zi). These are included in various formulas for allergies and colds including **Ephedra Decoction** (Ma huang tang), **Minor Blue Dragon** (Xiao qing long tang), **Xanthium Powder** (Cang er san) and the famous Chinese patented formula called Bi Yan Pian.

Besides these, there are highly effective herbs for treating a variety of upper respiratory conditions. These include herbs that expel Cold Phlegm, such as platycodon root (Jie Geng) which, because it has a neutral energy, is effective by itself for clearing the Lungs, and pinellia (Ban Xia), which is one of the most effective herbs for clearing Phlegm Dampness and mucus. Pinellia is used in **Citrus and Pinellia Combination** (Er Chen Tang), available as a patented product, a commonly used formula for drying and eliminating Cold Mucus. Other herbs are especially used to expel Hot Phlegm, such as peucedani (Qian Hu), fritillaria (Chuan Bei Mu) and trichosanthes root (Tian Hua Fen). Herbs that inhibit the cough reflex include apricot seed (Xing Ren), aster root (Zi Wan), coltsfoot flowers (Kuan Dong Hua) and loquat leaves (Pi Pa Ye).

WATER 水

Water embodies the latent potential of all life forms. It is a reservoir from which the potential for all life - past, present and future - emanates. In TCM, the Water element embodies the inherited constitution, or Ancestral Qi, that determines one's development, growth and strength. It is the Self which consists of the innate reserves inherited from one's forebears and from which emanates the primal spark utilized by the body to initiate and maintain all vital functions.

The important characteristic of Water is its ability to flow, making streams, rivers, ponds, seas and oceans of liquid flowing energy. Similarly, in the body the Water Element is that which circulates, lubricates, sustains and deeply nourishes. This includes the Blood, lymph and the flowing aspect of Qi in the form of bioelectrical nervous energy, as well as the fluidity of the endocrine system, all internal secretions, perspiration, tears, saliva, sexual secretions, lactation, the lubrication of the Lungs and all other mucus membranes of the body, and the moisture required for proper elimination from the Large Intestine and the Bladder. The fluid aspect of the Water Element is also responsible for maintaining lubrication, agility, suppleness and softness of the joints, muscles and the skin.

In TCM, the Kidneys, as the Yin Organ of Water, embody all of its aspects, including the regulation of the endocrine system. Obviously this goes beyond the role of the Kidneys per se and includes the small pea-like glands attached to them called the Adrenal glands. These regulate most of the endocrine functions, especially the sympathetic and parasympathetic nervous systems, through their secretion of Yang-stimulating adrenaline-type hormones and Yin-nourishing, cooling anti-inflammatory cortical hormones.

Symptoms of Water imbalances include urinary diseases, edema, lower back and joint pains. It also includes a myriad of conditions normally associated with the endocrine system such as impotence, infertility, mal-development, premature aging and fatigue. Further, there are a range of other conditions such as hair loss, premature graying of the hair and hearing problems that indicate Water imbalance (which is usually Deficient).

1) Yin Organ: Kidneys

As stated, the Kidneys are the root of Yin and Yang, regulating endocrine response throughout the body. They also regulate Water by maintaining the optimal balance of intracellular and extracellular fluid and the elimination of fluid waste through the urine. Still another important Kidney function is calcium metabolism and the maintenance of the bones.

2) Yang Organ: Urinary Bladder

The Bladder is more mechanically responsible for the elimination of Fluid waste.

3) Season: Winter

Winter is a time of storage and retreat. It is at this time that the life force lies dormant, collecting itself beneath the ground for the coming Spring. Kidney imbalances and symptoms such as lowered immunity, coldness and frequent urination frequently reveal themselves at this time of year.

4) Climate: Cold

Cold specifically taxes the reserves of the TCM Kidney-Adrenals; thus they respond adversely to cold foods and fluids and cold drafts, particularly directly on the lower back where the kidneys reside.

5) Direction: North

North, the direction of Winter, is associated with Coldness.

6) Time of Day: 3 - 7 P.M.

Bladder time is between 3 and 5 P.M. and Kidney time is between 5 and 7 P.M. Maximum benefits are achieved if corresponding teas are taken and/or acupuncture points are treated during the correlating biological time for the Organ. This is the time when each Organ flourishes, and any weakness in the Organ often results in an appearance or a worsening of symptoms during its time.

7) Color: Black

Individuals whose facial pallor emanates a dark or black color are considered to have Kidney-Adrenal Deficiency.

8) Flavor: Salty

Salt is necessary to retain sufficient fluid to support and maintain all the functions associated with Water. Since the human body is comprised of approximately 78% water, it is obviously a vital and necessary Element for our survival. A relatively small increase or decrease of the Water Element can put a severe stress on all homeostatic mechanisms. A sufficient amount of unrefined salt that naturally occurs with a variety of essential trace minerals is necessary to maintain proper Fluid balance. TCM recommends that herbal tonics for the Kidney-Adrenals be taken with a pinch of salt that helps potentize and carry the effects of the herbs into the Kidneys.

9) Sound: Groaning

When we become tired and fatigued, we develop a lower pitched sound that resembles a groan, indicative of Kidney Deficiency.

10) Smell: Putrid

This odor is difficult to distinguish from Metal but represents a further degree of decay and rottenness.

11) Body Orifices: Ears, Urethra, Anus and Genitals

Imbalances and diseases associated with these bodily areas can be indicative of a Water imbalance.

12) Body Parts: Bones and Bone Marrow

The Kidney-Adrenals are responsible for maintaining calcium balance in all the bones of the body, including the teeth. They also govern the bone marrow, which plays a vital role in maintaining the deep immune system of the body. The brain is considered in TCM to be one of the "curious Organs" and is called "the sea of bone marrow". Therefore the Kidney-Adrenals also govern the brain.

13) External Manifestation: Head Hair

The condition of the hair on the head is indicative of the condition of the Kidneys. If it is thin, dry and splits easily, it represents Deficiency. Premature graying or hair loss is a further indication of a Water depletion. It is not uncommon for women after childbirth, or for those under long term stress, to develop bald patches. This is usually caused by Blood and Kidney-Adrenal Deficiency. Further, individuals who experience traumatic shock often have their hair turn gray or fall out.

14) Emotion: Fear

Extreme fear or shock can injure the Kidney-Adrenals and precipitate chronic problems later in life. A common tragedy is the impaired and stunted growth syndrome that occurs as a result of childhood trauma and abuse. Besides this, there can be many other chronic Kidney imbalance symptoms that tend to manifest later in life.

15) Inner Resource: Will (*Zhi*)

An individual who lacks personal motivation or will power has a Water imbalance in the form of Kidney-Adrenal Deficiency. Water is the deep reserve that gives power to all activities and processes. In most cases, individuals who lack motivation and will power have Kidney Yang Deficiency. Following Five Element theory, Earth controls or subdues Water. The flavor associated with Earth is sweet so that an excess of sweet in the form of unrefined sugar in all forms, including alcohol, saps will power and establishes the basis for all physical and mental addictions.

It is becoming commonly understood that marijuana, an anti-motivational drug, diminishes our will and drive. From the TCM perspective, it is never appropriate to sedate or weaken the Kidney-Adrenals, which is exactly what marijuana does. The associated fear and insecurity that sometimes accompanies marijuana use further points to its debilitating effects on those whose Kidney Qi is already low. The hallucinations and vivid colors can be understood from the Five Element perspective that Water is unable, at least momentarily, to control Fire (hallucinations and visions). Finally, another long term side effect of continued marijuana abuse is impotence and infertility.

Balanced Water Type

Water represents the inner Self. Since it is one's very essence, it cannot be understood in any sense as Excess, but only as Deficiency. This is where the concept of Will, assigned to the Kidneys, is understood as the primary function of Water. It is through the will, or innate power of the body, that the Self is able to arise. Whatever we may understand as the singular characteristic of Water, it is in its flowing forth, supporting and empowering all psycho-physiological processes that it takes on its richest meaning. The most recurrent theme of ancient Taoism is the metaphorical description of the power of the flowing movement of Qi compared to water in a stream that ultimately bypasses and overcomes all obstacles in its path.

God and inner Self in Chinese medical philosophy are a dynamic expression of ephemeral being through eternity. In the individual personality, that divine expression is directed through the primal power of Will to initiate and maintain the initial lifespark impetus into full manifestation.

To describe the Balanced Water type, therefore, is to give embodiment to the perfect human which, at least on this daily level of survival, does not exist. Nevertheless, those who achieve the closest to the ideal of the Balanced Water type would manifest a high level of self awareness and confidence with a sense that they are acting from a place of deep strength and inner reserves. When emotional or physical stress does occur, the flowing nature of their highly developed Water Element seems to not leave any lasting scars. Further, because of the power of their perfected Will, they are able to manifest a high degree of stamina and endurance when challenged.

We find this expression of deep flowing strength in all areas of human occupation and endeavor. This includes their relationship with others which, because of their self-confidence and reliance, does not have the taint of deadly possessiveness and angry frustration that comes as a result of deep-seated fears. It is also present in the management of survival and economic endeavors. If there is one predominant positive characteristic to the Balanced Water type, it is the ability to be fully present for whatever presents itself with the appropriate degree of inner discipline. Because they are so closely attuned to their inner self, outer vicissitudes and shifts of fortune do not easily throw them into a state of insecurity and fear.

Yin Deficient Water Type

Water Yin Deficiency appears as a kind of auto-consumption, but in fact it is the very Essence that is unrestrainedly leaking out. Thus, there are symptoms of night sweats, insomnia, nervousness, anxiousness, irritability, thin or emaciated appearance, frequent urination and inflammatory conditions that are more localized in the extremities, such as a Yin Deficient sore throat or genito-urinary inflammation.

Unlike Excess conditions, Yin Deficient inflammatory symptoms do not arise from a whole bodily context of Excess, but rather from wasting and Deficiency that predisposes them to a recurring chronic expression. It is the lack of inner reserves that causes the Water Yin Deficient personality to have a comparatively low tolerance for physical or emotional stress, which is the precipitating cause for all Yin Deficient symptoms. Yet another defining characteristic is that Water Yin Deficient conditions tend not to readily respond to anti-inflammatory treatments with antibiotics, Vitamin C or Heat clearing alteratives.

With the inability to contain and restrain the Self, there is a kind of over-sensitivity, hollowness and inappropriateness to the Water Yin Deficient personality. The problem is that while there are many fitful and empty jabs at self expression, the Water Yin Deficient type lacks the stamina, endurance and, above all, inner focus to see things through to completion.

Obviously, one would use foods and herbs that embody the characteristic qualities of Yin such as moist, demulcent, solid, substantial and cooling foods. Oils and fats are Yin, so pork is the most Yin of animal foods, while okra and malva are the most Yin of vegetables. The best oil to use is ghee (clarified butter) as it increases metabolic fires without being heating to the body. Herbs that have demulcent, nutritive and tonic properties are indicated as well as demulcent astringents that prevent leakage of Qi and Fluids, such as Chinese schizandra berries (Wu Wei Zi) and cornus, or dogwood, berries (Shan Zhu Yu). One could think of a powerful tonic astringent, such as schizandra, as an herb that cements the aura of the personality and helps the body to contain its energy.

The primary formulas for treating Yin Deficiency are **Anemarrhena, Phellodendron and Rehmannia Combination** (Zhi bai di huang wan) and **Rehmannia Six Combination** (Liu wei di huang wan).

Yang Deficient Water Type

A Yang Deficient Water type includes Coldness, timidity, fatigue, lack of libido, back and joint pains, (especially the lower back and knees) and frequent urination. In this condition, there is an inability to circulate and maintain one's dynamic life processes on both the inner organic level as well as the outer level of procreation and lifework. An inability to exercise and/or a lack of exercise are primary aggravating factors with Yang Deficient Water types.

In general there is a diminished ability to maintain one's self both in terms of the normal use of the joints of the body as well as the ability to engage in creative projects. The Yang Deficient Water type seems unable to mobilize their resources and whatever energy they may have, either in their own maintenance and defense or the prerequisite attention, care and protection of others.

Sometimes this withdrawal from life appears as physical detachment, but there is no wisdom in renouncing that which one is unable to attain. As a result, Yang Deficient types are particularly susceptible to delusion based on falsely upheld spiritual values, a kind of 'sour grapes' attitude that allows for a particular form of arrogant self-righteousness which occurs in some forms of Yin Deficiency as well. At this stage, both the Yin and Yang Deficient personality is nearly lost to further enlightenment except through some awakening. Depending on how one uses the opportunity, physical crisis may either plunge one into utter despair or it can lead to a greater depth of letting go and serving the Soul's preeminent need to evolve into higher knowledge and truth.

Since a perfect balance of Yin and Yang and the Five Elements seems impossible, at least on this level of earthly existence, we must view imbalance as a stress or motivating force that drives us onward, to further and deeper levels of Self knowledge. From this perspective, besides showing who we are in relation to nature, Yin Yang and Five Element theories also reveal by implication, perhaps, who and what we are not.

For example, from the Five Element perspective, we are not simply a controlling and aggressive individual but someone with a Liver-Wood imbalance that can be corrected through any number of means from a simple change of diet to a profound psychological awareness, nor are we a sad and negative individual but someone influenced by an imbalance of Metal and Water. Our joy and happiness, therefore, also merely emanate from our Heart-Fire Element while our compassion and caring traits stem perhaps from our Spleen-Earth energy. In other words, these self analytical systems serve a function of aiding detachment to outer appearances. To be caught up in misidentifying with any of these qualities and Elements, is to be in a state of illusion or self-deception. The point then becomes that if we are not simply a bag of flesh and bones with a number of personal traits thrown in, who and what are we?

If our goal in life is simply and only to maintain harmony and balance between all of the Elements at all times, there would be no transcending purpose to existence and what we call life would be a rather boring and dull experience. In other words, from a practical Taoist perspective, the Five Elements can be used as a method of understanding and treating our imbalances as well as a psychological tool to help us transcend them.

The major formula for Kidney Yang Deficiency is **Rehmannia Eight Combination** (Ba wei di huang wan) and **Replenishing the Yang Decoction** (You gui yin).

INTERACTION OF THE FIVE ELEMENTS
In health there is a dynamic interaction between all Five Elements and the internal physiology, but in sickness an imbalance between one or more of the organic cycles will be evident and most usually affects an imbalance of either its parent, child, grandparent or grandchild through the Shen or Ko cycles. This will reflect itself both physically and on the mental and emotional levels.

For example, if Wood is in Excess, a condition of negative influence or control over Earth can affect poor digestion with a tendency towards indigestion, gas, acid belching and nausea. If Wood is Deficient, problems with the Liver can impair one's ability to gain weight and cause blood and lymphatic toxicity, weak digestion and infertility.

If there is Excess Fire, we may see symptoms of over-talkativeness, a tendency to inappropriate laughter and giddiness, feelings of excessive Heat with redness of the face, and heart and circulatory problems. Heart Excess can give rise to cardio-pulmonary disease, because the Heart-Fire overdominates the Lungs-Metal.

When Earth is in Excess, there may be symptoms of bloating with gas and constipation. Deficiency may cause weak digestion, difficulty assimilating food, fluids or, on the mental level, ideas. If Earth overdominates Kidney-Water, urinary problems may be aggravated. Problems with digestion can be exaggerated with strong cravings for sweet and a tendency towards mucus discharges. If the mucus discharges occur in the sinuses and Lungs, it is considered a problem between Earth and Metal. A discharge from the reproductive Organs involves the Liver and/or Kidneys as well.

A Deficiency in the Water Element indicates basic inherited weaknesses and retarded growth patterns. This can result in Kidney-Water's inability to nourish Liver-Wood, which may produce symptoms of body stiffness, dryness, impotence, infertility and headaches. The inability of Water to control Fire can cause an apparent excess of Fire, as in chronic fevers and certain heart and circulatory disorders. If Water is in Excess, it can dominate Fire, giving rise to heart problems resulting in severe edema and water retention.

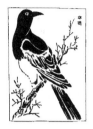

FOUR

FUNDAMENTAL SUBSTANCES

QI, BLOOD, FLUID, ESSENCE AND SHEN

The Fundamental Substances form the foundation of the body. They have their own particular origins, functions and purposes, and yet are mutually interactive and supportive. They include Qi, Blood, Fluids, Essence and Shen (Mind and Spirit).

"Qi" is the fundamental activating force and energy of life. It is a part of Yang and includes motivation and warmth for the body. Qi transforms, transports, holds, protects, raises up and warms. The concept of "Blood" is similar, though broader in definition to, Western medicine and includes circulation, stagnation and hemorrhage. "Fluids" describe all the various fluidic substances including saliva, sweat, urine, tears, lymph and other secretions. Both Blood and Fluids are a part of Yin and embody the ability to nurture, moisten and lubricate. The anabolic phase of generation, growth and development as well as the catabolic phase of aging, death and disease necessitate the dynamic interaction of Qi, Blood and Fluids.

Essence is the basis of reproduction, development, growth, sexual power, conception, pregnancy and decay in the body. It also forms the basic constitutional strength and vitality. When it manifests as Qi, it is known as Original Qi. Essence also includes semen and the reproductive capacity of the body. In its most broad and comprehensive sense, "Essence" refers to the overall hormonal strength that regulates normal growth, metabolism and sexuality. Although not a Fluid, it is Fluid-like and so is considered a part of Yin. It is stored in the Kidney-adrenals.

Shen encompasses both the Mind and the Spirit. It reflects the entire physical, emotional, mental and spiritual health of the body. It includes the capacity to think and act coherently, the force of the human personality, and the joy to live. It also includes the spiritual aspects of all the organs, especially the Yin organs. It is distinguished by the sparkle in the eyes, an overall vivaciousness and the will to live. Shen is housed in the Heart. Because of its active nature, it is a part of Yang.

Qi, Blood and Fluids are often termed the Chinese Three Humours. They represent broad categories of physiological functions for classifying and matching imbalances and diseases with corresponding herbal treatments. They are similar but not identical to the concept of "Tridosha", also called "Three Humours" (Water, Fire and Air), which forms the basic diagnostic approach of Ayurvedic and Tibetan medicine.

QI: THE PRINCIPLE OF UNITY
The Tao that can be told is not the eternal Tao.
The name that can be named is not the eternal name.
The nameless is the beginning of heaven and earth.
The named is the mother of ten thousand things.
Ever desireless, one can see the mystery.
Ever desiring, one can see the manifestations.
These two spring from the same source but differ in name;
this appears as darkness.
Darkness within darkness.
The gate to all mystery.[1]

Qi is the all-pervasive animating force of nature. Because it is the expression of both the quality and substance of all things, it is both quantifiable and ephemeral. It expresses itself both as a general quality of energy as well as the energetic manifestation of a specific part or organ.

In its cosmically supreme form, Qi is the subtle unifying energy of all phenomena. In nature it is expressed as movement, evolution, climate, growth, function and appearance. Within the realm of the body it is the energetic potential of each part, especially each of the vital Organs. In the plant kingdom it is perceived as the unique form, color, flavor, texture and unique biochemical configuration of each plant species. Similarly, we identify Qi as both the unique and particular qualities of manifestation throughout the human, animal, vegetable and mineral kingdoms, a continuum of mental, physical and spiritual qualities that Western philosophers and physicists describe as "energy". It is also known as "life force", "vital life force", in Ayurvedic medicine as "prana" and to the Japanese as "ki".

Qi is ever-changing and mutable. Thus it manifests differently according to circumstances and environments. Because Qi appears in various degrees of manifestation, both material and immaterial, it is beyond duality and forms the common thread from which all creation is manifest. The traditional symbol of Qi is the sun as the giver of life. It is by definition unlimited, and is sometimes equated with the concept of the Supreme Ultimate. Practically speaking, however, Qi manifests as essential vitality, digestive power, growth, reproductive energies, and so forth. Even the potential of our inherited constitution for ongoing health is an expression of a kind of "Inherited Qi".

Just as science has discovered that the DNA molecule is the all-pervasive code of life manifesting as different tissues and organs throughout the body, Qi, which is essentially one, manifests in different forms and qualities depending upon its functions within the body. In TCM, Qi has two major aspects in the body. In one, it represents a refined aspect, or Essence, which nourishes the body-mind complex. This Essence is expressed in different forms according to its location and function in the body. In its second aspect, Qi indicates the functional activities of the internal organs themselves.

THE FORMATION OF QI

Qi is basically generated in the human body from three sources: Pre-Heaven Essence, Post-Heaven Essence and air brought in and transformed by the Lungs. "Essence", or "Jing" as it is often called, represents the refined aspect upon which the grosser manifestation of the body is based. As such, it is considered precious and something to be guarded and protected.

"Pre-Heaven Essence" is an expression of the potential of the father, the mother and the grandparents as these unite to create a newly conceived child. Thus, Pre-Heaven Essence represents our essential "inherited" constitutional strength. This essence in the form of Qi, rather than fluid, is called Original Qi, Prenatal Qi or Inborn Qi.

"Post-Heaven Essence", on the other hand, represents what happens to us after birth. It is affected by what we acquire from air, food and water. Post-Heaven Essence is also influenced by various stresses, both emotional and physiological. This essence in Qi form is called Grain Qi, Food Qi or Central Qi.

Since our capacity to derive nourishment from air, food and water is dependent upon our ability to digest and transform these ingested materials into the fabric of our being, there is a close relationship between Pre-Heaven and Post-Heaven Essence as they manifest in the strength of our Lungs, Stomach and Spleen. In TCM, the Spleen represents our fundamental capacity to transform and transport food nourishment into cells throughout our body. Thus, the Chinese Spleen is a reflection of our essential metabolic strength. This is manifested in its ability to acquire energy from food, or Grain Qi. The Lungs in TCM are, among other functions, responsible for inhaling air and extracting energy from it, called Natural Air Qi, Gathering Qi or Pectoral Qi.

Thus, the process of Qi formation is as follows: Original Qi from the Kidneys goes to the area of the Spleen and Stomach where it combines with Grain Qi. This continues upward to the Lungs where it mixes with Natural Air Qi. From there it turns into Qi for the whole body, called True Qi, Normal Qi or Upright Qi. This last stage of Qi formation produces the Qi which circulates in the inner and outer layers of the body and nourishes the Organs. It does so by taking two different forms, as Nourishing Qi and Defensive Qi. Qi in the human body is generated from the following three sources: Pre-Heaven Essence which is inherited or innate constitutional potential from parents and grandparents and forms the Original Qi that resides in the Kidneys; Post-Heaven Essences which is what we acquire after birth from air and food; and Essence or Jing, refined aspects of the body upon which the grosser aspects of the body manifest.

THE CLASSIFICATIONS OF QI

ORIGINAL QI (YUAN QI)

Original Qi, also called Prenatal, Inborn, Primordial and Genuine Qi, is the most important and fundamental biological Qi category. It is pre-Heaven Essence in its Qi, rather than Fluid, form. Stored in the Kidneys, it also includes both the Original Yin and Yang Qi energies, and thus is the source of Yin and Yang in the body. Original Qi depends on nourishment from Post-Heaven Essence developed by the Spleen and Stomach into Grain Qi. Therefore, what we eat and drink and how well these substances are transformed in the body greatly influence the body's Original Qi and Yin and Yang energies.

Original Qi moves from the "life fire" or "vital gate" between the Kidneys (*ming men*) and circulates throughout the entire body to all the Organs, muscles, skin and so forth. It is thus the foundation of vitality, stamina and proper functioning of all systems in the body. Original Qi has several functions. It is the motivating power of the vital activities in the body, it is the basis for Kidney Qi and shares its role in providing the necessary heat for the body's functions. It is the activating force in changing natural Air Qi into True Qi in the body, it aids the production of Blood in the body through the transformation of Grain Qi in the Heart, and it spreads throughout the internal Organs and channels in the body, coming to rest at the Source points, as they are called in acupuncture.

Deficiency of Original Qi manifests as a fundamental weakness of any or all Organ functions. There may be chronic symptoms of low vitality, coldness, slow metabolism, slow growth and development, a reduction of physiological functions and a tendency to frequent illness with slow recovery. For instance, an individual who is born weak and malformed or has become weakened because of poor air, food, fluid and lifestyle habits, and has difficulty healing a broken bone later in life, is considered to have an Original Qi deficiency or impairment.

Original Qi Deficiencies are treated with good quality food, water, air, rest and appropriate tonic herbs, especially those prepared with food. Tonic herbs that may be used to nourish Original Qi include ginseng, codonopsis, astragalus, jujube dates, Dang Gui, Polygonum multiflorum, ophiopogon, lycium berries, schisandra berries and prepared rehmannia. In acupuncture, the Source points located on the twelve channels are needled, with moxabustion (penetrating warmth generated by burning Artemisia vulgaris near and over the selected points) at the navel and the Sea of Qi point, located an inch and a half below the navel.

GRAIN QI (GU QI)

Grain Qi, also known as Food Qi or Central Qi, constitutes the creation of Qi from food and drink. It represents the energy of digestion as it manifests in the Middle Warmer of the Stomach and Spleen. Food first enters the Stomach where it is "rotted and ripened", and is then transformed by the Spleen into Grain Qi. This Qi is not yet in a form the body can use, but must combine with Original Qi and rise to the chest to mix with Natural Air Qi to form the True Qi useable by the body.

NATURAL AIR QI (ZONG QI)

Natural Air Qi has several other names: Ancestral Qi, Pectoral Qi, Gathering Qi, Essential Qi and Chest Qi. All refer to the Qi produced by the combination of Grain Qi with air brought in by the Lungs. It is a subtle and refined form of Qi that nourishes the Heart and Lungs and promotes circulation of Blood and Qi. It regulates the rhythmic movement of the heartbeat and respiration. It also gathers in the throat, aiding speech and strength of voice. Further, Natural Air Qi flows downwards to aid the Kidneys, while the Original Qi of the Kidneys flows upwards to aid respiration. They therefore mutually assist each other.

If Natural Air Qi is weak, the feet and hands will be cold, speech impeded, respiration or heartbeat uneven, breathing shallow, heartbeat abnormal, circulation slow or poor, limbs cold or voice soft or weak. Thus, breathing exercises are very beneficial to strengthening Natural Air Qi.

TRUE QI (ZHEN QI)

True Qi, or Normal, Upright or Meridian Qi, is the final stage of Qi transformation. This is the Qi useable by the body and is the energy which penetrates and permeates the entire body and nourishes the Organs. It comes from the transformation of Natural Air Qi in the Lungs through the catalytic action of Original Qi. It takes two forms, Nutritive Qi and Defensive Qi.

NUTRITIVE QI (YING QI)

Nutritive Qi, or Nourishing Qi, has two main functions: to produce Blood and to nourish the entire body. When True Qi enters the Heart it is transformed into Blood. This Qi then circulates within the blood vessels and channels, moves the Blood and nourishes it. It is thus often called Nourishing Qi, or Nourishing Yin, since in comparison to Defensive Qi, it has a Yin rather than Yang function. This is the Qi activated by acupuncture.

DEFENSIVE QI (WEI QI)

Defensive Qi represents the surface immune system's ability to protect the body from attack of any exterior pathogens: Wind, Cold, Heat, Damp, Dryness and Summer Heat. It travels on the surface of the body between the skin and muscles, regulating the opening and closing of the pores and moistening the skin, muscles and hair. It is a more Yang form of Qi than Nutritive Qi, which is more Yin and serves to nourish the interior.

In addition, the circulation of Defensive Qi is associated with sleep. During sleep, Defensive Qi circulates in the interior of the body and during waking hours it circulates on the surface of the body. When Defensive Qi is weak, it may circulate longer on the surface of the body, thus shortening sleep duration. Frequently people awaken between 3-5 am when this occurs. Since the Lungs regulate the circulation of Defensive Qi, a weakness of the Lungs is most frequently related to a weakness of the Defensive Qi, and vice versa. Such a weakness often manifests as a tendency to catch colds and flu. Spontaneous daytime sweating may also occur since weak Defensive Qi may not properly open or close the pores.

The term "Upright Qi" is often used to describe the body's ability to resist Exterior Pathogenic Influences. It is not another type of Qi but describes the combination of Natural Air Qi from the Lungs with the deeper immune Qi originating from the combination of Essence and Original Qi transformed by Kidney Yang.

Qi Classification	Origin in the Body	Function
Original Qi (Yuan Qi)	Derived from Pre-Heaven Essence, stored in the Kidneys and is the foundation of all Qi in the body.	Source of Yin and Yang in the body, emanates from the "life gate" of the Kidneys to manifest as the essential vitality and stamina of the entire body.
Grain Qi (Gu Qi)	Emanates from the Stomach and Spleen and is derived from food.	Combines with both the Original and Air Qi to make True Qi which is the daily useable energy.
Natural Air (Zong Qi)	Lungs	Nourishes the Heart and Lungs, promotes circulation.
True Qi (Zhen Qi)	Exists in the Meridians and Internal Organs.	Final stage of Qi transformation. It penetrates and permeates the entire body and nourishes the Internal Organs.
Nutritive Qi (Ying Qi)	Derived from the True Qi in the Heart.	Produces Blood and nourishes the entire body.
Defensive Qi (Wei Qi)	Circulates on the surface of the body during the day and internally at night. It is regulated by the Lungs.	The surface immune system regulates the opening and closing of the pores of the skin, moistens the skin and hair, influences the duration of sleep.

THE FUNCTIONS OF QI

The basic functions of Qi in the human body are to transform, transport, hold, raise up, protect and warm.

QI TRANSFORMS

Qi is the transforming or changing power in the body. It transforms food into Qi, Blood or Body Fluid, and these can be changed into any of the others according to the body's needs. The waste from eaten food is transformed into feces, urine, tears and sweat. Qi is also the basic metabolic power of the body. Specifically, in the Spleen it transforms food into Food Essence, or Grain Qi; in the Heart it transforms Grain

Qi into Blood; in the Kidneys it transforms Fluids and in the Bladder it transforms urine.

QI TRANSPORTS

The movement of Qi is vital to life and promotes the functional activities in the body on all levels: voluntary and involuntary, mental, growth and development. There are four basic ways in which Qi moves: ascending, descending, inwards (entering) and outwards (exiting). For example, Spleen Qi transports Grain Qi upwards to the Lungs, Lung Qi transports fluids to the skin, Kidney Qi transports Qi upwards, Liver Qi transports Qi smoothly and evenly in all directions, Lung Qi transports Qi downwards, Stomach Qi transports Qi downwards and Large Intestine Qi and Urinary Bladder Qi transport feces and urine outwards respectively. This transporting function is also a regulating one, controlling and adjusting the movement, secretion and excretion of substances in the body.

QI HOLDS

Qi also has the function of holding, retaining or consolidating substances and Organs in the body. It helps keep Blood in its pathways and Organs in their proper positions, adjusts the appropriate flow of sweat, urine and saliva, prevents Body Fluids from escaping, and consolidates and stores sperm. Various Organs' Qi divides these functions: Spleen Qi holds in the Blood, fluids such as saliva and supports the Organs; Kidney Qi holds in sperm and, with Urinary Bladder Qi, the urine; and Lung Qi holds in sweat.

A weakening of the Qi holding function may result in hemorrhage, spontaneous sweating, polyuria, salivation, spermatorrhea, premature ejaculation and prolapses, such as the Stomach, Kidneys, Urinary Bladder, uterus or anus.

QI RAISES UP

Specific types of Qi rise in the body. Spleen Qi raises the Organs, keeping them in place, and its Grain Qi rises to the Lungs to form True Qi and later Blood. Kidney Qi rises to keep Essence and sperm in, and it rises toward the Lungs to receive the descending air. The Qi raising function is a further part of the holding and transporting functions.

QI PROTECTS

Qi protects the body from the invasion of Exterior Pathogenic Influences. It moves in the chest, abdomen and between the skin and muscles, and it regulates the pores and sweat glands.

QI WARMS

A function of Yang, the warming aspect of Qi maintains the normal Heat of the body and all of its parts. It is mostly a function of Kidney Yang, although Spleen Yang and Heart Yang contribute.

Overall, these various Qi functions appear in the body as follows: Kidney Qi transforms Fluids, moves Qi upwards, holds urine and warms the entire body. Spleen Qi transforms and transports food, holds the Blood in the vessels, raises the Organs, warms and supports overall metabolism. Heart Qi transforms Grain Qi into Blood, circulates Blood through the vessels and produces Fire. Liver Qi regulates and transports Qi smoothly and evenly. Lung Qi transports Qi downwards and, by ruling the pores of the skin, protects the body from external invasion.

If, for example, Kidney Qi is weak and unable to transform Fluids, there might be symptoms of edema or frequent urination associated with aching soreness of the joints and lower back. The individual will be highly reactive to cold temperatures. Formulas containing rehmannia, cinnamon bark and prepared aconite are indicated.

If Spleen Qi is weak there may be appetite disorders, tiredness, excessive bleeding (especially during menstruation), prolapse of the internal Organs and generally low energy and metabolism. In cases like these, formulas containing carminatives, such as citrus peel or cardamom, are given to promote digestion, and ginseng, codonopsis and astragalus are used to tonify Qi.

If Heart Qi is Deficient, anemia, coldness, cold hands and feet and pallid complexion may become evident. Formulas containing Dang Gui are used.

When Liver Qi fails to evenly regulate and transport Qi, emotional symptoms such as mood swings, anger and depression often occur along with a tight, constricted feeling in the chest. Formulas containing bupleurum are used.

If Lung Qi is deficient, there will be shallow respiration, tiredness and a tendency to catch colds frequently. Formulas containing astragalus root are used.

PATHOLOGIES OF QI

Several pathologies of Qi exist and involve either insufficient Qi or stagnant Qi in which Qi is either flowing improperly or is impeded. Deficient or stagnant Qi is usually associated with specific organs, such as Deficient Spleen Qi, or stagnant Liver Qi. Disharmonies of Qi are outlined in the Chapter on Patterns of Disharmonies.

METHODS TO BUILD AND STRENGHTHEN QI

BREATHING PRACTICES

Perhaps the best therapy to strengthen the Lungs is breathing exercises. There are several specific Yogic practices that have their counterparts in Chinese Taoism, called Qi Gong. They help to purify the body-mind and optimize energy in the main centers of the body. Several specific Yogic practices and Qi Gong exercises are detailed in the Appendix: Accessory Healing Therapies For the Herbalist.

QI MEDITATION: FILLING THE ESSENCE

Another method to strengthen Qi is meditation. After doing breathing practices, it is easier to concentrate and derive optimal benefit from meditation. One simple meditation involves bringing a slow breath down to the place known as the Sea of Qi, located an inch and a half below the navel. As you breathe, imagine that each inhaled breath feeds pure light energy into your body to gradually expand to form a luminous golden ball. Concentrate on the gradual expansion of this golden ball of light energy in the *'dan tien'* just below the navel as it encircles first the entire body, then the room and finally the world, to extend into space. Remain focused on this feeling of Qi abundance for at least ten to twenty minutes, then slowly visualize the contraction of the light back to its origin in the body.

OTHER

Other methods for circulating Qi include dance, Hatha Yoga, movement, play, sports, hiking, moderate aerobic exercises and other such activities.

Herbs and Foods are also an important source of Qi. A Qi Tonic soup can be prepared as follows: cook together 6 grams each of codonopsis, astragalus and dioscorea, 8 to 10 jujube dates, 3 grams of tangerine peel and a few slices of fresh ginger with brown rice, organic beef or lamb, potatoes, onions and carrots.

A Qi tonifying congee is made by combining 4 slices of astragalus, 6 to 9 grams of codonopsis and 10 to 15 red jujube dates in two quarts of water and 1 cup of sweet rice. Allow to cook slowly over low heat or in a crock pot for 6 to 8 hours. Have a bowl of this porridge first thing each morning.

BLOOD

Blood is a red liquid rich in nutrition which circulates within the blood vessels. It is different than the Western concept of blood in that its characteristics and functions are broader. Blood is a very dense and material form of Qi and, as such, is inseparable from it. Qi activates Blood, giving it life and movement. Blood is considered a Yin substance, as it is dense and fluid.

FORMATION OF BLOOD

Blood originates from two sources: Grain Qi created from food and fluids, and bone marrow formed from life Essence. The Stomach first receives and "ripens" food, and then the Spleen transforms it into a very refined substance, Grain Qi. Spleen Qi transports the Grain Qi up to the Lungs where it mixes with the pure aspect of air brought in by them. Lung Qi then propels this mixture to the Heart where the transformation into Blood is completed. From this we see an example of how Qi makes Blood move, and further understand part of the principle that the Heart governs Blood.

The second source of Blood is from bone marrow. Essence stored in the Kidneys produces Marrow which, in turn, generates bone marrow. Blood is then produced by the bone marrow. Thus, the Kidneys and the Spleen are both important sources for generating Blood.

The main source of Blood is food Essence developed in the Spleen and Stomach. Thus, the nutritional value of the diet, as well as the strength of the Spleen and Stomach, directly influence the formation of Blood. This is why the treatment of Blood Deficiency often includes tonics to strengthen the Spleen and Stomach functions, and why proper diet is so important in Chinese medicine.

ORIGIN OF BLOOD

The Stomach receives and 'ripens' food, the Spleen transforms it into Grain Qi and transports it to the Lungs. This mixes with the pure aspect of air, then the Lungs propel this mixture of Grain Qi and air to the Heart where it is transformed into Blood.

FUNCTIONS OF BLOOD

The main function of Blood is to nourish the body. It circulates continuously within the vessels traveling to the organs in the interior, and to the muscles, tendons, bones and skin in the exterior, providing nutrients to these areas. Blood also has the function of moistening the body. The Blood of various Organs ensures that the skin, hair, eyes, sinews and tongue are properly moistened.

Sufficient Blood is also necessary to provide a strong nourishing foundation for the Mind. When Blood is Deficient, the Mind lacks its foundation, resulting in restlessness, anxiety, slight irritability, a feeling of dissatisfaction and insomnia.

THE RELATIONSHIPS OF BLOOD WITHIN THE BODY

The normal circulation of Blood results from the mutual action of the Heart, Lung, Spleen, Liver and Kidney. The Heart circulates the Blood, Lung Qi enters the Heart to promote the movement of Blood and Qi, the Spleen keeps Blood flowing within the vessels, the Liver stores the Blood and helps it flow smoothly, and the Kidney Essence can be transformed into Blood. For example, a Deficiency of Heart Qi and Lung Qi may lead to stagnation of Blood of the Heart; a Deficiency of Spleen Qi may lead to hemorrhage; irregular Liver Qi may cause stagnation; and a Deficiency of Kidney Essence can lead to a Deficiency of Blood. Since Blood also nourishes Essence, Deficient Blood can lead to a Deficiency of Essence. Of all these, the Heart, Spleen and Liver are the most important and have special relationships with Blood.

HEART

The Heart governs the Blood. It is the place where Heart-Fire (Yang) transforms the mixture of Grain Qi and pure Air into Blood (Yin). It also is responsible for the circulation of Blood throughout the body to all the organs, muscles, tendons, sinews, skin and hair.

LIVER

When a person is active, Blood flows to the muscles and sinews to moisten them for flexibility and movement. When a person rests, Blood moves back to the Liver where it is stored and regenerated, thus the importance of rest and lying down when there is Deficient Blood (especially Liver Blood). Liver Blood functions to moisten the eyes, promoting good eyesight, and the sinews and tendons, supplying flexibility and suppleness of the joints. The Liver also has the function of smoothing and regulating the flow of Qi and Blood. Thus, it regulates the rate of Blood flow within the vessels according to different physiological needs such as activity or rest.

Liver Blood supplies the uterus with Blood and is extremely important for a regular and healthy menstrual function. Because the Liver also regulates the rate of blood flow, periods which are too light or heavy are often due to a disharmony of the Blood of the Liver. Deficient Liver Blood can lead to amenorrhea or scanty periods, while stagnant Liver Blood can cause painful periods.

SPLEEN

The Spleen is the origin of Blood, as it produces Grain Qi which transforms into Blood. The Qi of the Spleen is also responsible for keeping Blood in the vessels so that it does not extravasate. If Spleen Qi is Deficient, it cannot hold the Blood in its pathways and hemorrhaging, broken blood vessels and a tendency to easily bruise may result.

BLOOD AND QI
A traditional saying states that "Qi is the commander of the Blood. Blood is the mother of Qi." This refers to the inseparable relationship between Blood and Qi. Blood, a part of Yin, creates Qi, while Qi is responsible for Blood circulation. Grain Qi from food is the foundation of Blood; combined with oxygen from Lung Qi, it is essential for Blood production. Thus if Qi is Deficient, Blood will also eventually become Deficient. This is why Qi tonics are frequently given with Blood tonics when strengthening Deficient Blood.

Qi is the force which moves and circulates Blood, and it is Lung Qi which infuses the Qi into the blood vessels. If Qi is Deficient or doesn't move sufficiently, it stagnates. Because it can't then push the Blood, Blood stagnates also. Since Qi is in charge of holding Blood in the vessels, if it is Deficient, Blood may move out of its pathways, resulting in bleeding or hemorrhages.

In turn, Blood nourishes the Organs which produce and regulate Qi. It also provides a material foundation for Qi which prevents it from rising up or "floating", causing symptoms of Deficient-Heat. Thus, Blood, as mother, is essential for nurturing Qi, and Qi, as commander, activates the circulation of Blood.

BLOOD AND ESSENCE
Essence stored in the Kidneys is one of the sources for forming Blood. On the other hand, Blood nourishes and replenishes the Essence. Further, the Kidneys are the mother of the Liver according to the Five Elements, so Essence and Blood mutually influence each other. Thus, a Deficiency of one leads to a Deficiency of the other.

PATHOLOGIES OF BLOOD
There are three basic categories of Blood pathologies. These are Blood Deficiency, Blood Heat and Blood stagnation. In Blood Deficiency there is insufficient Blood to nourish and moisten the body. This usually affects the Organs with which it has special relationships. In Blood Heat, too much Heat in the body, usually in the Liver, causes Heat in the Blood and pushes it out of the vessels. Stagnation occurs from Blood moving improperly due to Coldness, Heat or stagnation of Qi, or injury. All of these are discussed in the Chapter on Patterns of Disharmonies.

METHODS TO STRENGTHEN BLOOD

A blood tonifying soup can be made from 15 grams of astragalus, 4 grams of Dang Gui and a few slices of fresh ginger combined with organic lamb (or beef). Various grains, such as rice, can be added along with vegetables, including onions, potatoes and carrots. This is the most effective formula for anemia or Blood Deficiency. The preponderance of the Qi tonic, astragalus, exemplifies the principle of Qi as the "commander" of Blood.

FLUIDS

The term Fluids (*Jinye*) refers to all liquids in the body other than Blood. It includes both intracellular and extracellular fluids, and undoubtedly includes what we know as the lymphatic system. Body Fluids are divided into two kinds. *Jin* are the clear, light and watery dilute Fluids which flow easily and quickly with Defensive Qi in the Exterior pores, skin and muscles. They are controlled by the Lungs, which disperses them, and the Upper Warmer, which controls their transformation and movement. Their function is to moisten and partially nourish the skin and muscles. They also become a component of Blood, helping to thin it and prevent its stagnation or coagulation. *Jin* manifests as sweat, tears, saliva and mucus.

Ye are the thick, heavy, turbid and dense Fluids which flow slowly with the Nutritive Qi in the Interior joints, viscera, bowels, brain and marrow. They are controlled by the Spleen and Kidneys, which transform them, and the Middle and Lower Warmer, which move and excrete them. *Ye* functions to moisten and nourish the joints, brain, bone marrow and spine.

Fluids also are needed to lubricate the eyes, ears, nose and mouth. Because it is difficult to separate these two types of fluids completely, they are combined into the one expression, *jinye*.

FORMATION OF FLUIDS

Body Fluids are formed from what we eat and drink. The process of forming Fluids occurs through several refining stages. Each stage further separates the Fluids into pure and impure portions. Thus the saying that there is "pure within the impure" and "impure within the pure". The pure parts are transported upwards in the body while the impure parts move downwards. The proper movement of pure and impure portions of body Fluids primarily occurs through the transformative function of the Spleen.

The initial formation of Fluids begins in the Stomach where food and drink are digested. Through the transformative function of the Spleen, they are then separated into pure and impure portions. The pure, or clear, portion goes from the Spleen up to the Lungs, which disperses part of them to the skin and sends part of them down to the Kidney. The impure or dirty part, transformed by the Spleen, is sent down to the Small Intestine where it is again separated into pure and impure parts. The pure part is sent to the Bladder while the turbid part goes to the Large Intestine. There some of the water is re-absorbed; thus the saying that the Large Intestine promotes the formation of Body Fluids. The Bladder also separates the fluids it receives into pure and impure portions. The pure part flows upwards to the surface of the body where it forms sweat, while the impure portion flows downwards and is transformed into urine.

The transportation and distribution of Body Fluid is mostly accomplished by the Spleen. The Lung disperses and descends downward to the Kidney, which governs water metabolism. Further, the Triple Warmer is the passage through which *jinye* moves. The Liver's function of smoothing and regulating the flow of Qi and Blood also has a part in transporting and distributing Body Fluids. Because the Heart controls the circulation of Blood, and Fluids are a component of this, the Heart also has a role in their distribution. Through the interaction of all of these Organs, Body Fluids circulate to perform their various functions.

The excretion of waste and excessive water in the body occurs according to its different physiological needs. Some is sent, through the water regulating function of the Lung, to the body surface where it is turned into sweat. Some is changed into urine by the Kidney's function of separating the clear from the turbid, and removed by the Urinary Bladder's function of storing and excreting urine. Others are transformed into nasal mucus, saliva and tears and are removed from the nose, mouth and eyes by their corresponding Organs. Further, exhaled air by the Lungs takes away some moisture.

FUNCTIONS OF BODY FLUID

Body Fluids have two functions. One is to moisten and partly nourish the skin, hair, muscles, eyes, nose, mouth, internal Organs, marrow, spinal cord, brain, joints and bones. The other is to seep into the blood vessels through the capillaries to become a component of Blood and nourish and moisten all areas of the body.

A few other functions occur through Body Fluids. When Body Fluids are metabolized, some waste forms and, along with other poisonous substances in the body, leaves through the sweat and urine. Thus, Fluids help maintain bodily cleanliness. Further, when the body gets hot, it sweats and releases heat; when it doesn't sweat, a portion of Fluids is excreted through the urine with other impurities. Therefore, Body Fluids also help maintain body temperature and detoxification.

THE RELATIONSHIPS OF FLUID WITHIN THE BODY

SPLEEN

Of the three major organs involved with Fluids, the Spleen is the most important. Because it begins the process of Fluid transformation, and regulates the direction of pure and impure Fluid transportation in all of its stages of production, the Spleen is intimately involved with water metabolism throughout the body. This reminds us that the functions of the Chinese organs occur throughout every cell of the body, not just in the "organ" itself as we are accustomed to thinking in the West. Thus, the Spleen is always treated in any type of Fluid pathology, commonly with mushrooms such as Fu Ling (Poria cocos). Note that the Spleen in Western physiology is a lymphatic organ also involved with lymphatic fluids.

LUNGS

The Lungs regulate the "water passages". They disperse part of the pure Fluids coming up from the Spleen to the space under the skin. Their descending action then sends the other pure portion down to the Kidneys and Bladder. Through their dispersing and descending functions they thus regulate the passage of water in the body.

KIDNEYS

Part of the pure Fluids that the Kidneys receive from the Lungs are vaporized and sent back up to the Lungs to moisten them, thus preventing them from getting too dry. Kidney Yang is also involved in the transformation of Fluids. First, it provides the necessary Heat needed by the Spleen to transform Body Fluids. This is why a Deficiency of Kidney Yang nearly always affects a Spleen Yang Deficiency, and Fluids accumulate as a result. Kidney Yang also aids the Small Intestine in separating Fluids into their pure and impure parts, and it provides Qi to the Bladder where it transforms Fluids into urine. Lastly, Kidney Yang aids the Triple Warmer in its transformation and excretion of fluids.

TRIPLE WARMER

The Triple Warmer aids the transformation, transportation and excretion of Fluids in all of its stages throughout the body. The Upper Warmer is likened to a "mist" since it assists the Spleen in directing the pure fluids upwards and the Lungs in dispersing them to the skin. The Middle Warmer is considered a "foam" or a "muddy pool" because it assists the Stomach in its digestive and churning functions and in directing the impure part downwards. The Lower Warmer is compared to a "drainage ditch" since here it aids the Kidneys, Bladder and Small Intestine in their function of transforming, separating and excreting Fluids. In TCM the Triple Warmer does not refer to a specific Organ but rather a coordinating function between all the Internal Organs.

QI AND BODY FLUIDS

The relationship between Qi and Fluids is similar to that of Qi and Blood. Qi produces Body Fluids, and they in turn help to nourish and moisten the Organs that regulate Qi. Fluids are primarily developed through the Spleen and Stomach, so when Qi is sufficient, the Spleen and Stomach function normally and Body Fluids are abundant. Likewise, when Qi is Deficient, the Spleen and Stomach are weakened and Body Fluids become insufficient. Body Fluids are also the carrier of Qi. Thus, any loss of Fluids may damage Qi. Excessive vomiting, profuse sweating or prolonged diarrhea can cause a severe loss of Qi.

Further, it is Qi that transforms, transports and excretes Fluids. Without this motivating force, Fluids accumulate and eventually stagnate in the body, causing a variety of diseases. Qi also holds Fluids in their proper place, just as it holds Blood in the vessels. When Qi is Deficient, Fluids may leak, resulting in symptoms such as profuse or spontaneous sweating (Lung Qi Deficiency), chronic vaginal discharge (Spleen and Kidney Qi Deficiency) and polyuria or urinary incontinence (Kidney Qi Deficiency).

BLOOD AND BODY FLUIDS

Blood and Body Fluids are both liquids with the functions of nourishing and moisturizing, although Blood is stronger, or more potent, in these functions. They both belong to Yin, and both are derived from Grain Qi. Fluids enter the blood vessels and become a part of Blood, while Blood extravasates out of the blood vessels and turns into Fluids.

Further, Blood and Fluids mutually nourish and supplement each other. The clearest part of Fluids enters into the process which creates Blood and is transformed into it, thus replenishing it. This is why a long term loss of Fluids can cause a Deficiency of Blood, as in excessive use of saunas or hot tubs, or chronic spontaneous sweating. Fluids also thin Blood so it doesn't coagulate or stagnate.

On the other hand, Blood supplements and nourishes Fluids. If Blood becomes Deficient or if there is excessive or chronic loss of blood, as in hemorrhage or chronic menorrhagia, Fluids can become depleted, leading to Dryness and further Blood Deficiency. This is why sweating and bleeding methods should never be used together. Thus, if a patient is bleeding or has severe Deficiency of Blood, sweating should not be induced. This is also why people with Blood Deficiency do not sweat easily. Therefore, if a patient sweats easily and profusely, bloodletting as a TCM therapy is contraindicated.

PHLEGM

Phlegm, or Mucus, is an important concept in Chinese Medicine, and refers to a pathological condition, rather than the necessary lubrication needed for joints, Organs and so on. When Body Fluids collect and congest, they can change into Phlegm. This initially occurs because the Spleen fails to transform and transport Fluids, but may also involve the Lungs and Kidneys if they fail to disperse and lower Fluids, or transform and excrete Fluids, respectively.

Phlegm is diagnosed with signs of a greasy or slippery tongue coating and a slippery or wiry pulse. There are two types of Phlegm, substantial and non-substantial. Substantial Phlegm is in the form of mucus secreted from the mucus membranes of the sinuses, lungs, bronchioles and reproductive organs. Non-substantial Phlegm can collect in the channels, joints and under the skin, causing lumps, nodules, numbness and bone deformities. It can also appear in the head, Stomach or Lungs, or obstruct certain Organs, such as the Bladder, Kidney or Gall-Bladder in which it forms stones. It is also responsible for a type of dementia called "invisible phlegm masking the orifices of the Heart."

While Dampness and Phlegm have similarities, they also have some differences. Phlegm is heavier than Dampness, but does not have its dirty, sticky or downward flowing characteristics. It originates only from an Interior dysfunction, while Dampness can occur from an Interior or Exterior dysfunction. It primarily affects the middle and upper part of the body, while Dampness mostly collects in the lower part of the body.

PATHOLOGIES OF FLUIDS

The formation, distribution and excretion of Body Fluids is a complicated process requiring the coordination of many Organs. Thus, pathological changes in any of the Organs may affect the normal metabolism of Fluids, especially those of the Lung, Spleen and Kidney, for they are the key Organs in maintaining the normal metabolism of water. Any disturbances in the transportation, distribution and excretion of Fluids may cause the stagnation of water. This manifests as phlegm-retention diseases and edema. On the other hand, pathological changes of Fluid also affect the functions of the Organs. For example, insufficient Fluids in the Lung causes dry cough, while excessive Fluids in the Lung can cause congestion with difficult breathing and cough.

An excess of Fluids is called "Dampness", and is the same as the Damp Internal Pathological Influence. The most common characteristic is a feeling of heaviness of the body or head. Fluid, or Damp, diseases include edema, phlegm-retention diseases, lymphatic problems and general fluid and cellular metabolism issues which, when not properly functioning, can also give rise to tumors, cysts and cancers.

A lack of Fluids is also considered a Fluid imbalance (Deficiency), since the body requires a certain amount of lubrication for normal function of the respiratory, alimentary and reproductive systems. Fluid is necessary for proper joint lubrication as well as a moistener for the intestines to promote proper bowel function. For this, demulcent herbs, such as psyllium seeds and husks, flax seeds and cannabis seeds are used.

Phlegm, the other type of fluid imbalance, can collect in the joints, skin, channels or Organs causing diverse imbalances. It forms when the Spleen, Lungs or Kidneys are unable to perform their transforming, transporting or excreting functions properly. The congested Fluids then transform into Phlegm, causing further bodily dysfunction.

Fluid imbalances can be divided into three categories: a Deficiency of Fluids, edema, and Phlegm blockage. Fluid Deficiency usually relates to a Deficiency of Yin or Blood, while edema or Phlegm always involve the Spleen, as its Qi is in charge of transforming and transporting Body Fluids. These are detailed in the chapter on Patterns of Disharmonies.

METHODS TO STRENGTHEN FLUIDS
To nourish Deficient Fluids, one essentially tonifies Yin. Include more Yin nourishing foods in the diet, such as glutinous sweet rice, okra and pork. Fish liver oils are also beneficial. Soups and stews that include small amounts of cooked Rehmannia glutinosa (Shu Di Huang), ophiopogon, lycium berries and American ginseng are also beneficial.

For breakfast make sweet rice congee using 1 cup sweet glutinous rice, two quarts of water, 3 grams each of prepared rehmannia, ophiopogon and lycum berries and 6 to 10 black jujube dates. To aid digestion add a dash of cardamon and ginger. Cook slowly over low heat or in a crock pot for 6 to 8 hours.

The most important activity to nourish Yin and Fluids is sleep and rest. Yin is especially increased with rest after eating. Avoid excessive activity, work, sex and most aerobic exercises. Swimming, walking and stretching exercises, such as Yoga, are beneficial.

ESSENCE ("JING")

As previously described, Essence is a highly refined substance, called *Jing*. It is the very foundation of life and the source of organic development. As such, it is considered a precious substance to be valued and guarded. While more than simply part of the Fluid element of the body, Essence is a highly refined and distilled substance that is Fluid. Even though it is both nutritive and supportive, its place of origin is within the complex realm of the endocrine system that the Chinese broadly classify as the Kidneys.

Essence encompasses the processes of reproduction, development, growth, sexual potency, conception, pregnancy and ultimate physical decay of the organism. It is the basic constitutional strength, vitality and resistance of the body. As part of growth from childhood, it is responsible for the growth of bones, teeth, hair, brain and sexuality.

In maturity, it controls reproductive function, fertility, conception and pregnancy. As Essence declines with age, there is a natural decline of sexuality, fertility, hair growth and coloring, skin smoothness and so forth. Thus, improper bone formation, retarded growth (mental or physical), delayed sexual maturation, premature aging, sterility or impotence are symptoms of Essence Deficiency.

Traditionally the natural flow of Essence in women is as follows: At age 7 Essence is abundant, influencing hair growth and adult teeth to replace the baby ones. At 14, the "Dew of Heaven", or menstruation, arrives and conception is possible. At 21, Kidney Essence peaks, growth is at its utmost and the wisdom teeth appear. At 28, the tendons, bones and muscles are their strongest while the hair grows its longest. At 35, Essence begins to decline, with the skin wrinkling, hair falling, and teeth loosening. At 42, the face darkens and the hair turns gray. At 49, the "Dew of Heaven" dries, resulting in menopause.

The Flow of Essence in Women

Age 7	Essence is abundant, causes hair growth and replacement of baby teeth.
Age 14	Menstruation begins, conception is possible
Age 21	Kidney Essence peaks, growth is fully realized and wisdom teeth appear.
Age 28	Tendons, bones and muscles are the strongest and the hair is the longest.
Age 35	Beginning of the decline of Essence, skin begins to wrinkle, hair falls and the teeth loosen.
Age 42	The face darkens, the hair turns gray.
Age 49	Menopause

In men the traditional flow of Essence is as follows: At age 8 Essence is abundant, influencing hair growth and the formation of permanent teeth. At 16 the "Dew of Heaven", sperm, arrives and conception is possible. At 24, Kidney Essence peaks, growth is at its utmost and the wisdom teeth appear. At 32, the tendons, bones and muscles are at their strongest. At 40, Essence begins to decline with the skin wrinkling, hair falling and teeth getting loose. At 48, the face darkens and hair turns gray. At 56, the "Dew of Heaven" dries up, resulting in infertility. At 64, the hair and teeth are gone.

The Flow of Essence in Men

Age 8	Essence is abundant, hair grows, permanent teeth develop
Age 16	Sperm develops and conception is possible
Age 24	Kidney Essence peaks, wisdom teeth appear, growth is at its maximum
Age 32	The tendons, bones and muscles are at their strongest
Age 40	Beginning of the decline of Essence, skin wrinkles, hair falls and teeth become loose
Age 48	Face darkens and hair turns gray
Age 56	Infertility
Age 64	Hair and teeth fall out

Essence has two sources, Pre-Heaven Essence and Post-Heaven Essence. Pre-Heaven Essence is a result of the combined potential of the mother, father and grandparents in the conceived child. It determines our unique growth patterns and reproductive capacity. This Essence in the form of Qi, rather than Fluid, is called Original Qi, Prenatal Qi or Inborn Qi. Because it is inherited from the parents, it is considered fixed in quantity and quality, although it can be affected and supplemented through Post-Heaven Essence. It represents the constitutional potential for strength, vitality and resistance throughout a person's life.

A litter of eight pups or kittens produces some that are innately more alert and curious, more interested in food, stronger and faster to grow and mature than others. These are blessed with greater Pre-Heaven Essence than the weaker members. Similarly, we must admit that certain of us are more prone to unstable health than others. In this way, we are each limited to some degree by the Pre-Heaven Essence bestowed upon us at birth. Inevitably, our limitations tend to become more evident with age.

Post-Heaven Essence, on the other hand, represents what happens to us after birth. It is affected by what we derive from air, food and water. Post-Heaven Essence is also adversely drained and affected by physical and emotional stress. Essence derived from outer nourishment assumes forms of Grain Qi, Food Qi or Central Qi. While Post-Heaven Essence is replenishable daily, Pre-Heaven Essence represents even subtler energetic resources that are not normally renewable on a regular daily basis except, perhaps, through regular and prolonged periods of focused breathing practices and meditation called "Qi Gong". Therefore in order to not dissipate our reserves of Pre-Heaven Essence, it is wise for us to eat and drink pure, wholesome foods and water and attend to our basic physical and psychological requirements, including proper sleep, exercise and recreation. In this way we optimize the quality and length of our lives. Herbs can contribute greatly to compensate for a lack of Pre-Heaven Essence.

While Essence is a part of Qi, there are significant differences. First, compared to Qi, Essence at best can be replenished very slowly. Further, Essence represents an inherited constitutional potential that resides in the greater definition of the TCM Kidney, while Qi is all-pervasive throughout the entire body-mind. Since another meaning for "*Jing*" is reproductive semen, the various hormonal secretions throughout the body become a material expression of Essence and are more fluidic in comparison to Qi, which is more purely energetic.

The potential of Essence is determined by observing overall patterns of health and disease from early childhood to the present. If a condition stems from birth or early childhood, or reflects an inherited tendency also manifested in the parents and grandparents, it is considered a problem of Essence. In general, such conditions are seldom cured and require a great amount of diligence to maintain stability. Such diligence is manifested not only in a healthy diet and lifestyle, but also through the regular integration of appropriate tonic herbs taken alone, in formula or regularly combined with food throughout life.

Further, the condition of the Kidneys reflects the state of Essence in the body. Any imbalance of their functions may indicate an Essence dysfunction. Likewise, if the Kidneys become weakened or depleted from excessive working, excessive sex, poor diet and/or lack of proper sleep, Essence also becomes depleted.

PATHOLOGIES OF ESSENCE

Because Essence is comprised of the fixed Pre-Heaven Essence and supplemental Post-Heaven Essence, it only manifests in imbalance as

Deficiency. Deficient Essence includes any disease or imbalance that is inheritable, as well as symptoms of improper growth, problems with development and maturation or reproduction problems. These are detailed in the chapter on Patterns of Disharmonies.

METHODS TO STRENGTHEN ESSENCE

If we understand Essence from only a physical perspective, we are limiting it to only having a Pre-heaven influence. Since Essence is a combination of both Pre-heaven and Post-heaven influences, we can understand ways by which Essence can be supported and possibly enhanced. To achieve this, we must assume Essence to be both physical as well as spiritual.

If we only limit Essence to a physical model, we must admit that there are individuals born with severe physical handicaps who are able to rise beyond their inborn Essence Deficiency to achieve greatness for themselves and others. We also see each day how individuals born with healthy Essence tend to dissipate it through self-abuse and lack of sufficient nurturing support from others; they end up broken and dejected with crippling psycho-physical imbalances stemming from damaged Essence.

In traditional society, Essence is supported and strengthened through practices of devotion and honor. Further, the honor and respect we give to others ultimately returns to ourselves a hundredfold while any disrespect or dishonor to others, especially those to whom we are close, returns to injure our spiritual Essence. The road to self respect for ourself or others begins with tolerance and forgiveness. Practically speaking, death or extreme alienation may make forgiveness difficult to achieve, except through letting go of old hurts and grievances within our own hearts.

Until we are capable of letting go, and to the extent that we are unable to release the negative imprint of past abuses, our Essence will be unable to emanate forth and manifest throughout our life as it should. One process of doing this is through adopting and forming new bonds with others who we see as worthy role models and a source of spiritual nourishment. This can be dangerous, if somehow the object of our newly found identification and devotion proves to be unworthy, so that the result is a further insult and injury of our Essence. Because of this, many feel safer to find or create an object of worship in the form of a chosen deity or religion. This is why for many people apocalyptic rebirth or "born again" experiences can allow one to contact Essential reserves to affect dramatic positive psycho-physiological changes.

For those of us who are capable of detaching and withdrawing from normal life for awhile, it is possible to find and reestablish contact with our inner Essence. This can be accomplished through a prolonged period of spiritual retreat, for instance, in a monastic setting or in nature through the Native American vision quest.

The thing that is seldom stated is that processes of forgiveness of self and others, letting go, spiritual renewal and retreat are recurring processes which we may have to undergo regularly until all trace of negative attachments that impair the full blossoming of Essence are completely eradicated. [2]

Essence can also be strengthened through prolonged and regular practice of Qi Gong. (A few specific Qi Gong exercises are given in the Appendix, Accessory Healing Therapies for the Herbalist.) Further, as Post-Heaven Essence nourishes and supplements Pre-Heaven Essence, a balanced diet rich in whole unrefined grains, legumes, vegetables, hard leafy greens, seaweed's and small amounts of organ meat and fruit also contributes to building Essence in the body.

SHEN (MIND AND SPIRIT)

Shen refers to the overall "Spirit" and the mental faculties of an individual. As Spirit, it encompasses a wide range of mental, emotional and spiritual aspects. Mentally, it relates to one's capacity to form ideas. Emotionally, Shen is the spark of interest and enthusiasm that is infectiously communicated to others, signaling innate vitality and flourishing life. Spiritually, it is the dynamic faith, vitality and force of the human personality that seemingly is able to surmount all obstacles and make things happen.

Shen resides in the Heart, and as one might imagine, encompasses more than physical heart functions. Folk wisdom of all countries attaches great emotional significance to the Heart as the seat of the emotions. In popular jargon we have terms such as "heartfelt gratitude" or "loving heart", so that the heart itself is drawn as a symbol of goodness and love. On the negative side we hear countless lovesick songs singing about a "broken heart", "cold heartedness" and so on. This connection seems ignored by medical doctors who quote statistics of heart disease as the number one killer in the Western world, as they reap heaps of scientific "kudos" and billions of dollars for complex heart bypass surgery and transplants. Fortunately, the Heart as described in TCM as the home of Shen can be neither bypassed nor transplanted. In the psycho-spiritual aspect of the Traditional Chinese Heart may lie the real cause for so much heart disease in Western countries.

Statistics aside, how many of us have known individuals who seem to eat all the wrong foods, even test with elevated cholesterol and triglyceride levels and yet outlive others who suffer unexpected heart attacks and strokes with no previous indications? If there is an epidemic of Heart disease in the West, perhaps we should look to the spiritual impoverishment of Western society as the cause rather than mechanical models of blocked arteries and defective valves. All we know is the many sad-hearted people who die of sudden heart attack and who have blocked arteries or a defective heart valve. What we do not know, and thankfully may never know, is how many people with partially impaired arteries and defective heart valves continue to live a life of profound spiritual life fulfillment because they have abundant Shen!

As the Heart rules the Mind, Shen influences our capacity to think clearly, behave appropriately, discriminate, be responsive, speak coherently and experience happiness and profound joy. The spiritual aspects of Shen influence that of all the organs, especially the Yin, receptive and transformative Organs. It differentiates into specific functions and qualities as follows: Spirit (Shen) resides in the Heart, the Ethereal Soul (Hun) in the Liver, the Corporeal Soul (Po) in the Lungs, the Will Power (Zhi) in the Kidneys and Thought (Yi) in the Spleen. Thus, Shen is the spiritual "power" behind all of the organs.

As a Fundamental Substance or quality of human existence, Shen has a material quality that is very much a part of the body. The origin of Shen is similar to Jing in that it is first transmitted to the fetus from the parents. In this, we might consider how the state of mind of the parents at the moment of conception and of the mother through gestation and pregnancy have a profound influence on the developing Shen of the fetus.

Regardless of the amount of Shen one is born with, it is after birth that Shen can be diminished or obliterated if nourishment of love and compassion represented by Heart Qi and Blood are not continued. The Fire Gate of Vitality (*ming men*) in the Kidneys also influences this as it manifests the level of will and determination that assists the Heart in housing the emotions and mind. If either Heart Blood or Qi or the Fire Gate of Vitality are deficient, then Shen becomes depleted.

When Shen is weak, Spirit and the mental capacities decline. There may be muddled thinking, forgetfulness, insomnia, lack of vitality, depression, lack of interest in life, unhappiness, confused speech or excessive dreaming. In the extreme, a Shen disharmony can result in irrational behavior, unconsciousness, incoherent speech, hysteria, delirium, inappropriate responses to people or the environment, or violent madness. Disharmonies of Shen can also occur from excessive Heat in the body. In this case it causes "reckless movement" with any of the above symptoms resulting.

In diagnosis of disease, the appearance of Shen is an important factor and is one of the first signs noted in examination of a patient along with tongue and pulse. No matter how ill a person is, if the eyes glitter and sparkle, there is luster in the face, the tongue looks bright and flourishing, or the personality is in "good spirits" or has vitality, then Shen is present and recovery is easier and more certain. On the other hand, no matter how simple the illness, if the eyes lack life or sparkle, the face is dull and cloudy or the person lacks interest in life, recovery may be difficult and the prognosis poor.

Sometimes during the last stage of a severe or terminal illness a person suddenly becomes alert, more positive and vital. It is termed "false Shen" because it is the last desperate spark of spirit manifesting before the life force separates from the body.

PATHOLOGIES OF SHEN

Because Shen is so closely linked to the Heart, it is not distinguished by pathologies of its own. Instead, symptoms are differentiated as the Heart pathology categories of Deficient Heart Blood, Heart Fire and Cold or Hot Mucus obstructing the Heart Orifices. However, one must keep in mind that Shen problems are spiritual problems and a true Chinese doctor must eventually develop the skills to address such spiritual issues on their own terms. This is done through shamanistic rituals, life counseling (compassionately listening and responding with the right word at the right time), prayer, affirmation, meditational practices that are given to the patient and recommendations to play more, change jobs, take a holiday and whatever else is needed to nourish the spirit and Heart. For physical herbal prescriptions, refer to those Heart categories for complete symptomology.

METHODS TO STRENGTHEN SHEN

Shen is fostered by tonifying Heart Blood and Qi, strengthening the Kidney's Life Gate Fire, and keeping Heat, Coldness and Fluids in balance in the body. Other methods include counseling, play, holidays (our Western term, vacation, means to vacate, while a holiday is a holy day), prayer, meditation, laughter therapy, living a fulfilling life path, being surrounded by loved ones as well as periods of solitude.

THE THREE TREASURES: QI, ESSENCE AND SHEN

Qi, Essence and Shen are known as the "Three Treasures" because they are the fundamental spiritual basis of a human being. They are part of the entire constitution and determine its physical and spiritual strength, manifesting as vitality, resistance, mental clarity, stability, expression, happiness, self-confidence and life outlook. Shen relates to the Heart, Essence to the Kidneys and Qi is produced by the Spleen and Stomach and relates to the Lungs.

Essence, Qi and Shen are each different states of condensation of Qi. Essence is the most coarse and dense, Qi is more refined and rarefied while Shen is the most subtle and immaterial. Thus, these substances represent the continuum between the psychological and spiritual, matter and energy, the physical and mental, the material and immaterial and so on. Of the three, Essence is the foundation for Qi and Shen. If inherited Essence is strong and well supported in life, so will be the other two and the life will be strong, both physically and mentally. Pre-Heaven Essence is the foundation of Qi and Shen while Post-Heaven Essence nourishes them.

Essence and Qi are the material foundation of Shen and determine the state of mind and spirit. A healthy mind and spirit are dependent on Essence, both inherited and created after birth, and Qi produced from food and fluids by the Stomach and Spleen. On the other hand, strong Shen is necessary to direct the Essence and make it effective in its functions. If Shen is weak, the person lacks will power and motivation and feels constantly tired. Both Essence and Shen have a common root in Qi.

The Three Treasures are often expressed in Chinese Medicine as Heaven, Person and Earth, corresponding to Shen, Qi and Essence respectively, and their corresponding organs of Heart, Stomach/Spleen and Kidneys. They are as follows:

SUBSTANCE	ORGAN	CORRESPONDENCE
Shen	Heart	Heaven
Qi	Stomach/Spleen	Person
Essence	Kidneys	Earth

In practice, these three fundamental substances are assessed according to their general and relative state. Essence indicates the inherited constitution and its current state, Qi denotes the state of energy produced on a regular basis and Shen represents the state of the person's emotional, mental and spiritual well-being.

Essence can, in large part, be determined from the patient's health and life history and the parents' and grandparents' health history. However, this may only inform us as to a potential that is waiting to find a hospitable environment and circumstance to become manifest. As we have seen, it is possible to suppress one's Essence through repression and inhibition. Qi is determined, to a great extent, by lifestyle and diet since childhood, and by the amount of exercise or physical play, since this is important for Qi circulation. Shen is observed by the degree of the personality's expressiveness and in the sparkle of the eyes which denotes vitality and life. On the other hand, lack of Shen is observed by the lack of expression and the appearance of dullness in the eyes, sometimes seen as a covering of mist or cloud. To some extent, the Three Treasures also have characteristic feelings and appearances on the pulse and tongue.

FIVE

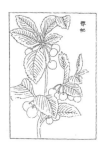

THE EIGHT PRINCIPLES

One of the most important and characteristic aspects of TCM is its clinical practicality. This is best exemplified in the classification of symptom patterns along with herbs and other medicinal substances and formulas. The Eight Principles describe this system as follows:

1. External	Acute diseases
2. Hot	Overly active metabolism
3. Excess	Sthenic
4. Yang	Hyper-metabolic (sthenic)
5. Internal	Mostly Chronic diseases
6. Cold	Low metabolism
7. Deficient	Asthenic
8. Yin	Hypo-metabolic (asthenic)

TCM classifies herbs as Hot or Cold in terms of their energies, External or Internal in terms of the depth of their penetration, Eliminating or Tonifying and the summation of the above as Yang and Yin. This is what makes TCM highly promising and effective in treating diseases which may not be amenable to other therapeutic modalities. Because of this, it is possible to form a treatment strategy based on direct observation and diagnosis.

There are essentially two approaches to diagnosis and treatment. One is based on treating the named disease, while the second approach treats according to pattern identification. This gives rise to the principle of *"one disease, many formulas, one formula, many diseases"*. What this means is that a specific named disease can only be treated according to a holistic differential diagnosis, which may require a decision between several formulas based on the accompanying patterns of the disease. It also means that a single herbal formula can be suitable for treating several diseases. To achieve this objective, TCM utilizes ten types of diagnostic strategies. These are:

1. Eight Principles (Ba gang bian zheng)
2. Symptom Sign Diagnosis (Zang fu bian zheng)
3. Six Stages based upon the Shang Han Lun (Liu jing bian zheng)
4. Four Stages of Heat (Wei q ying xue bian zheng)
5. Three Heater Discrimination (San jiao bian zheng)
6. Disease Discrimination (Bing yin bian zheng)
7. Qi and Blood Pattern Discrimination (Qi xue bian zheng)
8. Three Humor Diagnosis (Jin ye bian zheng)
9. Five Element Discrimination (Wu xing bian zheng)
10. Meridian and Connecting Vessel Discrimination (Jing luo bian zheng)

Most of these diagnostic strategies will be separately discussed, but they are not exclusive of each other and in practice tend to overlap. As Bob Flaws so aptly views it[1], each diagnostic approach is like a diagnostic "tool" that an experienced TCM practitioner may use according to which is better suited to understand the patient's condition. They can then arrive at the most appropriate diagnosis and therapeutic approach. Usually the Eight Principles form the primary understanding of the underlying imbalance and provide an effective holistic approach to treatment. Further, they provide the necessary overview, while Organ or Symptom Sign pattern diagnosis allows us to get even closer to the direct causes of a specific disease.

The Eight Principles were first elucidated by Zhang Jie Ben during the 17th century. It has since become the most fundamental process for TCM diagnostic evaluation. Actually it is mainly the first Six Principles, excluding Yin-Yang, which are determined through the use of the Four Methods of Diagnosis: Interrogation, Observation, Palpation and Audition. The remaining two Yin and Yang principles represent a summary of the previous six.

In Western medicine some corresponding diseases can be associated with each of the Eight Principles as follows:

External: acute conditions including colds, influenza, fevers, rashes, acute arthritic conditions and injuries.

Internal: chronic conditions such as constipation, gastritis, ulcers, urinary infections, cholecystitis, low energy, weakness, diabetes, hypoglycemia, cancer, epilepsy, gynecological conditions, infertility, impotence.

Excess: obesity, constipation, hypertension, high fever, severe infections, purulent discharges, manic behavior.

Deficiency: tiredness, weakness, weak digestion, low hydrochloric acid, hypo- thyroidism, hypo-adrenalism, anemia and wasting diseases such as TB and AIDS.

Hot: high fever, mild chills, thirst, flushed complexion, sensitivity to heat and hot weather, severe inflammatory conditions, infections, hepatitis and yellowish discharges from any mucus membrane or orifice.

Cold: severe chills, lack of thirst, pale complexion, sensitivity to coldness or cold weather, low hypothalamus function, weak digestion, hypoglycemia, lowered immunity, anemia, all hypo-conditions and clear or whitish discharges from any mucus membrane or orifice.

Yang: Generally, Yang represents a composite of any of the symptoms or conditions that are External, Excess or Hot. In addition, more fundamental endocrine imbalances associated with hypertension, hyper-adrenalism, hyper-thyroidism and an overbearing aggressive behavior are also considered Yang conditions.

Yin: Generally, Yin encompasses a composite of the symptoms or conditions that are Internal, Deficient or Cold. In addition, endocrine imbalances associated with hypo-thyroidism, hypo-adrenalism, hypo-glycemia, a pale complexion, fluid retention, timidity and a soft spoken voice are also categorized as Yin conditions.

Thus, Yin and Yang, as part of the Eight Principles, represent a composite of the previous External-Internal, Hot-Cold, Excess-Deficient determinations. For instance, an individual whose symptoms may be Hot, Internal and Excess would be considered to have more of a Yang condition because Internal is the only Yin indication. Another whose condition is Excess, Internal and Cold is Yin because the only Yang manifestation is Excess. This is important in determining the appropriate herbal treatment.

EXTERNAL-INTERNAL

External-Internal refers to the location of a disease or symptoms. It is differentiated as follows.

External Diseases

External conditions tend to be acute and located on the surface of the body. These include colds, flu, fevers, skin diseases and rheumatic conditions. Generally, these are subclassified as Wind-Cold or Wind-Heat.

The pathogenesis of External diseases begins with an invasion by one or more of the *Six Pernicious Influences*: Wind, Cold, Heat, Dampness, Dryness and Summer Heat (see Chapter 8 for a discussion of these). The effects of these can penetrate the upper respiratory passages including the nasal passages, the mouth and throat, the bronchioles and lungs, as well as the skin and hair. When this occurs, all physiological aspects associated with the Lungs can be affected. Besides the upper respiratory passages, the skin, body hair and the External immune system (Wei Qi), which are all governed by the Lungs, can be damaged. The resultant acute fever, cold or flu is an attempt by the body to throw off toxins and overcome negative pathological invasions.

The most definitive signs for External Wind-Heat or Wind-Cold are chills followed by fever, normal tongue fur and a floating pulse. In addition there may be symptoms of headache, nasal congestion, dilute clear or whitish discharge, white and thin tongue coating and a floating pulse. The difference between Wind-Cold and Wind-Heat conditions is that chills are more pronounced in Wind-Cold disease, and fever is more predominant in Wind-Heat conditions.

External Wind-Cold or External Wind-Heat also refer to various imbalances and diseases of the upper respiratory tract including colds, influenza, rhinitis and other respiratory allergies. Rheumatic conditions are also classified as External Damp-Wind-Cold or External Damp-Wind-Heat. Wind is a pathology that commonly accompanies External conditions. External Wind can refer to the proliferation of various bacteria and viruses. The fact that the Chinese character for Wind is a small insect suggests that perhaps they suspected the existence of external pathogens such as germs and viruses.

External can also refer to certain rheumatic disorders and skin conditions. These can be treated with herbs and formulas from the categories of Relieving Cold Wind Dampness or Relieving Hot Wind Dampness. In these cases the Wind-relieving properties alleviate pain because of their antispasmodic, analgesic effects. The method of treatment for External disease is diaphoresis (sweating). For this, one would select herbs and formulas from the categories of Cool Surface Relieving or relaxing diaphoretics, or Warm Surface Relieving or warming stimulating diaphoretics.

External Wind Cold includes symptoms of chills, fear of cold, avoidance of cold drinks, mild fever, headache, aching-stiffness, nasal congestion, allergies, colds and coughs with clear or white-colored sputum. The pulse feels floating, beating more on the surface than usual, tense and slow (around 60 beats per minute or less). The tongue has a thin white coat.

For External Wind Cold, external spicy warm diaphoretic herbs are used such as ephedra (Ephedra sinica), fresh ginger (Zingiberis off.), asarum (Asarum heterotropoides), cinnamon twigs (Cinnamomum cassia) or Western herbs such as sassafras (Sassafras albidum), onions, garlic (Allium sativum) and angelica (Angelica archangelica).

Formulas
External Cold Excess Condition: **Ephedra Combination** (Ma huang tang).
External Cold Condition in an individual who is neither too Excess or Deficient: **Pueraria Combination** (Ge gen tang).
External, Cold and Deficient Condition: **Cinnamon Combination** (Gui zhi tang).

Another external, spicy, warm formula: **Schizonepeta and Ledebouriella Combination** (Jing fang bai du san) which is especially useful for acute skin diseases such as boils, urticaria, eczema, dermatitis and conjunctivitis.

Formulas used in Ayurvedic Medicine include Trikatu, consisting of equal parts of powdered black pepper (Piper nigrum), pippali long pepper (Piper longum) and ginger (Zingiberis officinalis). Sito Paladi is also used. It consists of powders of cinnamon bark (1 part), cardamom (2 parts), black pepper (4 parts), black bamboo tabasheer (8 parts) and raw brown sugar (16 parts).

Western herbalism uses a formula called Composition Powder, which consists of bayberry bark (4 parts), white pine bark (2 parts), ginger (2 parts), cayenne pepper (1/2 part) and cloves (1/2 part).

External Wind Heat has more inflammatory or feverish symptoms including high fever, sore throat, eruptive skin rashes and thirst with a craving for cool drinks. These conditions can also be indicative of influenza, colds, upper respiratory problems, hot eruptive rashes and acute inflamed joint pains. The pulse is floating but fast (80 or more beats per minute), which indicates Heat. The tongue will have a thin coat, slightly yellow and dry.

Chinese herbs for External Wind Heat include cool, spicy diaphoretic herbs such as chrysanthemum flowers (Chrysanthemum morifolium), Bo He mint (Mentha haplocalyx), bupleurum (Bupleurum falcatum), burdock seed (Arctium lappa) or Western diaphoretic herbs such as mint (Mentha piperita), lemon balm (Melissa officinalis), feverfew (Chrysanthemum parthenium), elder flowers (Sambucus canadensis) and catnip (Nepeta cataria).

Formulas
Wind-Heat conditions: **Lonicera and Forsythia Combination** (Yin qiao san) is used to disperse Wind Heat. It clears acute inflammatory symptoms and relieves toxicity. It is indicated for symptoms of fever with slight or no chills, headache, thirst, cough, sore throat. The pulse is floating and rapid and the tongue has a thin, white or yellow coat. Yin Qiao is commonly indicated for the treatment of influenza, colds, coughs, acute bronchitis, upper respiratory tract infection, measles and other eruptive skin diseases, epidemic parotitis (mumps), acute endometritis, and early stage encephalitis or meningitis.

Wind Heat: **Morus and Chrysanthemum Combination** (Sang ju yin) is an External cooling diaphoretic formula which has similar indications to **Yin Qiao.**

In Ayurvedic Medicine sweet basil (Ocimum basilicum) tea is used, while in Western herbalism elder flowers (Sambucus nigra), mint (Mentha piperita), yarrow (Achillea millifolia) and boneset tea (Eupatorium perfoliatum) are given.

Internal Diseases
Internal syndromes describe conditions affecting the vital energy, Blood, Internal Organs and bone marrow. These conditions can be Hot, Cold, Excess or Deficient. In general, Internal tends to represent a more chronic pattern while External is acute.

TCM teaches that Internal diseases can be caused by the *Seven Emotions*: Joy, Sadness, Anger, Grief, Melancholy, Fright and Fear. There is a physiological relationship between the emotions and the immune system which is of tremendous importance. Negative emotions tend to make us vulnerable to chronic disease and vice versa. Other factors which cause Internal diseases include improper diet, trauma, and bites by animals or insects.

Internal Wind refers to diseases that affect the nervous and circulatory systems with joint or muscle spasms, spasmodic pains, tremors, epilepsy, coma and apoplexy. As with all Differential Diagnostic treatments, a unique treatment approach may be necessary based on individual combinations and variations

Formula
Big Pearl for Internal Wind (Da ding feng zhu) for Internal Wind with prostration, clonic convulsions caused by Yin Deficiency.

Internal Heat includes symptoms of constipation, acute abdominal pains, abdomen sensitive to deep palpation, internal inflammation, nervousness and restlessness. The pulse is deeper and more rapid. The tongue is scarlet, with a dry, yellow coat. Some pathological conditions include cholecystitis, hepatitis, urethritis, cystitis and nephritis. Alterative, heat clearing, antibacterial and antiviral herbs with a bitter flavor are used.

Formulas
White Tiger Decoction (Bai hu tang) for symptoms of high fever, aversion to heat, severe headache caused by fever, red complexion, deep, rapid and possibly full pulse, scarlet tongue with a dry yellow coat. It is used for children's fevers, encephalitis B, epidemic meningitis.

Coptis and Scute Combination (Huang lian jie du tang) is used as a general detoxifying formula. It is employed for infections and inflammations, high fever, irritability, boils, dryness of the mouth and throat, insomnia, spitting of blood, nose bleeds caused by Excess Heat, and cancer.

Anemone Combination (Bai tou weng tang) clears Heat, relieves toxicity and is used for bacterial and amoebic dysentery.

In Ayurvedic Medicine, neem (Azadirachta indica) and guduchi (Tinospora cordifolia) powders can be used. In Western herbalism, a combination of echinacea (Echinacea spp.), golden seal (Hydrastis canadensis), chaparral (Larrea divaricata) and garlic (Allium sativum) are used, either as a powder or alcoholic extract.

Internal Cold manifests symptoms of Coldness with a decided preference for warmth, warm food and drinks, pale complexion, loose stool, pale urine, clear mucus discharges, low vitality, apathy and slow speech. The pulse is deep and slow (around 60 or less beats per minute). The tongue is pale with a white coat. Herbs for Internal Cold include ginger (Zingiberis officinalis), cayenne (Capsicum frutescens), black pepper (Piper nigrum), prepared aconite (Aconitum praeparatum), cinnamon (Cinnamomum cassia), cloves (Caryophylus aromaticus), deer antler (Cornu cervi), epimedium (E. grandiflora), eucommia bark (E. ulmoides), and dipsacus (D. asperi, which is used to help relieve back pain) and cistanches (Rou cong rong, which further helps lubricate the intestines and promotes peristalsis).

Formulas

Aconite, Ginger and Licorice Combination (Si ni tang) which is used for Internal Coldness, to restore the Yang (vital function) and revive an individual from collapse, shock or heart failure.

Regulate the Middle Pill (Li zhong tang or Ren shen tang) dispels Internal Coldness as it improves digestion and raises metabolism.

Jade Screen Powder (Yu ping feng san) is used to warm the interior and tonify Qi to strengthen the External immune system. It is used for individuals who are weak and tend toward frequent colds and flu.

Internal Deficiency includes symptoms of fatigue, shortness of breath, involuntary sweating, dizziness, poor memory, timidity, soft spoken voice, lack of appetite, loose stools, pallor and palpitations. The pulse is deep, slow, thin and faint. The tongue appears pale with scalloped edges and a thin white coat. Deficiency symptoms involve Deficiency of Qi, Blood, Yin or Yang.

Formulas

For Qi Deficiency: Four Major Ingredients (Si jun zi tang) for improving digestion, tonifying Qi of the Spleen and Stomach; **Ginseng and Astragalus Combination** (Bu zhong yi qi tang), which is considered the supreme tonic for Qi tonification and for counteracting fatigue, with some detoxifying properties.

For Blood Deficiency: Dang Gui Four Combination (Si wu tang), which is the major formula used to tonify Blood.

For Qi and Blood Deficiency: Eight Precious Herbs (Ba zhen tang); or **Ginseng and Dang Gui Ten Combination** (Shi quan da bu tang) which is an important tonic for Qi, Blood and Yang Deficiencies.

In Ayurvedic medicine **Chyavanprash Compound** is used to tonify Qi and Blood. It is comprised of tonic herbs such as shatavari (Asparagus racemosa), ashwagandha (Withania somnifera) and shilajit (mineral pitch).

For Yin Deficiency: **Rehmannia Six** (Liu wei di huang tang); **Sweet Wormwood and Tortoise Shell Formula** (Qing hao bie jia tang); or **Anemarrhena, Phellodendron and Rehmannia Six** (Zhi bai di huang tang).

For Yang Deficiency: **Rehmannia Eight** (Ba wei di huang tang); or **Replenishing the Right Pills** (You gui wan).

Internal Deficiency Causing Parasites: Mume Formula (Wu mei wan), which is warming and tonifying to the Internal Organs and helps to overcome parasites.

Internal Excess may exhibit symptoms of edema (Excess Dampness), obesity, fullness of the abdomen, stagnation of Qi, Blood, Fluids (lymphatic) and Food. The pulse is deep and full and the tongue is enlarged with a thick coat. Excess commonly transforms to Heat, which produces symptoms of constipation, red complexion, bad breath, abdominal pain, yellow coated tongue and a bounding, rapid and/or full pulse.

Formulas
Major Rhubarb Combination (Da cheng qi tang), which is a strong purgative formula; or **Minor Rhubarb Combination** (Xiao cheng qi tang) which is a milder purgative.

In Ayurvedic medicine, a classic formula for all excesses is **Triphala**, which consists of equal parts Beleric, Emblic and Chebulic Myrobalans. This is an especially valuable formula because of its ability to detoxify and eliminate all Excesses without causing further weakness and Deficiencies. In Western herbalism laxative formulas are employed which combine one or more herbs such as rhubarb root (Rheum palmatum), cascara bark (Cascara sagrada), buckthorne (Rhamnus cathartica), senna (Cassia acutifolia), with cholagogues such as barberry bark (Berberis sp.), dandelion root (Taraxacum off.) , antispasmodics such as wild yam root (Dioscorea villosa) with warming carminatives such as ginger (Zingiberis) to prevent intestinal spasm.

Half External-Half Internal refers to conditions that are a mixture of External-Internal, Hot-Cold and Excess-Deficiency. This condition is characteristic of the Xiao Yang Stage of disease (Lesser Yang) (see Chapter 6: *Six Stages of Disease*) which requires harmonizing formulas with opposite properties. Most often these include formulas with bupleurum because this herb, while classified and used to relieve External Heat, also helps regulate and release Qi stagnation. Most, if not all, Bupleurum formulas combine treating both Internal and External, Hot and Cold, Excess and Deficient symptoms. Consequently, there are many formulas in this category.

Formulas
Minor Bupleurum Combination (Xiao chai hu tang), which has both External and Internal, warm and cool, tonifying and detoxifying herbs; **Major Bupleurum Combination** (Da chai hu tang) is a purgative formula that harmonizes Internal and External, Cold and Hot and Excess and Deficiency simultaneously even though its primary emphasis is to purge and eliminate Liver stagnation. For some who are prone to Yin Deficiency, bupleurum can bring up inappropriate feelings of anger.

HOT-COLD

Besides the attack of External climatic Heat or Cold, this category refers to the body's innate metabolism. Low metabolism accompanied by symptoms of Coldness, pale complexion, lethargy, weak digestion, low immunity and hypo-conditions such as hypo-thyroidism or hypo-adrenalism represents Cold and is a part of Yin. High metabolism with symptoms of Heat and inflammation, ruddy complexion, an aggressive manner, a loud voice and hyper-conditions such as hypertension represents Heat and is a part of Yang.

Cold can be caused either by an Excess of Cold and Yin or a Deficiency of Heat, or Yang. Heat can be caused by either an Excess of Heat, or Yang, or a Deficiency of cooling or calming elements, all under the category of Yin.

Cold

Coldness represents a waning of organic metabolic function while Heat is a catabolic increase. When there is a lack of protective Yang, there will be symptoms of intolerance to cold, cold extremities, cold-phobia and preference for warm climates, warm food and drinks. Lack of Yang will also cause symptoms of pale complexion, impotence, frigidity, lack of appetite, a weakened immune system, slowness of speech and slow movements. The tongue will appear pale with a white coat, possibly with scalloped edges. The pulse is slow (60 beats per minute or slower). For Excess Cold one would use Internal Warming herbs and stimulants such as cinnamon bark (Cassia cinnamomum), dry ginger (Zingiberis officinalis), prepared aconite (Aconitum praeparatum), cayenne pepper (Capsicum frutescens), Ayurvedic Trikatu or the Western use of cayenne and ginger contained in Composition powder. All of these relieve Coldness and stimulate Yang. Excess Yin also includes edema and Dampness and may be treated with diuretics and/or Internal warming herbs as well as aerobic exercise.

Formulas
Aconite, Ginger and Licorice Combination (Si ni tang); **Ginseng and Ginger Combination** (Li zhong tang) or **Aconite, Ginseng and Ginger Combination** (Fu zi li zhong tang), prepared aconite (Fu Zi) and cinnamon bark (Rou Gui) is added to any formula to make it warm.

For Western and Ayurvedic herbs refer to Internal Cold.

Heat
Heat can be a sign of Excess with stagnation, or Yin Deficiency. Excess symptoms are fuller while Deficient Heat arises from a state of auto-consumption. Excess Heat symptoms are accompanied by a preference for cool weather together with cool foods and drinks, thirst, Dryness, constipation, darker more condensed urine, possibly high fever and restlessness. The pulse will be fast (80 or more beats per minute), the tongue is red with a yellow coat.

Yin Deficiency presents with signs of wasting Heat symptoms, termed "false Yang", caused by an overstressed psycho-physical system. These include emaciation and weakness with malar flush, night sweats, five palm Heat, restlessness with little energy or energy in spurts, a red tongue with no coat and a fast but empty pulse.

Eight Principles delineates four types of Heat:
External Heat with high fever, mild chills, sweat, thirst, headache, sore throat, yellow sputum, floating and rapid pulse, normal to thin coated tongue, or dry with a slightly yellow coat.
Internal Heat with high fever, lack of chills, thirst, constipation, dark urine, abhorrence of heat and preference for cold (weather, drinks and food), irritability, sweat, rapid pulse, the tongue is red

with a yellow coat.

Excess Heat with high fever, flushed complexion, excessive thirst, constipation, scanty and dark urine, bitter mouth taste, psychosis, irritability, strong smelling breath, delirium, pulse is rapid and full, the tongue is red with a yellow dry coat.

Deficient Heat or Yin Deficiency with low afternoon fever, night sweats, flushed complexion, insomnia, feverish feeling in the hands, feet and chest, irritability. The pulse is rapid and thin and the tongue is red with little or no coat.

Treatment

External Heat: Use herbs and formulas described in the External Wind Heat category, such as **Lonicera and Forsythia combination** (Yin qiao san), and Western herbs such as boneset (Eupatorium perfoliatum) and red clover blossoms (Trifolium pratense).

Internal Heat and Excess Heat: One would use purgatives, cholagogues, alteratives and Heat clearing herbs such as gentian root (Gentian scabrae), coptis (Coptis chinensis), scutellaria (Scutellaria baicalensis), dandelion (Taraxacum officinalis), isatis (Isatis tinctoria), honeysuckle flowers (Lonicera japonica) and forsythia flowers (Forsythia suspensa). If there is constipation, purgative herbs such as rhubarb root (Rheum palmatum) and the mineral mirabilitum (Sodium sulphate) are employed. In Western herbalism, Heat-clearing herbs are called alteratives and include red clover (Trifolium pratense), dandelion root (Taraxacum off.), echinacea (Echinacea species), golden seal root (Hydrastis canadensis), gentian root (Gentian lutea) and burdock root (Arctium lappa).

Formulas

Gypsum Combination (Shi gao tang); **Gentiana combination** (Long dan xie gan tang); **Forsythia and Rhubarb Combination** (Liang ge san), used to clear Heat from the Upper and Middle Warmers while promoting bowel movement; and **Coptis and Scute Combination** (Huang lian jie du tang).

Deficient Heat: Characteristic of Yin Deficiency, the principle is to tonify Yin and clear the Deficient Heat. Quite often these people show a greater than average resistance to antibiotic therapy, which makes their infections particularly troublesome to treat. Not only is plenty of sleep and rest imperative, but they require more neutral to cool-natured tonics, either alone or in judicious combination with Heat-clearing herbs for effective treatment. In this case you want to tonify the Yin with appropriate Yin tonics, such as Chinese ophiopogon root (Ophiopogon japonicus), lycium berries (Lycium chinensis), unprepared Rehmannia glutinosa (Sheng Di Huang) and asparagus root (Tian Men Dong). Milder Qi tonics with Yin nourishing properties can also be used, such as polygonatum (solomon's seal root).

In Western herbalism nutritive demulcent or emollient herbs are employed such as marshmallow root (Althea officinalis), alfalfa syrup in a base of blackstrap molasses and honey, evening primrose oil, slippery elm bark (Ulmus fulva), Iceland moss (Chondrus crispus), usnea (Usnea barbata) or comfrey root (Symphytum officinalis). Ayurvedic herbs and formulas, such as Shilajit (a type of mineral-rich pitch secreted from certain rocks in the Himalayan mountains), Chyavanprash - a complex formula of over 40 herbs with at least 50% Amla (Emblic myrobalans), and Shatavari (Asparagus racemosa) are specifically used to clear Deficient Heat.

Formula **Anemarrhena, Phellodendron and Rehmannia Combination** (Zhi bai di huang tang).

SUMMARY OF HOT AND COLD SYNDROMES

	Cold	Hot
Preference	Prefers warmth	Prefers coolness
Thirst	Less thirst	More thirst
Complexion	Pale	Ruddy or flushed
Extremities	Cold	Hot
Stool	Loose	Dry or Constipated
Urination	Clear, long	Deep colored, scanty
Vitality	Low	High, Anxious
Tongue	Pale, white coat	Red, yellow coat
Pulse	Slower than 60 beats per minute	80 or more beats per minute

Difficulties in Determining Cold and Heat Syndromes

As with all conditions, it is not uncommon for there to be a combination of both pathologic Cold and Heat simultaneously. It is logically impossible for Cold and Heat to be in the same physical area of the body. In fact, a noticeable presence of either Cold or Heat likely indicates the presence of the opposite in another bodily area. With combined Hot and Cold syndromes, treat that which is most severe as the primary condition.

This situation of mixed symptoms is commonly seen in clinical practice. In such cases, it is best to combine the appropriate formulas and herbs to treat the specific symptoms involved.

Heat in the Upper Warmer and Cold in the Lower Warmer: Symptoms may include conjunctivitis, sore throat, toothache, headache, feverish feelings in the head and chest, sour and putrid vomitus, with cold spasmodic pains in the stomach, waist and legs with loose stool and clear urine. Depending on the nature and severity of the symptoms, either emphasize clearing Heat in the Upper Warmer, or tonifying Yang Deficiency and digestion in the Lower Warmer.

Cold in the Upper Warmer and Heat in the Lower Warmer: Symptoms include pale face and lips, clear or white runny nasal mucus or phlegm in the Lungs, Bladder or vaginal infections, bleeding or hemorrhoids. In this case, clear Heat from the Lower Warmer, vitalize and build Blood and Qi and clear Dampness from the Upper Warmer with warming Phlegm-dissolving herbs.

Cold in the Middle Warmer with Heat in the Lower Warmer: Symptoms include cold stomach pains, clear, watery vomitus, hiccup with dry stool or constipation, frequent passing of dark or blood-tinged urine, leukorrhea and painful genitals. Here we may have a condition where Heat congestion in the Lower Warmer causes Cold congestion and indigestion in the Middle Warmer (Stomach). The treatment principle is to clear Heat from the lower abdomen and at the same time warm the digestion.

External Cold and Internal Heat: Symptoms include: Minor chills, sore, swollen throat, thick yellowish phlegm, floating pulse with Cold cramping abdominal pains, loose stools, early morning diarrhea, clear, long urine and white and greasy tongue coat. With External Cold and Internal Heat we need to Warm the Exterior and clear Internal Heat.

External Heat and Internal Cold: Symptoms include: clear, copious or scanty and frequent urination, loose stools or diarrhea, sluggish digestion, flush, red skin eruptions or sore throat. Clear External Heat and use mildly supportive herbs for the Interior. Only after all External symptoms have been resolved can we move aggressively to warm the Interior.

DEFICIENCY AND EXCESS

Deficiency and Excess tell about the patient's strength and weakness. An individual who is Deficient tends to have a lowered immune system and sensitivity to External pathogenic factors. For these, the Deficiency assumes a chronic predisposition with hyper-sensitivity to stress, climate and foods as the primary acute manifestation. Further, patients whose symptoms emanate from a pattern of Deficiency generally take a longer time to recover.

On the other hand, Excess patients may develop dangerously acute symptomatic reactions to stress, climate and foods. Considering that such acute External reactions constitute an attempt on the part of the body to eliminate the toxic Excess, too much elimination all at once can overload and cause vital eliminative systems to malfunction, such as the Liver and Kidneys. On a more long-term chronic level, the Heart is overworked which can lead to heart failure. In general, Excess patterns are easier to treat because Excess is easily eliminated through fasting, vegetable diet and detoxifying herbs.

Many of the formulas and treatments have already been discussed in previous sections of Internal Excess and Internal Deficiency.

Deficiency

A state of Deficiency can include a lack of Qi, Blood, Yin, Yang or Essence. Tonic herbs and formulas are indicated for each of these deficiencies. Many have been previously presented in the section on Internal Deficiency.

Formulas
Qi Deficiency: Four Major Herbs (Si jun zi tang).
Blood Deficiency: **Dang Gui Four** (Si wu tang).
Qi and Blood Deficiency: Eight Precious Herbs Combination (Ba zhen Tang).
Qi, Blood and Yin Deficiency: Ginseng and Dang Gui Ten Combination (Shi quan da bu tang).
Collapsed Qi, and Blood Deficiency: Ginseng and Astragalus Combination (Bu zhong yi qi tang).
Yang Deficiency: Vitality Combination (Zhen wu tang) and **Rehmannia Eight Combination** (Ba wei di huang tang) for Spleen and Kidney Yang Deficiency.
Yin Deficiency: Rehmannia Six (Liu wei di huang tang), **Anemarrhena, Phellodendron and Rehmannia Combination** (Zhi bai di huang tang) and **Sweet Wormwood and Tortoise Shell Combination** (Qing hao bie jia tang).

Ayurvedic herbs used include shatavari (Asparagus racemosa) for Blood, Yin and hormonal Deficiencies, ashwagandha (Withania somnifera) for Qi and Yang Deficiency, shilajit for Yin Deficiency and Chyavanprash for general Deficiency of all systems.

Western herbs include bitter tonics taken before meals to improve appetite and digestion, and herbal preparations made with a base of raw sugar, blackstrap molasses, barley malt and honey. A Qi and Yin tonic syrup is made with a combination of equal parts Iceland moss (Cetraria islandica) and Irish moss (Chondrus crispus). Slippery elm gruel (Ulmus fulva) is made by combining slippery elm bark powder, grated ginger root and honey (or barley malt syrup) with cow's or goat's milk. This is a rehabilitation food that is served as a warm porridge. American ginseng (Panax quinquefolium), is generally considered a Yin tonic, but it also has some Blood and Qi tonic properties. It can be decocted and made into a syrup using barley malt, maple or rice syrup. The powder can also be combined with honey or barley malt syrup and taken in teaspoonful doses. A Yin and Blood tonic is Comfrey Mucilage made with comfrey root (Symphytum officinalis), honey and glycerine.

Excess

Excess represents toxic stagnation which can include stagnation of Qi, Blood, Fluids, Cold and food. Consider herbs and formulas that remove stagnation, detoxify, eliminate and clear Heat (alteratives, cholagogues, purgatives), as well as herbs and formulas that promote the circulation of Qi (carminatives and digestives) and Blood Regulation (emmenagogues).

Toxicity is anything that the body-mind is unable to use or is no longer needed. There can be physical toxins from food, air and water, and mental toxins that are generated hormonally and through other subtle internal secretions as a result of psychological stress.

The Five Stagnations described above are listed according to their accumulation in the Triple Warmer or "three jiaos". The Triple warmer is an Organ function representing the coordination and functional activities of the three major areas of the body. The Upper Warmer is located from the top of the head to the sternum, the Middle Warmer is situated from base of the sternum to the navel, and the Lower Warmer includes the area from the navel down.

Five Stagnations
1. Qi Stagnation

In general, Qi stagnation is characterized by pains that move or come and go, while the pulse is similar to Blood Stagnation. It can be "difficult" or "choppy" (thready, slow and short, entering and exiting with difficulty), "knotted" (slower than 60 BPM with occasional irregular pauses), "accelerated" or rapid (faster than 80 BPM with irregular pauses).

a) **Upper Warmer**: Emotional and mental symptoms, depression, hysteria, headaches, dizziness, vertigo, chest pains that change location or recur irregularly.

b) **Middle Warmer**: Belching, gas, tight stomach, full feeling in the abdomen and pains that move or come and go.

c) **Lower Warmer**: Stiffness, heaviness, tightness in the lower abdomen and lower extremities, pains that move or come and go.

Formulas: **Bupleurum and Peony Combination** (Jia wei xiao yao san) and **Bupleurum and Chih shih Formula** (Si ni san or Frigid Extremities Powder).

2. Blood Stagnation

The pulse can feel "difficult" or "choppy", "knotted", "accelerated" or rapid. The tongue appears purplish with purple maculae especially on the sides of the tongue. There are sharp, intractable pains anywhere in the body, perhaps as a consequence of a trauma or operation. Degenerated spinal disks and scar tissue are also considered Blood Stagnation. Older people can have liver spots on the skin or varicosities.

a) **Upper Warmer**: Discoloration, venous protrusions, blueness, heaviness of the head and arms. Other symptoms include a heavy feeling in the head, neck and shoulders, pains, angina, congestive heart failure, TB, lung congestion, breast lumps or bleeding in the lungs called "dry blood".

b) **Middle Warmer**: Lumps and tight, sharply painful areas in the abdomen.

c) **Lower Warmer**: the lower abdomen may have noticeable lumps, often associated in women with gynecological problems such as cysts and fibroids.

Formulas
Dang Gui Four (Si wu tang) and **Cinnamon and Poria Combination** (Gui zhi fu ling tang).

In Ayurvedic medicine a useful preparation given for Blood stagnation is **Guggul** (Commiphora mukul). It is prepared from the resin of a species of myrrh and is particularly indicated for increased bodily stiffness, arthritis and rheumatic complaints. In Ayurveda these are associated with symptoms of aging and described as a tendency for the body to accumulate toxins called *Ama*. Today *Ama* is generally equated with the accumulation of cholesterol and high blood lipids which gradually impair circulation.

3. Fluid Stagnation

The tongue is swollen, there is generalized edema, especially on the face, leukorrhea, enlarged glands or nodules and the pulse feels slippery, or rolling. Fluid stagnation is often associated with Qi deficiency or low energy.

a) **Upper Warmer**: Edema, Dampness of the head, chest, sinus and nasal drainage, cough with phlegm, exceptionally wet tongue with scalloped edges, pericarditis, pleurisy, Fluid stagnation in the brain and breast lumps.

b) **Middle Warmer**: swollen abdomen (pot belly), watery or gurgling sounds in the abdomen and ascites.

c) **Lower Warmer**: Edema, pitting, Dampness in the lower pelvic area (such as leukorrhea, and enlarged buttocks), fibroids and cysts. Cancer is also thought to be in part due to Fluid stagnation.

Formulas
For Removing Phlegm Stagnation: Citrus and Pinellia Combination (Er chen tang or Two Cured Decoction).
For Removing Damp Stagnation: Poria Five Herbs formula (Wu ling san).

4. Cold Stagnation

Symptoms include generalized feeling of coldness, cold extremities, cold phobia, the complexion and tongue are pale and the pulse is slow (less than 60 BPM).

a) **Upper Warmer**: coldness of the head, arms, chest and back, pale complexion.

b) **Middle Warmer**: cold digestion, bloating and anorexia.

c) **Lower Warmer**: coldness of the extremities, impotence, frigidity, diarrhea, gas and bloating.

Formulas
Aconite, Ginger and Licorice Combination (Si ni tang) and **Aconite, Ginseng and Ginger Combination** (Fu zi li zhong tang).

5. Food Stagnation

Generally Phlegm and food stagnate in the Middle or Lower Warmers. The abdomen and pulse feel large and full, the pulse is slippery or gliding, and the tongue is greasy, swollen, perhaps with a thick yellow or white coat.

a) **Middle Warmer:** greasy coated tongue, epigastric spasms and abdominal fullness.

Formulas
For Removing Middle Warmer Food Stagnation: Citrus and Crataegus Formula (Preserve Harmony Pill or Bao he wan).
For Removing Lower Warmer bowel stagnation with constipation: Major Rhubarb Combination (Da cheng qi tang); **Minor Rhubarb Combination** (Xiao cheng qi tang); and **Rhubarb and Mirabilitum Combination** (Tiao wei cheng qi tang, or Stomach Regulating Purgative Decoction).

In addition, detoxifying formulas without specific laxative effects such as **Coptis and Scute Combination** (Huang lian jie du tang) can also be considered.

In Ayurveda medicine, Triphala is used to clear stagnation of the Middle and Lower Warmers. It is the most commonly used and valuable of all traditional Ayurvedic preparations. It consists of three fruits with mildly cleansing and strengthening properties. Each fruit is capable of eliminating an Excess of each of the three corresponding Humours (Vata, Pitta and Kapha). Beleric myrobalan eliminates excess Water, benefiting the heart, circulation and lungs; Chebulic myrobalan eliminates excess Air which benefits the intestines, lungs and nervous system; Emblic myrobalan (amla) regulates Fire and is the second highest known source of natural vitamin C next to acerola berries.

A further unique aspect of this important substance is that the vitamin C in amla does not dissipate either under high heat or reasonable aging. This is because it is bound up with certain tannins. Besides being detoxifying, especially to the liver, amla is also highly nutritious. With each of the three substances in Triphala assigned to balance each of the Three Humours, Triphala itself is considered balancing to all three humours and safe to take year-round for eliminating all excesses while imparting strength to the entire gastrointestinal tract. It is the safest and best mild purgative to take on a regular basis and will cause no laxative dependency.

Western herbs include detoxifying and alterative herbs such as burdock root (Arctium lappa), dandelion root (Taraxacum off.), sarsaparilla (Smilax off.), chaparral (Larrea divaricata); purgative or laxative herbs such as rhubarb root (Rheum palmatum), buckthorne bark (Rhamnus cathartica), cascara bark (Cascara sagrada); Blood moving or emmenagogue herbs such as wild ginger (Asarum canadense), blue cohosh (Caulophyllum thalictroides), motherwort (Leonurus cardiaca); and Qi regulating carminative herbs such as green citrus peel (Citrus reticulata) and ginger root (Zingiberis off.).

Overall: Qi Stagnation
This is called the "mother of all stagnations". It is usually caused by a disharmony of the Seven Emotions (see Chapter 8 for a detailed discussion of these).

Organ	Vice	Virtue
Liver	anger, frustration	benevolence, forgiveness, esteem, respect
Heart	over excitement (over achieving)	compassion, care for one's self
Lung	grief, sadness	conscientiousness, correctness, feeling good about one's self
Spleen	obsession, over thinking	empathy, centeredness
Kidney	fear, paranoia, worry	courage, wisdom

In ancient times, part of a physician's job was to help change vices into virtues. This was called "culturing the virtue", and healing occurred when the vices were changed to their corresponding virtues. Taoism, the underlying philosophy of Traditional Chinese Medicine, also focused on changing personalities. The Seven Emotions - fear, anxiety, pleasure, anger, sympathy, fright and sadness - were all considered the main part of Chinese medicine until the early 1800's. During the Han dynasty the Five Elements were used to transform the emotions, and the famous clinician, Sun Szu Miao, used one Emotion to overcome another.

Formulas
For treating stagnation diseases affecting all three "jiaos" (Triple Warmer) **caused by the Seven Emotions: Citrus and Perilla Combination** (Fen xin qi yin).
For Removing all Five Stagnations: Stagnation Relieving Pills (Yue qu wan).

YIN AND YANG
Yin and Yang are a summation of the Eight Principles. They include Yang Excess, Yang Deficiency, Yin Excess and Yin Deficiency and are defined and treated as follows.

Yang Excess: This the same as Excess Heat with symptoms of high fever, restlessness, red complexion, loud voice, aggressive actions, strong odors, yellow discharges, rapid pulse and hypertension, for instance. Herbs that detoxify, drain Fire and Heat and promote bowel movements are most useful here. These can include the formulas and herbs given earlier under the categories Internal Heat and External Heat.

Yang Deficiency: This manifests symptoms of lethargy, coldness, edema, poor digestion, lower back pain, the type of constipation caused by weak peristaltic motion, and lack of libido. Here there is a lack of heat and activity to perform adequate functions in the body. This is the same as the category of Internal Cold. Refer to that section for herbs and formulas.

Yin Excess: This is the same as Internal Dampness described under the Pernicious Influences. These imbalances include symptoms of excessive fluid retention, lethargy, a plump or swollen appearance and overall signs of Dampness, and yet these people may have adequate energy. Spicy, warm-natured herbs, such as ginger (Gan Jiang) and cinnamon (Rou Gui), and diuretics, such as Fu Ling mushrooms, can help promote the elimination of excess water in such cases.

Yin Deficiency: This is the same as the category Deficient Heat mentioned earlier. These diseases involve emaciation and weakness with wasting Heat symptoms, termed "false Yang". Such individuals are nutritionally depleted to the point that they begin to manifest false Heat symptoms, but in the context of Deficiency rather than Excess. For instance, an individual who is emaciated, runs on nervous energy, talks fast but peters out quickly, sleeps poorly, and has little stamina and low resistance is experiencing Empty Yin, or Yin Deficiency. Refer to that category for herbs and formulas to treat this condition.

COMBINATIONS OF PATTERNS

Obviously there can be combinations of more than one imbalance. Some examples of these would be:

External-Excess-Heat: Skin eruptions, rashes, boils, eczema, strong body odor, possibly heavy or no sweating, restless sleep, anxiety, mucus is yellowish, or even red tinged with blood, breathing is loud and strong, pulse is floating, rapid, full and/or tense, urination is scanty, darker colored, tends to be constipated or have diarrhea. If they have a fever it tends to be high. This is "Yang within Yang".

Therapeutic principle: clear External Heat, eliminate toxins, dry upper and lower Damp Heat. The herbal properties should be cool or cold, emphasizing the use of cooling diaphoretics, antispasmodics, diuretics, nervines, expectorants, antipyretics, alteratives, febrifuges, purgatives and astringents.

Formulas
Lonicera and Forsythia combination (Yin qiao san).
Western herbalism gives detoxifying and eliminative diaphoretic Heat clearing herbs.

External-Excess-Cold: Cold, stiff, slow moving, lowered immunity, aversion to Cold, Wind and Damp, lack of sweating, lower fevers with a tendency towards chills, complexion is pale, puffy and swollen, tends to drowsiness and sleepiness, mucus is clear or cloudy white, breathing is strong and labored, tendency towards frequent urination which is light colored, stool is normal to loose, the pulse is floating and full and the tongue is pale, scalloped, moist with a white coat.

Therapeutic Principle: Release Cold Exterior and dry Damp, employing herbs that have diuretic, warming, stimulant, expectorant, carminative and astringent properties.

Formulas
Ephedra Decoction (Ma Huang tang) and **Minor Blue Dragon Combination** (Xiao qing long tang) for acute upper respiratory conditions.

Ayurvedic and Western compounds previously described can also be used. These include Trikatu Formula, Sito Paladi and Composition Powder.

External-Deficient-Heat: A frailer individual, who is thin, restless, anxious, frequent mood changes, low immunity, aversion to heat and wind, thirst, spontaneous perspiration, night sweats, low grade fever, restless sleep, acute or chronic recurring sore throats, urination is thin, yellowish, possible recurring bladder infections, stool is watery, slightly yellowish or dry and constipated, the pulse is floating, fast, thin, weak and the tongue is reddish body with a thin or shiny coat. This is a Yin Deficient condition.

Therapeutic Principle: Clear External Deficient Heat, strengthen immunity and moisten Dryness. Use herbal formulas that are cool, nourishing, nutritive tonics.

Formulas
Decoction of Polygonatum Rhizome (Jia jian wei zhu tang).

Ayurvedic medicine uses **Shatavari** (asparagus racemosa) combined with ghee, while Western herbalism gives **Comfrey mucilage** (described earlier).

External-Deficient-Cold: Cold, aversion to wind, frail, anemic, pale complexion, thin, insecure, sad and depressed, low immunity, clear or whitish mucus, no thirst, acute conditions that may arise quickly but with mild or subnormal fevers and chills, shallow breath, urination is clear, copious and frequent, stool is loose, tending to sleep a lot. Pulse is floating, slow and thin and the tongue is pale, moist, scalloped with a thin, white coat.

Therapeutic Principle: Warm Coldness, tonify Qi and the immune system. Use warming surface relieving diaphoretics, warming stimulants and tonics.

Formulas
Jade Screen (Yu ping feng san); **Cinnamon Combination** (Gui zhi tang) for acute upper respiratory conditions; **Minor Bupleurum Combination** (Xiao chai hu tang); and **Bupleurum and Cinnamon Combination** (Gui zhi chai hu tang).

Ayurvedic medicine gives **Sito Paladi or Chyavanprash**, while Western herbalism uses a tea of slippery elm, marshmallow root, cinnamon, ginger and honey, or garlic tea with honey.

Internal-Cold-Deficiency: A frail individual with Coldness, timidity, low energy characterized by symptoms of hypo-thyroidism or hypo-adrenalism, pale complexion, anemic, lack of thirst, recurring colds and flu, sleeps easily, thin, clear mucus discharges, lack of thirst, lips are pale and wet, breathing is shallow and weak, low libido, aching lower back and joints, menstruation is pale, very light, late or irregular, urination is frequent and copious, possibly with nighttime urination, stool tends to be light and loose, pulse is hollow, slow and weak, tongue is pale, scalloped and wet, with a thin white coat. This is "Yin within Yin", or a Cold condition.

Therapeutic principle: Warm Internal Cold and tonify Qi and the immune system using warming diaphoretics, Qi and Yang tonics and diuretics.

Formulas
Aconite, Ginseng and Ginger (Fu zi li zhong tang); **Aconite, Ginseng and Licorice** (Si ni tang); **Ginseng and Ginger combination** (Li zhong tang); and **Rehmannia Eight** (Ba wei di huang tang).

In Ayurvedic medicine **Chyavanprash** is given, a complex preparation comprised of 50% amla fruits and approximately 48 herbs, prepared with honey, raw sugar and ghee. It can be taken as a paste in warm milk. **Trikatu** is also used for Coldness and to warm digestion, while **Sito Paladi** is used for colds and flu.

Western herbalism gives alfalfa prepared into a syrup with honey and molasses (a similar product is sold in Homeopathic pharmacies, called "Alfalco"). Further, **Composition Powder** is given for acute problems, and a paste of freshly mashed garlic cloves and honey or barley malt syrup can be given in teaspoon doses several times daily as needed.

Internal-Cold-Excess: Presents symptoms of Coldness, pale complexion, flacidity, severe edema, slower moving, melancholic, alternating moods, aversion to cold and dampness, poor digestion with a tendency towards gas and bloating, a tendency towards clear or white mucus and allergies, cold extremities, short menstrual cycle, slow bleeding perhaps with dull pains, urination is copious, light colored, possible nighttime urination, stool is loose, pulse is deeper, slow and slippery or gliding. This is Excess Cold Dampness that can lead to Yang Deficiency.

Therapeutic principle: Warm Internal Cold, warm digestion, clear Dampness, tonify Yang with the herbal properties of Internal warming stimulants, carminatives, diuretics and Yang and Qi tonics.

Formulas
Aconite, Ginger and Licorice Combination (Si ni tang); **Vitality Combination** (Zhen wu tang); and **Ginseng and Ginger Combination** (Li zhong tang) possibly with prepared aconite (Fu Zi) and cinnamon bark (Rou Gui).

Ayurvedic medicine uses **Chyavanprash, Trikatu or Hingashtak**, while Western herbalism might prescribe a tea of prickly ash, angelica, lovage, elecampane, ginger, cinnamon and parsley root.

Internal-Heat-Excess: Tendency towards constipation, with a possible tendency to have blood in the stool, urine, vomit, nasal secretions, strong body odors, aversion to heat, irritable and aggressive temperament, active, energetic, restless with a tendency towards insomnia, loud, commanding voice, strong appetite, thirst, heavy coarse breathing, a tendency towards infections and inflammations, strong sexual drive, eyes may be yellow or reddish colored, lips dry and cracked, heavy menses, possibly early and long lasting, urination is dark colored, stool is either hard and solid or possibly constipated, or hot, yellowish diarrhea. This is a "Yang Heat" condition.

Therapeutic Principle: Clear Internal Excess Heat, eliminate toxins and cool the Blood and Liver. Use herbal formulas which are cooling alteratives, cholagogues and purgatives.

Formulas
Coptis and Scute Combination (Huang lian jie du tang); **White Tiger Decoction** (Bai hu tang); **Major Rhubarb Combination** (Da cheng qi tang); **Minor Rhubarb Combination** (Xiao cheng qi tang); **Rhubarb and Mirabilitum Combination** (Tiao wei cheng qi tang).

Ayurvedic herbalism uses **Triphala, Guggul** or **Castor oil**, while Western herbalism gives blood purifying formulas such as equal parts dandelion root, sarsaparilla root, burdock root, barberry root, red clover, sassafras bark, prickly ash bark, and a half part each of lobelia and ginger.

Internal-Heat-Deficiency: Symptoms of Coldness, paleness and Deficiency, low immunity, thin constitution, restlessness, lack of stamina, Heat sensations but with an overall tendency to feel cold with a consequent aversion to heat, cold and wind, thirst, night sweats, restless sleep, dryness, weak digestion, low grade infections, burning sensation in the palms, soles of the feet or chest, menstruation is light but short, some pain but irregular, pulse is rapid, thready and weak, tongue is red with a thin body, lack of coat and is shiny. This is a Yin Deficient condition.

Therapeutic principle: Clear Deficient Heat, nourish and moisten Yin using herbal properties of Yin tonics, demulcents, alteratives, nervines and nutritive tonics.

Formulas
Rehmannia Six (Liu wei di huang wan); **Sweet Wormwood and Tortoise Shell Formula** (Qing hao bie jia tang); and **Anemarrhena, Phellodendron and Rehmannia Combination** (Zhi bai di huang tang).

Ayurvedic herbalism gives **Shatavari** (Asparagus racemosa) combined with ghee, while Western herbalism uses **Comfrey mucilage.**

PATTERNS THAT CHANGE

The various syndromes can transform into each other. For example, either External-Internal, Hot-Cold, Excess-Deficient can change into each other depending upon the stage of the disease. When an Internal syndrome changes to an External one, it is considered a positive direction because the Internal toxins of the body are being eliminated from the deeper layers. However, an External disease changing to an Internal one is a negative direction reflecting a worsening of the overall condition. Thus, it is important to treat the current condition accurately.

SUMMARY OF FORMULAS FOR THE EIGHT PRINCIPLES

External-Excess-Heat	Lonicera and Forsythia
External-Excess-Cold	Ephedra Decoction Minor Blue Dragon
External-Deficient-Heat	Decoction of Polygonatum Rhizome
External-Deficient-Cold	Cinnamon Combination Jade Screen Minor Bupleurum Bupleurum and Cinnamon
Internal-Deficient-Cold	Aconite, Ginseng and Ginger Aconite, Ginseng and Licorice Ginseng and Ginger Rehmannia Eight
Internal-Excess-Cold	Aconite, Ginger and Licorice Vitality Combination Ginseng and Ginger
Internal-Excess-Heat	Coptis and scute White Tiger Major Rhubarb

	Minor Rhubarb
	Rhubarb and Mirabilitum
Internal-Deficient-Heat	Anemarrhena and Phellodendron
	and Rehmannia Six
	Rehmannia Six
	Sweet Wormwood and Tortoise Shell
Half External/Half Internal	Minor Bupleurum
with Coldness	Cinnamon and Bupleurum
	Minor Blue Dragon
with Excess	Major Bupleurum
with stagnation	Bupleurum and Peony
	Bupleurum and Chih Shih
	Bupleurum and Citrus
Yin Deficiency	Rehmannia Six
	Turtle Shell Formula
	Restore the Left (Zuo gui yin)
	Ginseng and Ophiopogon
Yang Deficiency	Rehmannia Eight
	Vitality Combination
	Restore the Right (You gui wan or You gui yin)
	Ginger, Licorice, Aconite and Ginseng
	Dragon Bone, Oyster shell, Ginseng and
	Aconite

Root and Branch

There often exists a combination of acute and chronic symptoms simultaneously. This is exemplified by the concept of **Root and Branch**. The **Branch** represents the more superficial acute symptoms while the **Root** is the underlying Excess or Deficiency. Acute External conditions should be treated before treating Internal Deficiencies. An example is an individual with Internal Deficiency who develops acute symptoms of cold, fever or flu. The cold, fever or flu would be considered the outer Branch symptoms while the Internal Deficiency is the Root.

Generally, the principle of treatment is to treat the outer Branch symptoms either before or at least simultaneously with the Internal Deficiency. For this we can use **Cinnamon Twig Combination** (Gui zhi tang) or **Jade Screen** (Yu ping feng san), which contains the tonic herbs astragalus and atractylodes alba, along with the surface relieving Ledebouriella (Fang Feng).

On the other hand, a surface skin rash can be the Branch of Internal Excess Heat of the Liver with Lower Bowel stagnation. For this, use a formula that combines both purgative properties through the use of rhubarb root and Heat clearing herbs such as phellodendron, gardenia bud, coptis and/or scutellaria. Such a Damp Heat rash on the surface will clear up with Internal clearing herbs. If, however, it is an acute rash suddenly erupting such as measles, the strategy is to quickly get it to erupt and ripen using warm surface relieving diaphoretics.

Other applications of the Root and Branch treatment principle involve the specific disease syndromes that may include more than one Organ system. For instance PMS can be caused by Blood stagnation which is the Branch, while the underlying root may be Liver Qi stagnation. Applying the principle of Root and Branch, one would use herbs and formulas to relieve Blood stagnation while at the same time using formulas to relieve Liver Qi Stagnation.

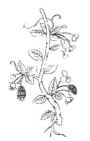

SIX

THE SIX STAGES of DISEASE & THE FOUR LEVELS of DISEASE

THE SIX STAGES OF DISEASE CAUSED BY EXTERNAL COLD

The theory of Six Stages was developed during the Han Dynasty by Chang Chung-Ching (AD 142-220). They were first described in his *Shang Han Lun*, (Treatise On The Treatment of Acute Diseases Caused by Cold), a highly revered work regarded as one of the first clinical manuals on the practice of Chinese herbalism. Each stage with its characteristic symptoms describes the progress and treatment of diseases caused by Cold, from the initial invasion at the three Yang stages to the subsequent degenerative consequences of the three Yin stages.

Over millennia, the application of the principles and formulas of the Shang Han Lun has expanded to include a wide range of conditions. As a result, the 107 formulas comprise the basic set that represents the foundation of both Traditional Chinese and Japanese-Chinese herbalism called "Kampo".

It is especially poignant to realize that this important work was written as a result of Chang's tragic experience of losing three-quarters of his family from a plague. During that time, he observed the ineffective treatment of many of the herb doctors of the time, with their inability to effectively respond to the changing character of acute disease. A study of the principles of the Six Stages allows us to respond appropriately to the often sudden changes associated with External diseases such as colds, coughs, allergies, influenza and communicable diseases caused by External Cold. At a later period, the Four Levels of Disease caused by Heat was formed to better understand and treat more complicated viral diseases. The Six Stages are as follows:

	Yang Stages	Yin Stages
Tai Yang	(Greater Yang)	Tai Yin (Greater Yin)
Shao Yang	(Lesser Yang)	Shao Yin (Lesser Yin)
Yang Ming	(Sunlight Yang)	Jue Yin (Absolute Yin)

The original purpose of the Six Stages was to develop an approach to treating External diseases that tended to progress from an acute Yang stage to a more degenerative and chronic Yin stage.

Still another practical application of the Six Stages is in acupuncture. For instance, the Small intestine meridian, which runs upward along the the arm to the side of the head, is called the **Upper Tai Yang**, while the Bladder meridian, which runs from the inner canthus of the eye down the back to the end of the small toes, is called the **Lower Tai Yang**. However, in practice, one seldom uses points on the corresponding meridians to actually treat related Organ disharmonies, so the association of the Organ meridians with the Six stages in acupuncture is more nominal than practical.

Furthermore, the order of the Six Stages tends to be more theoretical than actual. Usually febrile diseases begin with the Tai Yang stage and most commonly pass to the Yang Ming and more rarely through the Shao Yang stage. This demonstrates that diseases may not necessarily follow the sequence described in the Six Stages. In fact, a disease can arise in any one of the stages and proceed to any of the others. However, it is considered more dangerous if an acute febrile disease progresses to a deeper Yin stage, while it is a sign of improvement if a Yin stage disease moves to a more superficial Yang stage. This retracing describes what many Western herbalists and homeopaths regard as the "healing crisis".

Today it is more common to apply the diagnostic principles, treatment strategies and formulas of the Six Stages to the treatment of febrile, acute diseases. Chronic and degenerative diseases, on the other hand, are approached by other strategies such as the Three Humors, Eight Principles and Symptoms Sign or Zang Fu diagnosis.

THE THREE YANG STAGES

TAI YANG STAGE (Greater Yang)
This stage occurs when an External disease first attacks the body's defenses. Symptoms are the result of a superficial attack of External Wind, Cold, Heat and/or Dampness. They include general body-aches, with body stiffness, sweating, **fever with chills** and possible headaches with accompanying neck and shoulder stiffness characteristic of the early stages of cold and flu.

Early symptoms are often described as shivers "up and down the spine;" this describes the Bladder meridian that parallels the spinal column on the back, and the Small Intestine meridian that goes along the outer arms to the upper back and shoulders. Such vulnerability to

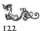

External Evils will not occur if one is not already in a weakened state, and one's pores (ruled by the Wei Qi that controls their opening and closing) are not able to sufficiently ward off Cold and Damp conditions. If we give purgatives during this stage, we weaken the body from within and allow the invading External Pathogens to penetrate deeper. Therefore, diaphoretic, or sweating, therapy is indicated.

Treatment for Tai Yang Stage imbalances

Principle: To induce diaphoresis and to eliminate External symptoms. Use herbs with a spicy-acrid, light and diaphoretic nature. They are generally not boiled; they should be infused in a covered pot to retain their volatile oils. **Precaution**: Do not sweat to exhaustion.

Formulas

Generally, formulas are taken from one or a combination of three 'formula families' as follows:

Ephedra Decoction (Ma huang tang)
Actions: This formula is a warm stimulating diaphoretic which dispels External Wind-Cold. It is also anti-asthmatic and used for individuals with fever, colds, asthma and upper respiratory problems with Excess conformation.

Cinnamon Twig Combination (Gui zhi tang)
Actions: This formula is a warming diaphoretic and tonic, regulating the constructive or nutritive energy (Ying) and the immune system (Wei). It is for more Deficient type individuals with Tai Yang imbalances.

Pueraria Combination (Ge gen tang)
Actions: As a diaphoretic, it treats External Wind-Cold-Damp and is antispasmodic, relieving stiffness and pain of the shoulders and neck. While Ephedra Decoction is for Excess, and Cinnamon Twig Combination is for a Deficient condition, Pueraria combination is for an individual with average constitution with Tai Yang imbalance. It is also indicated for shoulder and neck stiffness without a cold or fever.

Shao Yang Stage (Lesser Yang)

This stage is characterized by diseases that have symptoms of both External and Internal, Excess and Deficiency, Heat and Cold. Such symptoms are characteristic of diseases like malaria and typhoid fevers that show alternating heat and chills, and a cyclic recurrence of symptoms. Symptoms may tend to be lingering, there may be thirst but no desire to drink, diminished appetite or lack of appetite, nausea and vomiting, feeling of fullness and discomfort in the chest, aching body and limbs, bitter taste in the mouth, dizziness, restlessness, irritability and insomnia. The tongue body may be normal to red, the coat thick, greasy-white or grey. The pulse is bowstring or tense.

This state is a deeper penetration of an External Pathogenic Influence where it penetrates to the level of the Gall Bladder and Triple Warmer meridians. As the second stage, Shao Yang may differentiate itself by a tendency towards the Tai Yang or the Yang Ming stages, with the prevailing characteristic of lingering vacillation or alternation of symptoms being the most predominant characterisic; whichever stage it overlaps will display signs of that other stage as well.

Reflecting this, Shao Yang formulas have been adopted for the treatment of acute diseases that tend to linger and recur such as intermittent fever, malaria, bronchitis, asthma and more chronic conditions. Because Shao Yang formulas treat opposite complexes simultaneously, they are considered harmonizing formulas. The most widely used Shao Yang formula is:

Minor Bupleurum (Xiao chai hu tang)
Actions: This formula treats the Lesser Yang (Xiao Yang) channel, the Gall Bladder and Triple Warmer, harmonizes and regulates the Liver and Spleen functions, and addresses combined symptoms of Yin-Yang or External and Internal simultaneously.

Other formulas include:
Major Bupleurum (Da chai hu tang)
Actions: It treats Lesser Yang (Xiao Yang) channel, the Gall Bladder, Excess conditions, is laxative and purges Internal Heat.

Bupleurum and Cinnamon Combination (Chai hu gui zhi tang)
Actions: It is antipyretic, treats upper respiratory problems, is carminative, hepatic, is neuromuscular for intercostal neuralgia, headache, arthralgia, nephritis and pyelitis and is a nervine tonic. This is a combination of both **Minor Bupleurum Combination** and **Cinnamon Combination** which makes it particularly useful when there is more Coldness and Deficiency.

Bupleurum and Chih shih formula (Si ni san or Frigid Extremities Powder)
Actions: It regulates the Liver and Spleen and eliminates Internal Heat. This formula is specific for a combination of

stagnation of Heat in the Liver with Coldness in the fingers and toes.

Bupleurum and Dang Gui Formula (Xiao yao san or Rambling Powder)
Actions: This formula harmonizes Liver and Spleen, Regulates Qi, tonifies Blood, is anti-depressive, promotes digestion, and clears Heat. This formula is harmonizing, relieving Liver stagnation and treating symptoms of moodiness and depression. It is particularly useful for PMS and physical and emotional symptoms associated with menopause.

Bupleurum Formula (Yi gan san)
Actions: This is an antispasmodic formula, calming Liver Wind and tonifying Liver Blood and Qi. This is used for treating excitability, nervousness and anger caused by Liver stagnation.

Yang Ming Stage (Sunlight Yang)

This stage includes the Stomach and Large Intestine meridians. The primary indications are high fever without chills. If there are minor chills present, it signifies the struggle of the body attempting to overcome an External Pathogenic Influence. Other primary characteristics are high fever with a preference for cold drinks and food, tendency to less clothing irrespective of weather conditions, extreme thirst and excessive perspiration. The tongue body is red while the coat is yellow. The pulse is rapid and overflowing. In Eight Principles this would also be classified as Internal Hot Excess.

Yang Ming is further subdivided into Yang Ming Stage Channel Evil and Yang Ming Stage Organ Evil, which is considered more severe. Yang Ming Stage Organ Evil has accompanying constipation as a definitive symptom. Both stages require the use of bitter, cold and purgative herbs and formulas. Yang Ming stage is also associated in Japanese Kampo with the Five Stagnations, which further extends the principle to include a variety of acute and chronic imbalances.

1. **Abdominal swelling with constipation**: Use rhubarb formulas such as: **Major Rhubarb Combination** (Da cheng qi tang).
   Actions: This formula is used to purge Heat from the Stomach and Intestines and relieve constipation.

Minor Rhubarb Combination (Xiao cheng qi tang)
Actions: A less drastic purge than Major Rhubarb Combination, it removes Heat from the Stomach and Intestines.

2. **High fever with thirst**: This is a Yang Ming stage imbalance with the Heat originating in the Stomach. For this Qi level Heat stagnation, gypsum formulas are indicated such as:

> **White Tiger Decoction** (Bai hu tang)
> **Actions**: It eliminates Heat in the Qi (secondary defense) system and the Yang Ming channel and promotes the secretion of Body Fluids. White Tiger Decoction with 6 grams of ginseng added is used to support the righteous Qi by counteracting the cold energy of gypsum.

3. **Heat stagnating in the chest with irritability**:
> **Gardenia and Prepared Soybean Decoction** (Zhi zi dou chi tang)
> **Actions**: This is anti-inflammatory, clears Heat, relieves fever and irritability, is a mild sedative, relieves insomnia and restlessness and a full sensation in the chest.

4. **Heat caused by stagnation of Blood**: This may include a variety of gynecological symptoms such as fibroids, ovarian cysts and endometriosis. Formulas for stagnant Blood include purgative formulas such as:

> **Rhubarb and Moutan Combination** (Da huang mu dan pi tang)
> **Actions**: A laxative, it clears stagnant Heat in the Intestines, reduces swelling and disperses lumps. This is used for lower abdominal stagnant Blood and gynecological problems especially associated with the lower left abdomen (this is a Kampo indication that seems to suggest Blood Stagnation affecting the descending colon and the left ovary).

> **Persica and Rhubarb Combination** (Tao ho cheng chi tang)
> **Actions**: This dispels Heat and Blood stagnation in the Lower Warmer. In contrast to the previous, this formula is especially appropriate for problems in the lower right abdomen (a Kampo indication associated with Blood stagnation affecting the ascending colon and the right ovary).

> **Cinnamon and Poria Combination** (Gui zhi fu ling wan)
> **Actions**: It promotes blood and lymphatic circulation, thus removing stagnant Blood, and softens and resolves hard lumps such as cysts and fibroids. This formula generally improves female health and is commonly used for Blood stagnation with symptoms of fibroids, infertility and painful menstruation.

Clematis and Stephania Combination (Shu jing huo xue tang)
Actions: It opens circulation of the channels and collaterals, stimulates blood circulation, removes Blood stagnation, is antirheumatic, removes Damp stagnation and is for stagnant Blood causing arthritic and rheumatic pain.

5. Stagnant Excess Water with irregular urination: Use diuretics such as **Poria Five Herbs formula** (Wu ling san).
Actions: It is diuretic, clears edema, diaphoretic, digestive and strengthens the Spleen.

THE THREE YIN STAGES

The Three Yin Stages represent deeper stages of penetration of Cold with Internal weakness and Deficiency. Because of this they require internal warming and tonic formulas. Many of these, such as **Ginseng and Ginger Combination**, **Vitality Combination** and **Aconite, Ginger and Licorice Combination** are useful for all three stages.

Tai Yin Stage (Greater Yin)

Tai Yin refers to the Channels of the Spleen (Lower Tai Yin) and Lungs (Upper Tai Yin). Upper Tai Yin Lung symptoms include cough, asthma, hemoptysis, sore throat, chest fullness and pain along the Lung channel including the shoulder and the anterior aspect of the arm.

Spleen Deficiency includes Deficiency of Qi and Yang with Spleen Dampness. Symptoms include belching, vomiting, epigastric pain, abdominal distension, loose stool, jaundice, fatigue and coldness. The tongue body is pale and possibly swollen with scalloped edges and very wet. The pulse will be slow, weak or soft and slippery.

Overall, the predominant symptomology is associated with Dampness caused by Spleen Yang and Qi Deficiency. This Dampness can be in the Lungs causing congestion, asthma, bronchitis, or it can be reflected in any mucus membrane. This can include other symptoms such as vaginal discharge, cloudy urine and weeping eczema.

Originally, one of the causes leading to the Tai Yin stage imbalance was the over-use of bitter, cold-natured herbs for treating the External Yang stages of disease. An excess of bitter, cold-natured herbs can injure the Spleen and Stomach, subsequently damaging the normal fire of the digestive organs. Internal warming therapy is indicated to help restore the normal Spleen Yang and Qi.

Formula
Ginseng and Ginger Combination (Li zhong wan or Regulate the Middle Pill).

Actions: It is tonic, warming and tonifying to Spleen and Stomach Yang, strengthens the digestion and raises digestive metabolism.

Shao Yin Stage (Lesser Yin)

The Shao Yin stage is a still deeper stage of imbalance corresponding to the Kidney and Heart Organ Channels. The Kidneys are considered the root, or deepest source, of Yin and Yang in the body. Since Kidneys include both Kidney Yin Deficiency (Hot pattern) and Kidney Yang Deficiency (Cold pattern), Shao Yin stage imbalances have both a Cold and Hot pattern with completely different treament strategies.

Shao Yin Cold Pattern: This includes symptoms of Coldness, chills, aversion to cold, fatigue and lethargy, loose stools, aversion to cold drinks and foods and preference for warm substances, lack of thirst, abundant pale urine. The tongue is pale and the pulse is deep and thready.

Formula
Aconite, Ginger and Licorice Combination (Si ni tang)
Actions: It is for Yang exhaustion of the Lesser Yin (Xiao Yin) stage and Yang Deficiency caused by excessive perspiration.

Shao Yin Heat Pattern: This has classic symptoms of Yin Deficiency with sensations of heat, fever, insomnia, dry mouth, thirst, scanty, dark urine, red tongue with little or no coat and a thin, rapid pulse.

Formulas
Coptis and Gelatin Combination (Huang lian e jiao tang)
Actions: It purges Fire and nourishes the Yin.

Anemarrhena, Phellodendron with Rehmannia Combination (Zhi bai di huang wan)
Actions: To nourish the Yin of the Kidney and reduce Deficient Fire.

Jue Yin Stage (Absolute Yin)

The last Yin stage is indicated by thirst, difficult urination, and physical collapse. It is associated with the Pericardium and Liver. Internal warming herbs and tonics, such as those previously described, are used as appropriate. There are two forms:

a) With parasite infection:
Lower Warmer Deficiency and Coldness impairs the digestive function and causes roundworms to travel upwards to warmer parts of the digestive tract.

Mume Formula (Wu mei wan)
Actions: It is a warming stimulant and tonic for the Internal Organs, tonifies Qi, is anthelmintic and removes parasites.

b) With coldness, headache and dry mouth:
Evodia Combination (Wu zhu yu tang)
Actions: It warms the Liver and Stomach and is anti-emetic.

SUMMARY OF THE SIX STAGES

STAGE	SYMPTOMS	TREATMENT
Tai Yang Greater Yang	Fever with chills, general body aches & stiffness, headaches sweating or lack of sweating, pulse is felt more on the surface and the tongue has a normal appearing thin, white coat.	Diaphoretic formulas such as: **Ephedra Decoction** (Ma huang tang) **Cinnamon Twig Combination** (Gui zhi tang) **Pueraria Combination** (Ge gen tang).
Shao Yang Stage Lesser Yang	Variously combined symptoms of Hot and Cold, External & Internal, Excess and Deficiency. Reflects a deeper penetration of the disease with more lingering and recurring symptoms, aching extremities, dizziness, restlessness, irritability, insomnia, bitter taste in the mouth, chest discomfort, thirst or lack of thirst. Pulse is bowstring or tense and the tongue may be either normal or redder with a thicker greasy white coat.	Bupleurum formulas are used such as: **Minor Bupleurum** (Xiao chai hu tang) **Major Bupleurum** (Da chai hu tang), **Bupleurum and Cinnamon Combination** (Chai hu gui zhi tang), **Bupleurum and Chih Shih** (Si ni san) **Bupleurum and Dang Gui** (Xiao yao san), **Bupleurum Formula** (Yi gan san).
Sunlight Yang (Yang Ming)	Fever without chills, preference for cool drinks, extreme thirst, excessive perspiration. The pulse is rapid and full and the tongue is red with a yellow coat.	High fever, thirst, abdominal discomfort use **White Tiger Decoction** (Bai hu tang); for abdominal swelling use **Major Rhubarb Combination** (Da cheng qi tang) or **Minor Rhubarb Combination** (Xiao cheng qi tang); for Blood Stagnation use

STAGE	SYMPTOMS	TREATMENT
		Rhubarb and Moutan Combination (Da huang mu dan pi tang), Persica and Rhubarb Combination (Tao he cheng qi tang), Cinnamon and Poria Combination (Gui zhi fu ling wan), Clematis and Stephania Combination (Shu jing huo xue tang); for stagnant fluids and irregular urination use Poria Five Herbs Formula (Wu ling san).
Greater Yin Stage	Affects the Spleen and Lung channels. Overall symptoms are Qi Deficiency and Dampness. Symptoms range from Upper Warmer symptoms of cough, asthma, hemoptysis, sore throat, chest fullness; to Middle Warmer symptoms of belching, vomiting, abdominal pain, loose stool, jaundice, fatigue and coldness; to Lower Warmer symptoms of cloudy urine, vaginal discharge and weeping eczema. Pulse is slow, weak, soft or slippery. The tongue is pale with scalloped edges.	Ginseng and Ginger Combination (Li zhong wan or Regulate the Middle Pill).
Shao Yin Stage (Lesser Yin)	Affects the Heart and Kidney organ meridians. There are two patterns: Shao Yin Cold pattern shows a marked aversion to cold, chills, cold drinks and foods, loose stools, lack of thirst, abundant pale urine. The tongue is pale and the pulse is deep and thready. Shao Yin Heat Pattern exhibits symptoms of Yin Deficiency with Heat, fever, insomnia, restless sleep, dry mouth, thirst, scanty and dark urine, rapid pulse, red tongue with little or no coat.	For Shao Yin Cold use Aconite, Ginger and Licorice Combination Si ni tang). For Shao Yin Heat use Coptis and Gelatin Comb. (Huang lian e jiao tang) or Anemarrhena, Phellodendron with Rehmannia Six (Zhi bai di huang wan).

THE FOUR STAGES OF DISEASE

Caused by External Heat

While the theory of Six Stages is based on diagnosing and treating diseases caused by External Cold, the Four Stages, evolving through the Ming (1368-1644 A.D.) to the Qing dynasties (1644-1911 A.D.), was first expounded by Ye Tian Shi (1667-1746) in his book, *Discussion of Warm*

Diseases. It describes the treatment of virulent diseases caused by External Wind Heat. As such it provides a more relevant diagnostic and treatment protocol for the treatment of infectious and feverish diseases.

The Four Stages are as follows:

1. **Wei Fen**: This is the superficial defensive energy corresponding to the immune system.
2. **Qi Fen**: This includes the secondary defense system involving the Lungs, Spleen, Large Intestines, Stomach and Gall Bladder.
3. **Ying Fen**: This is the nutrient system, which also relates to the central nervous system.
4. **Xue Fen**: This involves the invasion of Heat into the Blood and Vital Essence.

The characteristics and herbal treatment for each of the Four Stages is as follows:

Wei Fen Stage (Wei Qi Stage Heat)

Generally this stage represents the early stages of febrile and infectious diseases with symptoms of fever, chills, sore throat, slight fear of wind and cold, red-tipped tongue and floating and rapid pulse. In the Eight Principles this corresponds to External Excess Wind Heat syndrome, so it is of a Yang character.

Formulas
Lonicera and Forsythia Combination (Yin qiao san)
Actions: It is diaphoretic, disperses External Wind-Heat, is alterative, antibiotic and antiviral, clears Internal Heat and relieves toxicity.

Morus and Chrysanthemum Combination (Sang ju yin)
Actions: It is a cooling diaphoretic, dispels Wind-Heat, is antitussive and relieves cough.

Qi Fen Stage (Qi Stage Heat)

This is similar to the Yang Ming stage of disease. It is deeper than Wei Fen and its symptoms include high fever, profuse sweating, extreme thirst, flushed face, scanty urine, constipation, yellow-coated tongue and slippery, rapid or full pulse. There is a strong desire for cool water.

Formulas
Ginseng and Gypsum Combination (Bai hu jia ren shen tang)
Actions: To eliminate Heat in the Qi (secondary defense) system and the Yang Ming channel and to promote the secretion of Body Fluids.

Ephedra, Apricot, Gypsum and Licorice Decoction (Ma xing shi gan tang)
Actions: Clears External conditions and is anti-asthmatic.

Ying Fen Stage (Ying Stage Heat)
The last two stages of the Four Stages represent acute stages that are not often seen clinically, and are generally better referred to Western medical treatment whenever possible. Another consideration is that formulas for these two stages typically rely on the use of rhinoceros horn, which is ecologically unacceptable at present. Alternatively, practitioners may substitute the indicated amount of rhinoceros horn with double or even triple the amount of water buffalo horn or cow's horn.
Symptoms of Ying Fen include high fever, restlessness, insomnia, delirium, loss of consciousness and/or coma.

Formula
Clear the Nutritive Level Decoction (Qing ying tang)
Actions: Clears Heat from the Nutritive Ying level and nourishes Yin and Vital Essence.

Xue Fen Stage (Blood Stage Heat)
This stage involves severe damage to the Vital Essence and Blood, so that in addition to severe high fever and coma, there are symptoms of bleeding such as epistaxis and hematuria. The tongue has a deep red color verging on cyanotic (blue), and the pulse is feeble and rapid.

Formula
Rhinoceros and Rehmannia Combination (Xi jiao di huang tang)
Actions: Treats severe fevers and Heat in the Blood system and removes Blood stagnation.

Following is a chart outlining the most predominant symptoms associated with each of the Four Stages of Heat:

STAGE	SYMPTOMS	CONDITION
Wei Level	High fever and slight chills, sweating, thirst, headache, sore throat, yellow phlegm; floating and rapid pulse; pink tongue with a slightly yellow coat.	Heat stroke, Summer Heat, External Heat attacking the body. This stage corresponds to Eight Principles' External Heat category.
Qi Level	High fever, lack of chills, irritability,	The External Pathogenic Factor has

excessive perspiration, excessive thirst, constipation, abdominal pain, red face, fear of heat, cough, yellow phlegm, dark urine; full and bounding pulse; the tongue is red with a yellow coat.

penetrated the surface and manifests as a high fever and inflammation affecting the internal Organs. This stage corresponds to the Eight Principles' Internal Heat category.

Ying Level   Late afternoon and tidal fever, insomnia, irritability, delirium, skin blotches; the pulse is rapid and thin; the tongue is dry and scarlet.

Deeper penetration of Heat that affects the Mind and Spirit. This stage correspond to the Eight Principles' Yin Deficient Heat.

Xue Level   High fever, delirium, coma, insomnia, (Blood level) signs of bleeding such as vomiting blood, nose bleed, blood in the stool, bruising under the skin; the pulse is rapid and thin, the tongue is dark red with prickles or a brown burnt coat.

Heat has penetrated to the deepest level where it drives out the Blood causing hemorrhage, affects the Spirit, with tremors and spasms and so gives rise to Liver Wind. This also corresponds to a deeper stage of Yin and Blood Deficiency.

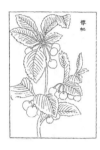

SEVEN

THE ORGANS

The Organs are a central concept to Chinese Medicine, as they perform the essential functions of the body, including assimilating, eliminating, storing, circulating, preserving, and transforming. When each of these processes is functioning properly, the body is in balance and health. When they aren't, there is disharmony, and thus imbalance and disease. The concepts of harmony and balance are at the core of Chinese medicine and represent a theoretical concept which goes beyond the body to include the emotions, mind, family, society, nature and the universe.

The theory of the Organs developed from several sources, but primarily through observation and experience. Because of spiritual beliefs, bodies were generally not dissected in ancient times; rather, intuition and keen observation were applied to directly perceive energetic imbalances in the body through the four diagnoses of looking, listening, smelling and palpating. Further, long-term medical experiences contributed information; for example, herbs used to strengthen the Essence of the Kidneys were found to also accelerate healing of the bones. Given this historical development of the Oriental medical understanding of the body, it is quite remarkable that they arrived at many similar conclusions about the **actions** of the Organs as we know them in Western medicine.

The understanding of the Oriental Organ functions is much broader and encompasses much more than the organic functions we define in Western medicine. In fact, Chinese medicine acknowledges two Organs which have no precise physical counterpart in the body: the Pericardium (the sac of fluid surrounding the Heart), and the Triple Warmer (which describes the relationship of all physiological processes in the upper, middle and lower parts of the body). Thus, to step into a broader understanding of the Chinese Organ processes, it is better to temporarily lay aside Western concepts of internal organs.

In Chinese Medicine, the Organs encompass a broad range of functions that include spiritual, mental and emotional aspects, as well as their physical functions. Further, each has its correspondences in environment, climate, color, sense organ, tissue and more. In fact, many of the Organs' operations occur on a cellular level, such as Spleen Qi corresponding to the function of the mitochondria in the cells, or Kidney Yang relating to ATP in the body.[1] Thus, the Chinese Organs function on a level throughout the entire body and are not limited to the visceral organ itself.

The Chinese Organs are divided into Yin, Yang and Extraordinary Organs. The Yin Organs, or the "five viscera" or solid Organs, are considered more important than the Yang Organs. They are vital since they perform the important functions of producing, transforming, regulating and storing the Fundamental Properties of Qi, Blood, Fluids, Jing and Shen. The Yin Organs include the Heart, Pericardium, Spleen, Lungs, Kidneys and Liver.

The Yang Organs, or the "six bowels" or hollow Organs, function to receive, break down and absorb the parts of food and fluid to be transformed into Fundamental Substances, and to transport and excrete waste products. In relation to the Yin Organs, they are more external in the body and not as vital, since they transform substances but do not retain them. The Yang Organs include the Small Intestine, Triple Warmer, Stomach, Large Intestine, Urinary Bladder and Gall Bladder.

The Yin and Yang Organs are paired together, as stated previously in the Five Elements Chapter. This forms an interior-exterior relationship in the body called the "Husband-Wife" Law that also extends to their respective meridians. They are as follows:

Yin Organ	Yang Organ
Heart	Small Intestine
Lung	Large Intestine
Spleen	Stomach
Liver	Gall Bladder
Kidney	Urinary Bladder
Pericardium	Triple Warmer

The six "extraordinary" Organs in the body are considered to be miscellaneous, or "curious", because their functions are different from those of the six bowels, or Yang Organs. They include the Brain, Uterus, Marrow (or Medulla), Bones, Blood Vessels and Gall Bladder. The Gall Bladder is both an extraordinary Organ as well as a Yang one because its Yang function of breaking down impure food is also supplemented by its curious one of being the only Yang Organ which contains a pure substance, bile.

Patterns of disharmony for any of the Organs are determined by the relationships between Qi, Blood, Fluids, Pernicious Influences and the Organs. These patterns, along with their signs and descriptions, are thoroughly discussed in the chapter on Differential Diagnosis.

THE YIN ORGANS (ZANG)

HEART

Ancient Chinese medical texts, particularly the *Su wen* of the Yellow Emperor's Classic, compared a person to a social organization. Thus, a societal role was assigned to each Organ. The Heart is the Emperor, the embodiment of Heaven on Earth. Here peace, order and rulership radiate from the center, commanding all the Organs. As such, the Heart has a dual function: to govern Blood and to house the Spirit, or Mind (Shen).

Governs Blood

The Heart regulates the circulation of Blood throughout the vessels, Organs and body tissues. It is also the location where Grain Qi is transformed into Blood. Heart Qi is the driving force of the heart beat; when it is functioning properly, the Blood flows smoothly and the pulse is even. Heart Qi also keeps normal strength, rate and rhythm of the heart beat. When Heart Qi or Blood are Deficient, blood circulation is poor and the hands and feet become cold, for instance. A healthy Heart also helps determine a strong constitution, along with Kidney Essence, by giving vigor and strength.

Controls the Blood Vessels

The Blood vessels are the ducts through which Blood flows, propelled by Heart Qi. They show the condition of Heart Qi and Blood: when both are strong, the vessels are in good condition and the pulse is full and regular; if either are weak, the pulse can be weak, irregular or thin.

Houses the Spirit / Mind (Shen)

The Spirit/Mind complex is called **Shen** in TCM. The Shen are the messengers of Heaven and are innumerable in number, like drops of water in the ocean. The Shen radiate enthusiasm, exuberance, creativity, social communication and interaction. The emperor (Heart) radiates the Shen throughout the body. Blood is the commonality here, as the Heart's ability to house the Shen depends on adequate nourishment from the Blood. Further, the emperor rules the body, through the circulation of the Blood throughout the organism and maintenance of its conduits, the blood vessels. The Spirit/Mind complex incorporates many characteristics and functions: mental functions, memory, consciousness, spirit, thinking and sleep. While seemingly diverse and unrelated, these functions are all encompassed in Shen, and can be divided into two categories, mental and spiritual. Thus the Mind and mental faculties reside in the Heart. The ability to think sharply, a clear and balanced consciousness, intellectual power, competent long term memory and good sleep are all signs of strong and abundant Heart Blood. If the Western mind considers that adequate blood flow and quantity are necessary to nourish the brain for these thinking processes to occur, then perhaps these relationships with the Heart can be better understood.

The connection between Blood and the Mind is very important. Blood is the root of the Mind: it embraces and anchors it. When it is sufficient, mental faculties are strong and the person is happy, peaceful and joyful. When it is Deficient, mental faculties are weak, resulting in symptoms such as mental restlessness and disturbance, insanity, abnormal behavior, excessive dreaming, dream-disturbed sleep or insomnia, anxiety and depression. On the other hand, long term dwelling on unhappiness, sadness and emotional problems can cause a Deficiency of Blood and induce palpitations, memory problems and unclear thinking.

The Spirit encompasses the entire mental, emotional and spiritual complex. Shen is the vital force of life, the passion for living. It is the organizing principle of all elements and Organ complexes. It incorporates the ability to love ourselves and others, to have trust, to be self-confident and to have direction and purpose in life. It also includes our ability to feel, to intuit, to be in touch with our Spirit, our Divine Light. When we are out of touch with our Spirit, our inner direction and guidance, our joy of life, or we lack trust, self-confidence, or love, we can become restless, agitated, anxious, worried and sleep poorly. These qualities can be seen in the eyes: if they sparkle and shine, the Spirit is strong; if they are dull and lifeless, the Spirit is clouded.

The metaphors, "open your heart", "wearing her heart on her sleeve", "He is lion-hearted", "follow a path with heart", "heartfelt", "heartbreak" or "my heart feels broken" all reflect states of Shen which we commonly experience and acknowledge. They can physiologically affect the body by stagnating circulation or depleting Blood, creating cold extremities, a pale and lusterless complexion, tightness in the chest and a lack of emotional warmth. On the other hand, hyper-excitability, hyperactivity, excessive laughter, extreme talking or inordinate partying and looking for thrills without balance for other life activities can lead to hysteria, nervous breakdowns, manic-depressive behavior, unfocused life direction, anxiety, abnormal behavior, mental restlessness, palpitations and pressure in the chest region.

The state of the Heart also influences our ability to form meaningful relationships or to be able to relate well to others. On the other hand, relationship problems can weaken the Heart and Mind, especially if they occur for a long time. The primary relationship is first with ourselves, our inner Spirit. Thus, spiritual practices are important for nurturing the Heart. The virtues of Shen include being joyful, blissful, grateful, happy, empathic, sympathetic, compassionate, loving, kind and merciful, while its vices include being overly excited and over-stimulated, dejected, dissatisfied, self-pitying, thoughtless, ungrateful, bored, tedious, apathetic and indifferent.

Because of the tremendous impact of Shen on health, it is always the first aspect to be taken into account when healing the body: harmonizing the Spirit is the highest goal. In ancient times as now, the highest level physician is able to heal through observation of and counseling with the Spirit; middle level physicians need to ask questions and use physical therapies to heal, whereas lower level physicians must touch the body to diagnose and treat the person. Our growing understanding today of the mutual impact and interrelationship of the mind and body is giving us the experiential foundation to understand and follow what the Chinese have done for thousands of years.

Opens into the Tongue

Branches from the Heart meridian ascend and connect with the tongue; thus, conditions of the Heart can be seen by observing the tongue. When Heart Blood and Qi are abundant, the tongue will be pale-red and bright and have a normal shape; when insufficient, the tongue will be pale and white with a thin shape; when stagnated, the tongue will be dark purple and show echymosis; when there is Heat in the Heart, there can be red and painful tongue ulcers. The area of the tongue specifically correlating to the Heart is the tip. When there is too much Heat in the Heart, the tip is red. Injuries to Heart Qi can cause an indentation to the tip of the tongue.

When the Heart doesn't function normally to control the Mind, then speech abnormalities can occur, such as stuttering, tongue rigidity, delirium or aphasia. The Heart also influences talking and laughter, so a Heart disharmony can result in excessive or inappropriate laughter, fast talking or talking incessantly, while lack of desire to talk shows Deficient Heart Qi. On the other hand, professions requiring a lot of talking, such as sales and teaching, can injure the Heart Qi over time. Thus, it is said that the Heart controls speech.

Manifests in the Face

The face is rich in blood vessels, which are controlled by the Heart; shen is reflected in the face through its color and luster. When the Heart functions well, Blood is plentiful and the face will be a normal color with sheen and moisture. When Heart Blood is insufficient, the face will be pale and lusterless. If Heart Blood is stagnant, the face will be purple.

Sweat is the Fluid of the Heart

Sweat is one of the Body Fluids, and Blood and Body Fluids mutually interchange. Thus, when Blood is too thick, Body Fluids enter to thin it down. On the other hand, someone who is Deficient in Blood should not be allowed to sweat excessively as this this will further deplete the Blood. This can cause palpitations and continuous violent beating of the heart. Deficient Heart Yang can cause spontaneous sweating, while Deficient Heart Yin can cause night time sweating. Because the Heart governs Blood, and Blood mutually interchanges with Body Fluids, including sweat, the Heart, being part of the Fire element, is related to sweat.

The Heart Loathes Heat

Again being the Yin Organ of the Fire Element, Heat is the most injurious Pernicious Influence to the Heart. Although TCM says Exterior Heat cannot invade the Heart itself, it also invades the Pericardium, the extension and protector of the Heart. When this happens, coma, delirium or aphasia can occur.

Dreams

When Heart Blood is plentiful, the Mind is rooted, and it is easy to fall asleep and sleep soundly. When Deficient, the Mind "wanders", causing inability to fall asleep, restless sleep or insomnia, dream-disturbed sleep or excessive dreaming. Dreams are, thus, generally related to the Heart.

Emotion: Joy

Joy is the emotion of the Heart, as has already been discussed under the topic of the Mind. Both lack of joy and excessive joy (in the sense of over-excitement) can injure the Heart and, likewise, a Heart disharmony can cause joylessness or elation.

PERICARDIUM

As Emperor, the Heart needs to be protected and gaurded. It also needs a way to communicate its authority to the rest of the organism.

this is the role of the Pericardium, or Heart Protector. Physically, the Pericardium is the sac, or outer shield, sourrounding the Heart. Its function is to both protect and maintain the Heart, and to form the system of connections through which the Heart may relate to the rest of the body.

As the Heart Protector, it guards against the invasion of External Pernicious Influences into the inner sanctum of the Heart. The main attacking Influence here is Heat. When pathogenic Heat attacks the Pericardium it results in high fever, coma and red tongue.

LUNGS

The Lungs hold the office of Minister or Chancellor in the body. It is physically closest to the Heart, and the heartbeat is dependent upon respiration from the lungs. Thus, the Lungs hold a privileged place. The Lungs control vital energy in the body. They extract Qi from the air during respiration and transfer it through the respiratory passages to the Blood, with which it is then circulated throughout the body. The Lungs also have direct contact with the outer environment through breathing, and because they are considered to be directly related to the skin. Because of this, they are the most prone to External Pernicious Influences, and thus they are often called a delicate Organ or the "princess" of the Organs. The Lungs are also the uppermost Organ in the body and consequently are often termed a "lid" on the other Organs.

Rule Qi

Through respiration the Lungs inhale pure air, circulate it throughout the body and then expel dirty air. This keeps the metabolism in the body functioning smoothly. The Lungs also assist in the formation of Qi. The essence of food and drink is sent by the Spleen to the Lungs, where it combines with inhaled air to form Natural Air Qi. The Lungs then spread it throughout the body by way of the Heart channels to nourish all tissues and promote normal physiological activities. When there is an imbalance of this function, cough, shortness of breath, asthma or chest distention may result.

Control Channels and Blood Vessels

Through their function of circulating and disseminating Qi, the Lungs have a broad role in maintaining vessel health. Qi is the motivator of movement, and thus is related to Blood flow. Further, Nutritive Qi flows with Blood in blood vessels and channels. Because the Lungs rule Qi, they direct circulation of Qi in blood vessels and channels, creating warmth throughout the body.

Control Dispersing and Descending

The Lungs disperse or spread Defensive Qi, food essence and Body Fluids all over the body to the space between the skin and muscles. Through this function, likened to a mist, the Lungs nourish the body and warm and moisten the muscles, skin and hair. They also control equal distribution of Defensive Qi and control the normal opening and closing of the pores. When impaired, a person is easily susceptible to invasion of Pernicious Influences, and thus colds and flu. Further, the pores become blocked when the condition is one of Excess, resulting in no sweating; or they become over-relaxed from a condition of Deficiency, allowing sweating to occur spontaneously. In addition, if the Lung function of dispersing Body Fluids is impaired, they collect under the skin and edema arises, especially of the face.

The Lungs, being the uppermost Organ in the body, have a descending function. If impaired, cough, shortness of breath, asthma, and a stuffy sensation in the chest appear. If they affect its paired Organ, the Large Intestine, constipation can occur from lack of Qi moving the stool downward. Other than helping to circulate Qi, they are also associated with water metabolism by causing water in the Upper Warmer to descend into the Kidney and Bladder. This keeps urination smooth and water metabolism normal. If this function becomes disturbed, dysuria, edema and phlegm-retention diseases result.

This association with water metabolism can be better understood by likening it to a finger on a straw full of water. If the finger is withdrawn, the water runs out uncontrolled. Thus, pregnant women or those whose Lung Qi is Deficient often have urine leakage after jumping, coughing or sneezing. On the other hand, if this function is impaired, the "finger" may not withdraw appropriately, causing urinary retention or scantiness. Thus, through this function it is said the Lungs regulate the water passages.

The dispersing and descending functions are mutually interdependent: if one is impaired, the other is affected. Their coordination keeps breathing even and circulation good. If impaired, stuffiness of the chest, difficulty breathing, cough and asthma can appear.

Control Skin and Hair

Because the Lungs connect to the exterior of the body and they function to disperse Qi and Fluids to the body surface, they control the skin and body hair. The distribution of Fluids to the skin and hair keep them moist and nourished. If functioning properly, the skin will have luster, the hair will be glossy and the opening and closing of the pores and sweating will be normal. If impaired, skin and hair will be dry, rough, and even flaky, and the hair will look withered and dry. Further, the pores will not open or close properly, causing lowered immunity, lack of sweating or spontaneous sweating. In the latter case, some Defensive Qi is actually lost with the sweat.

Open to the Nose

The nose is the doorway to the Lungs, and it also is in contact with the external environment. Its functions of respiration and sense of smell are dependent on Lung Qi. If it's Qi is strong, nasal breathing will be clear and open and sense of smell normal. If impaired, the nose will be blocked and there will be loss of sense of smell, watery nasal discharge and sneezing. If there is Heat in the Lungs, there may be nosebleeds with the alae nasi flapping rapidly.

House the Corporeal Soul (Po)

The Po are seven "spiritual entities," one for each of the bodily orifices. They are the most exterior and material of outwardly observable of all spiritual aspects and lack self awareness. They have no existence independent of the body, but are linked to its seven orifices. The Po are closely connected to the Lungs and respiration. In Greek, spirit means "breath" and soul means "wind or vital breath". In Sanskrit, *prana* means "vital life force" and is intimately linked with breathing and air. In Latin, spirit means "to breathe" and "breath, air, life, soul", resulting in our terms "inspire" and "inspiration". Thus the Po, or Corporeal Soul, is a manifestation of the breath of life and the vital energy of the body, Qi, and it is the material and physical manifestation of a human being's soul.

The Corporeal Soul, closely linked to Essence, is related to sensation and feelings and is most active during the day. It takes Qi into the body by breathing and then sends it to the Organs and channels. Even in a coma, the Po keep the body alive through automatic regulation of bodily rhythms, respiration, metabolism and general homeostatis. even though consciousness (Shen) isn't present. During gestation, Po controls Hun, and at birth, Hun becomes independent. At death, Hun returns to Heaven while Po dissolves the physical body and returns to the earth. Death is deliverance from the constraint of Po, the physical body, and thus is considered the great liberation.

The Po are tied to Time and Space and experience things in the moment. They are said to experience pain but not suffering, as pain is in the moment while suffering is one's response to it. When our awareness is in the present, we experience each moment as unique and complete. This is the virtue of the Lungs. When we hold onto things of the past, we experience sadness and ultimately grief.

Sadness and grief, the emotions of the Lungs, suggest loss of something or somebody we were not yet ready to let go. While an important and necessary emotion, prolonged grief injures the Lungs, resulting in a suppressed immune system and leading to colds, flu, pneumonia and asthma. The breath is directly affected by emotions, and through them, the Lungs are also affected. When we are sad, crying, angry, joyful, excited or fearful, our breathing changes.

Po is connected to the ability to receive and let go, and deals with what is "mine" and what isn't. Thus, it is involved with the intake of life-giving energies and the discharge of toxic ones. Attachment, possessiveness, unchecked desires, miserliness, hoarding, selfishness, defensive pride, stoicism, greed, envy, defensiveness, self-pity and extreme sensitivity or lack of sensitivity all come under this category, as a type of mental or emotional constipation (the metaphor for the Lungs' connection with the Large Intestine). Often these behaviors arise from feeling a lack of worthiness, deprivation or from unfulfilled needs. Thus, the person overcompensates and holds on to fill the inner void.

On the other hand, generosity, charity, giving, openness, receptivity, surrendering, non-attachment, sensitivity and thinking of others all reflect a healthy flow of outward energy and a strong sense of worthiness and self-fulfillment. When we feel we have what we need on all levels - physical, emotional, mental and spiritual - we are open to receiving and giving, or letting go without attachment or sense of loss.

The virtues of Po include being reverent, conscientious, ethical, upright, honest, careful, prudent, sensible, honorable, modest, respectful, correct, righteous and cautious, while its vices are being excessively sad, sorrowful, grieving, unethical, immoral, corrupt and wicked.

Loathe Cold

Because of the direct connection of the Lungs with the external environment and their function of regulating the pores and disseminating Defensive Qi, they are extremely susceptible to attack by Pernicious Influences, especially Cold.

Govern the Voice

The throat is said to be the door of the Lungs and home of the vocal cords. Further, Lung Qi provides strength, clarity and tone of voice. When healthy, the voice is clear and strong; if impaired, the voice may be low, weak or muffled by mucus. Thus, many common throat disorders are treated by attending to the Lungs.

Emotion

The emotions of the Lungs are grief and sadness. An excessive expression of these emotions injures Lung Qi and leads to Lung ailments such as asthma, pneumonia, flu and lowered immunity to colds.

SPLEEN

The Spleen, along with the Stomach, is the primary Organ for digestion in the body. It is the crucial link between taking food and drink into the body and transforming them into Blood and Qi, truly an alchemical process. Thus, it rules transformation and transportation, which can be loosely translated as metabolism and absorption. The Spleen, together with the Stomach, are the officials in charge of the storehouses and granaries and thus are considered the root of Post-Heaven Qi, or the source of all Qi produced by the body after birth. Thus, it is of central importance in the health of the body. While Kidney Jing is the hand of cards we are dealt in this life, the Spleen represents how we play that hand of cards.

Rules Transformation and Transportation

The Spleen receives the partially digested food from the Stomach and transforms it into Grain Qi. It then transports it upwards to the Lungs where it is mixed with Air Qi. This mixture travels to the Heart where it is transformed into Blood. Further, the pure part absorbed by the Spleen is transported to all parts of the body so that all the Organs, limbs, bones, hair and tendons are nourished. Thus, it is said the Spleen provides the material basis for the acquired constitution and that it functions as the root of Qi and Blood in the body. To tonify Blood and Qi in the body, therefore, we tonify the Spleen. If the transforming and transporting functions are normal, then digestion, appetite, absorption and bowel movements will be good. If imbalanced, there may be poor appetite, indigestion, abdominal distention or pain, anorexia, lassitude and loose stools.

The Spleen also functions to separate, move and transform water in the body. It is in charge of separating the usable and the unusable from the fluids ingested. It then "raises" or distributes the pure to the Lungs, and the dirty to the Intestines where it is further separated. This function occurs at the same time it is transforming, transporting and distributing nutrients. Thus, these functions influence each other, and an imbalance in one will affect the other. If the Spleen's transforming function occurs improperly, however, the Fluids can congeal to form Phlegm or cause edema. Thus, whenever there is Dampness or Phlegm in the body, the Spleen is at cause and is treated.

Controls Blood

Not only is the Spleen the root of Blood in the body, it is also in charge of keeping the Blood flowing in the vessels. The particular aspect of Qi that commands Blood in this way is Spleen Qi. When weak, Blood can escape its pathways, leading to hemorrhages, vomiting of blood, blood in the stool, blood under the skin, menorrhagia, uterine bleeding and possibly chronic bleeding.

Rules the Muscles, Flesh and Limbs

When the Spleen functions properly to distribute food essence throughout the body, the muscle tone is good, the muscles are strong and the limbs have strength to move. If the Spleen doesn't function well, the muscles become thin or atrophy, the arms and legs get slack or weak and the person feels tired.

Opens to the Mouth and Manifests in the Lips

Digestion begins in the mouth; thus the Spleen has a functional relationship with the mouth and lips. If the Spleen is strong and vigorous there is good appetite, the mouth is able to distinguish the five tastes, and the lips are red and moist. A dysfunction of the Spleen leads to poor appetite, the inability to distinguish tastes or a sticky, sweet taste in the mouth and pale, dry lips.

Controls Raising of Qi

The tendency of Spleen Qi is to ascend. It not only sends Grain Qi up to the Lungs, it also lifts and holds the Organs in place. If Spleen Qi is Deficient, chronic diarrhea along with prolapse of various Organs, such as Bladder, Stomach, Uterus, Kidney and the anus, can occur. The Spleen also functions to raise the clear Yang to the head. If Dampness obstructs the Spleen, the clear Yang can't ascend, resulting in fuzziness and heaviness of the head.

Loathes Dampness

The Spleen likes dryness but loathes Dampness. If there is a dysfunction of the Spleen's ability to transform and transport Fluids, Dampness can collect causing urinary problems, vaginal discharges, abdominal distension and Phlegm. On the other hand, excessive Dampness in the body can impair the function of the Spleen.

Emotion: Worry

Worry, brooding, obsession, sympathy and nostalgia are the emotional qualities of the Spleen. Indulgence in or prolonged experience of any of these emotions leads to poor digestion, gas, bloating, ulcers, decreased appetite and stagnation of Qi. Worry is often due to unexpressed needs, while "venting your Spleen" is stating them. Nostalgia can be an escape from the present and a compensation for what is missing in one's life now, which can include lack of emotional nourishment or a need for identity.

Sympathy can over-extend our energy reserves from caring too much for others' problems, resulting in low energy and the inability to digest what we need in our own lives. This can occur initially from a lack of self-assertion, sense of self or insecurity. When we feel at home in ourselves and live in the present, we can "digest" life's experiences and then are centered in ourselves.

Houses Thought (YI)

Yi is not a spiritual entity, but a quality of mind, a central channel of expression. It has been roughly translated as Idea or Thought. Yi is the intellectual function of the body complex which includes absorbing and remembering information, focusing, memorization, concentration, studying, thinking and organizing ideas. The virtues of the Spleen embody being bright, brilliant, intelligent, sharp, quick, clever, smart, alert, attentive, able and capable; its vices comprise being melancholic, witless, dense, dull, blunt, absent-minded, forgetful, oblivious and distracted. Yet Yi is more than that. It is also purpose, intention, engagement and reliability. In our lives it can mean we are either moving in an appropriate direction with purpose, or we are changing and wavering along the way.

If Spleen Qi is strong, study, memorization, thinking and concentrating occur with ease. If impaired, thinking can be fuzzy, memory dull and concentration poor. On the other hand, extreme studying, concentrating, thinking and mental work for prolonged periods, all of which generally involve excessive sitting, causes Fluid metabolism to slow and Fluids to collect in the lymph, resulting in swollen abdomens and heavier hips. Quite often the propensity to think excessively is actually an escape from feeling our bodies and emotions, especially if we don't know how to resolve uncomfortable issues. Being lost in thought, absent-minded, preoccupied or forgetful can also indicate one is self-absorbed.

Energy is required for concentration and thinking, and in Western terms it might indicate having adequate blood sugar to nourish the brain. Both energy and blood sugar levels are determined by Spleen functions. When blood sugar is depleted from excessive thinking, it impairs the Spleen and sets up food cravings. This can be interpreted as the Spleen's signal to refuel and the body's desire for stimulation. These are generally satisfied by snacking on sugar, chips and other nutritionally deficient foods, which further depletes the Spleen and, coupled with the usual lack of exercise from mental preoccupation, causes weight gain. A vicious self-perpetuating cycle occurs, and over time makes it more difficult to concentrate, think and focus.

In the original Five Element system, the Earth element was in the center of the circle surrounded by all the other elements. Earth is the ground, the pivotal center, the source of life for all others. Thus, the Spleen has a similar place in the psyche. Ultimately, it represents our connection to the outside world, or Earth itself. Being in harmony with ourselves is being at home with ourselves, unobsessed, integrated and at ease.

When we are not self-fulfilled or integrated, we can become self-absorbed, consumed with nostalgia, obsessed or worried. All of these stress the Stomach and Spleen, resulting in gastric ulcers and poor digestion. Often such concerns are over those on whom we depend for nourishment. When we are obsessed with others or frequently crave sympathy and support or approval, we aren't nourishing ourselves. Instead the "I need" becomes foremost in our thoughts, and really reflects a lack of proper nourishment, Blood and Qi.

Feeling nourished is important on all levels for proper Spleen functioning. Metaphorically, nourishment means being able to take the world into ourselves, being able to assimilate our experiences and having adequate emotional, mental and spiritual as well as physical nourishment for all levels of our being. When we cannot "stomach," digest, or assimilate what happens in our lives, we often escape through nostalgia and reminiscing about past 'better' times. This is a way of compensating for a present lack of nourishment in our lives.

Further, feeling under-nourished on any level of being can actually reflect low self esteem. Insecurity and lack of self assertion result, creating more malnourishment because we can't act to get our needs met. We then get anxious and turn to sweets to feed the emptiness within. This only perpetuates the issue. The solution is to listen to one's body and emotions and act on them. This is coming home, to center, to the earthy part of ourselves and nourishing it. When we balance and center within, we are connected without.

LIVER

The Liver is the General for the body, able to conceive plans (strategies), put them into action and call the troops back for rest when needed. This requires vision, regulation and the ability to exert one's volition. Thus, the Liver's main function is to regulate the smooth flow and proper direction of Qi and Blood throughout the body. It also stores the Blood and regulates the amount of Blood circulated by the Heart.

Smoothes and Regulates the Flow of Qi and Blood

Just as a tree spreads out freely in all directions, so does the Liver (a part of the Wood Element) promote unrestrained and regular movement of Qi and Blood throughout the body. In its ideal state Qi flows, disperses and circulates freely, easily, softly and gently. When imbalanced its flow is irregular, goes in a wrong direction, or gets "stuck". This creates stagnation, pains which come and go or change location, rebellious Qi and similar symptoms.

There are three aspects to this function: regulating the smooth flow of Qi and Blood in regard to digestion, the emotions, and the secretion of bile. Keeping Qi and Blood moving normally is essential for normal bodily movements and nourishment. If impeded, pain and distention in the flanks, the breasts and the lower abdomen result, and moveable lumps without pain occur in the breasts and lower abdomen. Further, Qi is the driving force of Blood. If flowing irregularly or improperly, Blood becomes stagnant and leads to sharp pain in the breast and hypochondria, fixed masses in the abdomen and breasts, with localized pain and irregular menstruation, dysmenorrhea and amenorrhea.

The Liver function of ensuring the smooth and regular flow of Qi helps the Stomach to ripen and rot food and the Spleen to extract food essence. If imbalanced, Stomach Qi may ascend rather than descend, causing belching, sour regurgitation, nausea and vomiting, and the Spleen Qi may descend rather than ascend, resulting in chronic diarrhea and abdominal distension. Further, the proper discharge of bile is controlled by the regular flow of Liver Qi. This is necessary for good digestion of foods and fluids. If obstructed, a bitter taste in the mouth, vomiting of yellow fluid, belching, distention of the flanks, loss of appetite or jaundice may result.

The Liver harmonizes the emotions with the Mind by maintaining a happy state, sensitivity, ability to reason, an even disposition and a sense of being at ease. If Liver Qi is obstructed, it directly affects the emotions, causing emotional swings, irritability, frustration, and depression. It also causes distention in the breasts, a sensation of oppression in the chest, hypochondriac pain, belching, sighing, dullness, feeling of a "lump" in the throat and PMS symptoms. On the other hand, tension, stress, constantly going without rest, repressed anger and prolonged frustration in life can lead to Stagnant Liver Qi.

Furthermore, the Liver's function of regulating the smooth flow of Qi and Blood also acts to remove stagnant Qi from the Triple Warmer and to dredge the water passages. Impairment of this function may lead to edema.

Stores Blood

The Liver stores Blood and regulates its smooth flow, just as a General deploys his forces and gathers them back to rest. There are two aspects to this: Blood volume and menstruation. When the body rests, most Blood returns to the Liver to be stored and replenishes the person's energy. When the body is active, Blood is moved freely outward by the Liver to the necessary locations and in the needed amounts to nourish and moisten the muscles and tissues. If impaired, lack of Blood occurs, leading to improper nourishment where needed, causing dry eyes, blurred vision and fatigue. This function also directly affects our resistance to invading External factors, as proper distribution of Blood to the skin and muscles aids the body's ability to resist attacking Pernicious Influences. If impaired, the necessary nourishment of skin and muscles fails to occur, and the body becomes more susceptible to External invasions.

The storage and regulation of the smooth flow of Blood directly affects healthy menstruation. If this Liver function is flowing properly, menstruation is normal. If impaired, irregular menses, amenorrhea or dysmenorrhea may result. Additionally, if there is Heat in the Blood, excessive menstruation may occur. This function is extremely important in women's health. Most gynecological problems are due to a malfunction of Liver Qi or Blood. Liver Qi stagnation can lead to Blood stagnation, causing dysmenorrhea, clotting and PMS, whereas Deficient Liver Blood can lead to scanty menstruation or amenorrhea.

Overall, there is an interconnecting relationship between the Liver and Blood. If the Liver function is abnormal, it may affect the Blood, much like a dirty container spoiling its contents. If the Blood is abnormal, however, it may also affect the Liver function.

Controls Tendons and Ligaments

Liver Blood moistens and nourishes the tendons and ligaments. This ensures smooth movement of the joints and good muscle action. If Liver Blood is insufficient, malnutrition of the tendons results, causing numbness of the extremities, sluggishness of joint movements, spasms, muscle cramps, difficulty in bending or stretching, tetany and tremors of the hands and feet.

Manifests in the Nails

The finger and toe nails are the "excretion" of the Liver, and thus show its state and condition. If there is Damp Heat or congestion in the Liver, the nails are yellowish with ridges. If there is Deficiency of Liver Blood, the nails are brittle, soft, thin, pale, dry and break easily. When Liver Blood is plentiful, the nails are hard, pink and moist.

Opens to the Eyes

The Liver "opens" to the eyes, the sense organ connected with it. Strong Liver Blood moistens and nourishes the eyes to provide good vision. If it is Deficient, dryness, blurred vision, night blindness, myopia, color blindness and floaters result. If there is Heat in the Liver, the eyes may be bloodshot, red or swollen and feel painful or burning. If there is Internal Liver Wind, the eyeballs may turn upwards and move involuntarily. In addition, as tears are the Fluid of the eyes, excessive tearing or lack of tears both show an imbalance of the Liver.

While the Liver is the main Organ connected with the eyes, others help determine their state. Shen, or Spirit, is reflected in the brightness of the eyes while Kidney Essence helps nourish them. Heart Fire leads to painful red eyes and Kidney Yin Deficiency can cause failing eyesight and dryness of the eyes.

Houses the Ethereal Soul (Hun)

Hun are three in number representing Heaven, Earth and Man, the number for humanity. Thus, the Hun make us human, unique. Hun are the Soul aspect and Yang in nature. Hun and Po are intimately linked; Po are the physical aspect of the Soul and are inextricably linked with it, while Hun are the ethereal aspect of the Soul. Po develop with the body, whereas Hun enter the physical body upon birth. At death, Po dissolve with the body, returning to the earth, while Hun return to Heaven, the world of subtle and non-material energies. Hun are also the Soul counterpart of Shen, the Spirit, or the individualized expression of the Shen. Hun actually reside in the Blood, another close relationship between Shen and Hun.

The Hun are rooted and nourished by Liver Yin and Blood. They are most active at night during sleep and help determine the quality of sleep experienced. If Hun are not rooted in the Liver due to a Deficiency of Liver Blood or Yin, then they wander, resulting in insomnia, dream-disturbed sleep, a feeling of floating before sleep or a vague fear of falling asleep at night.

Hun are responsible for balancing and harmonizing the Seven Emotions. Just as the Liver regulates Qi, it regulates the Emotions in a general way. What Emotion is expereinced is not important, but the free circulation of it is, and the harmonization of the Emotions thus prevents them from being blocked or repressed. Further, if the Liver is imbalanced between Yin Blood and Yang Qi, the Seven Emotions become imbalanced and cause illness.

The Hun pertain to the giving of images: intuition, inspiration, psychic abilities, creativity, speculation, imagination and vision. The opening to the Liver and Hun, the eyes, is the "window of the Soul," giving us the vision to foresee and plan. Hun are that quality of the psyche which offers the capacity to plan our lives and find a sense of direction and purpose. When Liver Blood is Deficient, we can experience a lack of direction in life and an inability to plan or envision what to do.

The Hun are also linked to self-awareness and its interaction with the environment. It expresses as socially appropriate actions or awkward social behavior, and accounts for healthy boundaries between self and others. Assertiveness is needed to state our boundaries, whereas a challenging of our boundaries can provoke anger, the emotion of the Liver. Repeated over-stepping of our boundaries over time by others can lead to frustration, resentment or even rage. The opposite can happen as well: an inability to get angry or defend yourself when appropriate can indicate a Deficient Liver. Furthermore, our ability to respect other's boundaries is reflective of a healthy and flexible Liver.

The virtues of Hun embody being courageous, brave, fearless, decisive, resolute, indomitable, expressing righteous anger, benevolence and human kindness. It requires a higher vision to see both sides of a question and move beyond self-awareness and self-preservation in favor of another person or the greater good. Their expression supports a healthy and supple Liver. The vices of Hun include being excessively angry, impatient, agitated, annoyed, frustrated, timid, cowardly, conceited, self-centered, and boastful. They harm the Liver by creating Liver Qi Stagnation, Liver Fire or consuming Liver Yin.

Hun provides resoluteness, creativity, an indomitable spirit and drive, life direction and growth. It is the motivation to grow and express one's true self, and it helps integrate all aspects of our being and personality regardless of the obstacles. Like a tree, a healthy Hun can grow around obstacles to achieve its vision and plan.

When our growth, inspiration, spiritual achievements, drive or plans are blocked or thwarted in any way, be it from lack of self direction or from outside influences hindering us, we become frustrated, annoyed, irritable, angry and eventually depressed. This can also occur when we do not express or assert our true inner self, feelings and needs. Resentment, guilt and depression arise when our expression is blocked. Often we turn to stimulants such as chocolate, coffee, colas, sugar, alcohol, smoking or drugs to escape the frustration and depression.

In modern times we now turn to anti-depressants to enable us to handle our stressful and often non-fulfilling lives with better "spirits". Instead, they help us further disconnect from our true feelings, and thus our power and energy to live our true purpose of being. They only help us fit the mold of expectations we live with rather than deal with the real issues: suppressed anger, lack of expression, not living one's true purpose in life or not listening to our deep instincts or intuition and acting on them.

So, often these are the real reasons behind women's gynecological issues, PMS, and cancers of the breast, ovaries and uterus. Stagnation of Liver Qi has a major influence on these issues, and suppression of anger and self expression stagnate Liver Qi. For men it can take the form of headaches, heart trouble, prostate cancer and explosive aggressive personalities. Shouting, the sound of the Liver, can represent the need to express and assert oneself.

Chronic fatigue can also be a suppression of this energy. The Liver is intimately linked with our overall sense of well being. When imbalanced, not only our emotions become depressed, but so does our energy. Often it is a signal that we are ignoring our growth: what true purpose, goal, direction or mission in life is being suppressed? The more this Hun expression is repressed, the more our energy becomes stagnant and less available to us, resulting in fatigue and feeling poorly most of the time.

Learning to give expression to one's Hun is extremely important to the health of the body. Using tools such as counseling, group therapy, exercise, listening to one's inner guidance and direction, sharing one's true feelings with family and community, creative expression and rites of passage such as vision questing are all healthy outlets for one's true inner feelings. They free the body's energy and give direction and purpose to one's life.

Loathes Wind
Climatic Wind can stir up Internal Wind in the body and affect the Liver and its regulating and harmonizing functions. This Wind can be likened to the nervous system. It is not uncommon for Liver disharmonies of headaches and stiffness of the neck to appear after being exposed for a while to windy weather.

Emotion: Anger
When our boundaries are crossed or an improper action occurs, our appropriate reaction is righteous anger. On the other hand, Stagnant Liver Qi, Liver Fire, or Deficient Liver Blood or Yin can lead to Heat in the Liver. The emotional result is anger. Inappropriate anger, frequently feeling angry and a propensity to frustration and irritability reflect Liver imbalances.

Connected to the left side, hypochondria, lower abdomen and external genitals
Although physiologically situated on the right side, the Liver is related to the left side of the body. This is because in the original Five Element System, when the Spleen was placed in the middle of the other Elements, the Liver was placed on the left side of the cycle. Thus, any left-sided symptoms, such as pains on the left side of the head, abdomen and tongue, especially reflect the Liver, while the right side reflects the Lungs.

The Liver meridians cross through the hypochondria, lower abdomen, groin and external genitals. Thus, symptoms or diseases that arise in these areas, such as masses, tumors and lumps, should be treated with an overall analysis of signs of the Liver.

KIDNEYS

The Kidneys are the only double organ in the body and here are found Jing, Yin, Yang, and Ming Men or "Life Gate Fire." The Kidneys are the original basis for life, like the foundation of a house because they store Jing, Pre-Heaven Essence. This refined aspect represents our essential "inherited" constitutional strength and forms the material foundation for Yin and Yang. Thus, the Kidneys are considered to be the root of Yin and Yang for the entire body. Kidney Yin provides the material foundation for Kidney Yang, while Kidney Yang provides the Heat and movement for Kidney Yin. Because they have the same source, they are interdependent; a depletion of one creates a Deficiency in the other. Thus, when strengthening Kidney Yin, one also tonifies Kidney Yang and vice versa. Further, the Kidneys are the source of Water and Fire in the body because of Essence being part of the Water Element; Fire is included because the Kidneys house the Life Gate Fire (Ming Men) of the body.

Store Essence and Govern Birth, Growth, Development and Reproduction
Pre-Heaven Essence is inherited from both parents at the time of conception and determines the constitutional strength and resistance of

the body. Essence transforms into Source Qi, which forms the material basis on which the human body grows, develops and reproduces. It also includes the Original Yin and Original Yang energies, and thus is the source of Yin and Yang in the body.

Essence encompasses the processes of reproduction, development, growth, sexual potency, conception, pregnancy, menopause and ultimate physical decay of the organism. It is the basic constitutional strength, vitality and resistance of the body. As part of growth from childhood, it is responsible for the growth of bones, teeth, hair, brain and sexuality. In maturity, it controls reproductive function, fertility, conception and pregnancy. As Essence declines with age, there is a natural decline of sexuality, fertility, hair growth and coloring, skin smoothness and so forth. Thus, improper bone formation, retarded growth (mental or physical), delayed sexual maturation, premature aging, infertility, sterility or impotence are symptoms of Essence Deficiency.

Pre-Heaven Essence can never be increased but is supplemented by Post-Heaven Essence derived from the Grain Qi produced by the Spleen and enhanced by the prolonged practice of Qi Gong. Post-Heaven Essence is transported to the Organs to provide for their physiological activities. When plentiful, the excess is stored in the Kidneys for future needs. When insufficient, the Kidneys draw on their stored Essence to provide for the Organs' needs. If this continues, they even take the inherited Jing, causing a depletion of Essence in the body. Thus, the Yin and Yang of each of the Organs depend on the Yin and Yang of the Kidneys, and in the treatment of prolonged diseases and deficiencies, the Kidneys are always treated regardless of the Organs involved.

Rule Water

The Kidneys regulate water circulation and help maintain Fluid balance in the body. They are the foundation of water metabolism in the body, furthered by the Spleen's function of transforming and raising pure Fluids and the Lungs' function of circulating and lowering Fluids to the Lower Warmer. The Kidneys also receive Fluids from the Lungs, extract some to be excreted and some to be vaporized, which they return to moisten the Lungs.

The Kidneys regulate water through their Yang aspect. It acts as a gate, opening to excrete waste Fluids, and closing to retain needed water by any of the Organs. When functioning normally, it results in normal urination. When the gate is closing more than opening, scanty dark urine and edema occur. When opening more than closing, profuse and frequent pale urination result. Further, the Kidneys provide the Qi to the Bladder to store and transform urine. They also provide Yang to the Intestines to separate the pure fluids from the dirty ones. The Kidneys further supply Yang to the Spleen to assist its function of transforming and transporting Body Fluids.

Control and Promote Reception of Qi
While the Lungs rule respiration, the Kidneys aid in inhalation by receiving the inhaled air and holding it down. This enables Natural Air Qi to penetrate the body deeply. If the Kidneys are Deficient, they cannot hold the Qi down and it "rebels", causing breathlessness, chronic asthma, panting or difficult breathing. The involvement of the Kidneys in any of these conditions can be concluded by determining if inhaling is more difficult or causes more problems than exhaling.

Rule the Bones and Produce Marrow
Both these aspects are derived from Essence which produces marrow that, in turn, creates and supports the bones. Marrow in Chinese Medicine encompasses bones, bone marrow, the brain and spinal cord. Marrow in the bones nourishes them and determines their strength, development and repair. If insufficient in children it results in soft, maldeveloped and weak bones or late closure and softness of the fontanel. In adults, it can produce weak legs and knees, brittle bones or stiffness of the spine.

In the brain, Marrow nourishes mental vigor and power, concentration, thinking, sight and memory, especially short term. Thus, the Kidneys represent the power behind the senses. If depleted, poor memory and concentration, dizziness, dull thinking and poor sight occur. The teeth are considered the surplus of the bones, so they are also nourished by the Kidneys. Disorders such as slowly growing teeth, loose or early loss of teeth and unhealthy teeth in general signal insufficient Kidney Jing.

Manifest in the Hair
Because Essence can turn into Blood, and Blood nourishes the hair, the condition of the Kidneys reflects in the hair of the body, especially head hair. When Jing is sufficient, the head hair is moist, glossy, thick, plentiful and retains its original color. When Blood or Essence are Deficient, then withered, thin, prematurely grey and frequent loss of hair or baldness occur.

Open to the Ears
The opening of the Kidneys is through the ears, since their Qi goes through them. Thus, their condition reflects the state of the Kidneys.

If Deficient, hearing problems, including deafness, frequent or chronic earaches and tinnitus, may occur.

Control the Lower Orifices
   The lower orifices include the urethra, anus and spermatic duct in men. Kidney Qi regulates the Fluids in the Lower Warmer, and controls the opening and closing of these orifices. If malfunctioning, urinary incontinence, diarrhea, spontaneous defecation while eating, or spermatorrhea may occur.

Emotion: Fear
   Fear, fright and paranoia all reflect a Kidney imbalance. Excessive or prolonged exposure to any situations creating fear or fright injures the Kidneys. On the other hand, depleted Kidneys can cause one to be more easily frightened, paranoid or fearful.

The Gate of Vitality (Ming Men)
   The Gate of Vitality was originally considered to be the right Kidney, which provided the Yang functions in the body, while the left was both Yin and Yang. Later, and continuing to today, it was considered to lie between the two Kidneys with the function of replenishing the Yang of the Kidneys. It is considered to be the root of Original Qi, which is Essence in its Qi form, and the seat of Fire in the body which provides the necessary Heat to all the internal Organs to perform their functional activities. This has a special influence on warming the Stomach and Spleen to aid digestion, warming the Lower Warmer and Bladder to promote transformation and excretion of Fluids, and warming the sexual function and Uterus to aid fertility, puberty, menstruation and sexual performance. If impaired, poor digestion, diarrhea, tiredness, feeling cold, cold limbs, Dampness, edema, impotence, infertility, lowered sexual drive and leukorrhea can occur.

House Will Power (Zhi)
   Zhi is not a spirit but a quality. Like the Kidney functions, Zhi gives support to all the five psychic energies of the other Organs. Since Shen keep all these psychic energies in balance, Shen and Zhi are in constant communication with each other. Zhi is the source of Will, the motivating force to get things done and to accomplish it. It creates power, skill and ability. It is resolve and determination, the deep inner power and endurance of a person. Zhi gives purpose to life and sustains the person to achieve those purposes. The combination of Zhi and Shen here creates a magnetic personality, full of charisma, vigor and sexual vitality. Thus, if the Kidneys are strong, so will be our will power,

and our Mind will stay focused and accomplish the goals it sets. However, if the Kidneys are weak, Will power will be lacking and the Mind will be easily swayed and discouraged. When one has purpose (Yi) then one has Zhi. To hold firm to a purpose and give it continuity indicates Will (Zhi).The virtues of Zhi include being strong in will power and being resolute, determined, firm, enduring and wise. The vices are being excessively afraid, apprehensive, scared, paranoid, suspicious, distrustful, anxious, insecure, fearsome, worried, concerned, stubborn, and obstinate. Strong resolution and Will need vigor and stamina to carry out the intended choices. It enables us to stand our ground or advance in the face of any fear or apprehension. If weak, we are easily bullied and overwhelmed.

The emotions and vices of the Kidneys can all get in the way of our Will and determination to succeed on a particular path or at a particular goal. When we resolve to accomplish something despite the obstacles, however, we are summoning our vital energy and the best of our Kidneys. This gives strength of character and power of personality. If we are held back by our fears, suspicions and distrust, we feel inadequate and inferior.

On the other hand, fear often results from a sense of inadequacy and inferiority. This indicates a lack of self-trust. It is these types of feelings and a lack of Will which can lead to a victim complex in which everything that happens is due to someone else or some outside circumstance rather than to our own lack of determination or following through on our choices. When we feel inadequate, we can panic or get paranoid. Procrastination and avoidance are further signs of a weakened Will, and can occur from fear, paranoia, suspicion or mistrust blocking us. On the other hand, audacity, foolhardiness and acting superior to others can signal an unchecked Will. Often these behaviors are aggressive cover-ups for a true inner feeling of inadequacy or inferiority.

The Kidney connection to fear is seen very tangibly in the body: when we are afraid, we often feel the urgent need to urinate or cannot hold our urine at those times. Fear and Anger are opposite sides of the same coin, which demonstrates the connection between the Kidneys and Liver. When fear is experienced, the weakened Kidneys cannot nourish the Liver and anger often results. On the other hand, anger can be a cover-up for underlying fears not acknowledged or expressed.

The Kidneys are the channel of life and death. The ultimate fear is the fear of death. Facing one's mortality and looking past it to discover and accept your destiny is the transformation of fear into Wisdom, the Kidney's greatest virtue.

Kidneys Loathe Dryness

Being an Organ that rules Water metabolism, the Kidneys loathe being dry. Kidney Yin can be damaged by prolonged exposure to dry weather, Internal Dryness caused by profuse and continued loss of Fluids from sweating or diarrhea, Deficient Stomach Yin, or tobacco smoking.

YANG ORGANS (FU)

While the Yin Organs store, the Yang Organs transport. Overall, the Yang Organs have the functions of excreting, digesting, receiving, rotting, ripening, transforming, transporting and waste management. With all Organs, except the Gall Bladder, this has to do with the direct interaction with food, drink and their waste products. These Organs include the Small Intestine, Triple Warmer, Stomach, Large Intestine, Gall Bladder and Urinary Bladder.

The Stomach is the most important of the Yang Organs, as it is in charge of the digestion. Along with the Spleen, it is known as the "Root of Post Heaven Qi" because the essence of the digested food and fluids ultimately becomes the Qi and Blood of the body. Thus, proper digestion is essential for the production of Qi and Blood and the subsequent nourishment of all the Organs in the body.

SMALL INTESTINE

The Small Intestine is like an officer who receives and then transforms food and drink. It receives the partially decomposed food from the Stomach and further digests and absorbs it by separating the pure part from the waste. The useful part is sent to the Spleen, which in turn transports and distributes it all over the body. The waste is sent into the Large Intestine where it is further separated into pure and impure portions before being excreted as waste. The impure waters are sent to the Urinary Bladder to be excreted from the body. When functioning normally, this occurs with smooth urination and normal elimination of feces. When in disharmony, water is mixed with waste, leading to dysuria, loose stools, constipation, diarrhea, intestinal rumblings and abdominal distension and pain.

Psychologically, the Small Intestine receives things, eliminates those that are not relevant and makes those that are thrive. Thus it is said to influence mental clarity and judgment, demonstrating its link with the Heart and Mind. It also aids in decision making by giving the powers of discernment and clarity. This is different than the Gall Bladder's role in decision making, as the Small Intestine gives the ability to discriminate and differentiate what is relevant from what isn't (separating the pure from the impure), while the Gall Bladder lends the initiative and courage to make the decisions.

TRIPLE WARMER

The Triple Warmer, also known as the Three Heater or Triple Burner, is an "Organ" unique to Chinese Medicine. It is best understood as a large bowel containing all the Internal Organs, a functional passageway uniting all the organs into a complete system and harmonious whole. All the physiological functions of the Triple Warmer encompass the sum total of activities of the Yin and Yang Organs in the body.

The Triple Warmer includes three Warmers: the Upper Warmer embracing the body cavity above the diaphragm which houses the Heart, Lungs, Pericardium, throat and head; the Middle Warmer which extends from the diaphragm to the umbilicus and houses the Spleen, Stomach and Gall Bladder; and the Lower Warmer which comprises the lower abdominal area below the umbilicus housing the Liver, Kidney, Urinary Bladder, Intestines and Uterus. The Liver is included in the Lower Warmer because of its close relationship with the Kidney rather than its physiological placement in the body. Pathologically, diseases of the Upper, Middle or Lower Warmer involve a dysfunction of the Organs contained within that Warmer.

The functions of the Triple Warmer control all the transformations of Qi in the body, ensuring their coordination and unity. It orchestrates the production of all types of post-natal Qi and their free circualtion from the deepest to the most superficial levels. The Upper Warmer directs respiration and disperses Natural Air Qi to all the Organs, tissues, and skin. Thus, it is likened to a "mist" which diffuses Fluids throughout the body. The Middle Warmer transforms and transports foods and fluids and sends the extracted nourishment throughout the body. It is equated to a "foam" or "bubbling cauldron", referring to digestive churning and fomentations. The Lower Warmer is a "swamp", gutter or drainage ditch, where the clear is separated from the turbid, the clear being transported upwards and the turbid being sent downwards and discharged from the body.

The Triple Warmer is the passage through which water, food and Fluids are transported; it is the communication channel and controller of the entire circulation of Body Fluids. These functions result from the combined functions of the Lung, Spleen, Kidney, Stomach, Intestines and Bladder. According to the Chinese, Fire controls Water, implying that the Fire Element, or Triple Warmer, controls the water passages functionally encompassed by the above Organs.

STOMACH

The Stomach, along with the Spleen, is in charge of the storehouses and grainaries in the body. It is in charge of receiving ingested food and drink and then "ripening" and "rotting" it through its digestive process. It then sends the pure portion to the Spleen for its metabolic processes, and the impure part to the Small Intestine for further digestion. Thus, Stomach Qi descends while Spleen Qi ascends when it directs Grain Qi to the Lungs and Heart. The Stomach hates to be hot or dry and likes moisture, the opposite of the Spleen.

Diet is the main cause of Stomach disorders. Foods which are heating, drying, greasy, spicy, or cold upset the Stomach. Poor eating habits, such as working, driving or standing while eating, eating at irregular times or over- or under-eating also disrupt the Stomach functions. Excessive worry or thinking either stagnates or depletes Stomach Qi. A disturbance of Stomach functions results in poor appetite, indigestion, food retention, and distension and pain in the epigastric region. If Stomach Qi does not properly descend, belching, burping, hiccuping, nausea or vomiting occur.

LARGE INTESTINE

The main function of the Large Intestine is to receive the contents of the Small Intestine, absorb excessive water from it and discharge the waste from the body through the anus. Thus, the Large Intestine is the officer in charge of passing and removing things. Dysfunctions have to do with disturbances in bowel movements, including the substance and amount of feces and the times of defecation. The Large Intestine also represents our ability to let go of things, either material or emotional.

Disturbances of the Large Intestine can occur from External as well as Internal causes. It is possible for the Large Intestine to be directly invaded by Exterior Cold by passing through the exterior layers of the body. This occurs from prolonged exposure to cold weather or environments and from lack of proper clothing. Sitting on concrete can also cause Cold to enter.

Internally, excessive consumption of cold damp foods and drinks such as iced drinks, ice cream, popsicles, raw vegetables and certain fruits causes Coldness in the Large Intestine, while prolonged eating of greasy, fatty and spicy foods produces Dampness and Heat. Just as sadness, grief and worry affect the Lungs, they also can affect the Large Intestine and cause Qi stagnation.

GALL BLADDER

The Gall Bladder is unique among the Yang Organs in that it stores a clean Fluid, bile, rather than deal directly with food, drink and their waste products. It also doesn't open directly to the exterior through the mouth, rectum or urethra. Thus the Gall Bladder is also considered an extraordinary Organ. Bile is a bitter fluid produced by the surplus of Liver Qi and stored in the Gall Bladder. It is sent downwards to the Small Intestine to aid with digestion. Liver Qi ensures the smooth flow of bile when it is functioning normally. If Liver Qi is Stagnant, bile does not flow smoothly, resulting in poor digestion and absorption, loss of appetite, diarrhea, nausea and belching.

The Gall Bladder is the officer in charge of making decisions, of being exact, just and decisive. Since bile is a pure substance, it is said to give the ability to judge clearly and purely. This capacity to make decisions links well to the Liver's capacity to plan one's life. The Gall Bladder also gives initiative to make the decisions and the bravery, determination and courage to carry them out. Thus, timidity, indecisiveness, lack of drive or initiative to make decisions and being easily discouraged reflect a Gall Bladder disharmony.

URINARY BLADDER

The function of the Bladder is to receive, store and excrete urine. Through water metabolism, Fluids are dissipated all over the body to moisten it and then accumulate in the Kidneys. There urine is produced out of the final portions of turbid Fluids sent from the Lungs, Small Intestine and Large Intestine. It is then sent down to the Bladder where it is stored until excreted. This function requires Qi and Heat provided by Kidney Yang, and is referred to as the Bladder's function of Qi transformation. Thus, dysfunctions of the Bladder involve urinary problems. On an emotional level, the Bladder relates to jealousy, suspicion and holding grudges. It also reacts to anger over time, which can cause bladder infections as a result of being "pissed off".

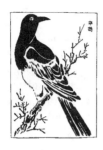

EIGHT

CAUSES OF DISEASE

Traditional Chinese Medicine regards balance as the basis of health. This includes balance between all aspects of life, including work and rest, emotions, diet, sexual activity and external factors associated with climate and weather. Apart from hereditary factors, sustaining a condition of imbalance is the cause of disease.

In TCM, there are several definitive causes of disease. These include environmental, emotional and lifestyle factors. Environmental causes are External, while stress-related emotional factors are Internal causes of disease. Further, causes that are neither External nor Internal include diet, lifestyle and miscellaneous issues such as parasites.

It is obvious that besides those diseases stemming from innate hereditary factors, External environmental causes or Internal stress-related emotional issues both cause lowered resistance and impaired immune function. Today, however, dietary indiscretions, such as the excessive intake of refined, processed and denatured foods and drinks consumed by the vast majority play a significant role in compromising the immune system and depressing organic processes that eventually lead to disease.

EXTERNAL CAUSES OF DISEASE

The External causes of disease are attributed to the Six Pernicious Influences. These are environmental factors which, when we are over-exposed to them, can invade the body and cause disease.

PERNICIOUS INFLUENCES

The body is a dynamic balance of Yin and Yang and its various subcategories, including the solid (Zang) and hollow (Fu) Organs. When this balance is upset, the body may not be able to adjust to environmental changes. Likewise, when normal environmental forces become excessive or occur unseasonably, and one's innate vital energy is weak, the body reacts adversely to external climatic and environmental conditions. This is described as the Six External Pernicious Influences, or adverse climatic

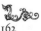

factors, invading the body and causing disease. These are: 1) Wind, 2) Cold, 3) Heat, 4) Dryness, 5) Dampness and 6) Summer Heat. The easiest way to understand the Pernicious Influences is to think of how their counterparts in weather manifest. For instance, wind moves things, changes direction, is fickle and alternates intensity. Water is damp and heavy, sinks to a lower level and slows things down. Coldness contracts and stops activity or movement. Heat circulates, activates and expands. Summer Heat is scorching hot, rising and dispersing. Dryness evaporates moisture. The correspondence between these weather patterns and how they manifest in the body is metaphorical, yet it demonstrates how the microcosm reflects the macrocosm.

Since the Pernicious Influences relate to the seasons, diseases caused by Wind relate to Spring, the Wood element and its two associated Organs, Liver and Gall Bladder. Thus TCM theory states that all Internal Wind emanates from the Liver and Gall Bladder. Heat and Summer-Heat relate to Summer and are associated with the Fire Element involving the Heart and circulation; and the Earth Element involving digestion, assimilation includes the Stomach and the Spleen. Traditional theory describes Fire as originating in the Heart. Dampness relates to both humidity and Winter weather, which stresses the Earth-Spleen function of assimilation and digestion. Dryness, associated with Autumn, can injure the Metal-Lung function. Finally, Cold is associated with Winter and can injure the Water-Kidney-Adrenals, which are the root of Yin and Yang for the entire body. The Six Pernicious Influences relate to the presence of these Influences in the dwelling and work place as well as outdoor climate.

The Six Pernicious Influences invade the body either singly or in combinations. A few examples of these include Wind-Cold type of rhinitis, Damp-Heat symptoms of itching and oozing skin rashes, or even a Wind-Cold-Damp arthralgia. Further, if the Six Pernicious Influences do not remain in balance, it is possible for them to transform and change. For instance, pathogenic Cold can transform into Heat after entering the body, Heat can change to Cold, and Summer Heat can consume Body Fluids (Yin) and transform into Dryness.

The Six Pernicious Influences usually invade the body through the skin, mouth, or nose, while Wind frequently invades through the back of the neck. Such illnesses are called External Pernicious Influences. They usually come on suddenly, with no warning, and accompany sudden acute illnesses. They are characterized by aversion toward the particular Influence (such as fear of heat or cold, dislike of wind or dampness), fever, chills, body aches and general tiredness.

When the Internal Organs are imbalanced, or there are pathological changes caused by bacteria, chemicals or other factors in the body, syndromes similar to Wind, Cold, Heat, Dampness, Dryness and Summer Heat may occur. Because their characteristics are similar, they are distinguished from the six External Influences and named Internal Pernicious Influences. In this case, the body manifests similar signs and symptoms to those of the External Influences with an important difference: the illness does not usually come on suddenly nor are there normally fever or chills. They are often related to chronic diseases. All Pernicious Influences, however, reflect their climatic conditions and are treated accordingly.

While the six Pernicious Influences can be the direct cause of disease, a Deficiency of Qi, Blood, Yang or Yin can often be the predisposing underlying cause. This, according to the theory of Root and Branch, designates the Pernicious Influence as the Branch and the underlying Deficiency as the Root. For example, when there is Blood or Yin Deficiency in the body (root), it can stir up Wind (branch); Qi or Yang Deficiency (root) makes the body more susceptible to Cold (branch); Yin Deficiency or Stagnation (root) can lead to Heat (branch); and Yin or Blood Deficiency (root) can result in Dryness (branch). Treatment of a Pernicious Influence must focus first on clearing the presenting branch symptom, if possible, and second on the underlying root cause. Formulas usually reflect this by using appropriate tonic herbs in smaller amounts than the primary herbs included for branch symptoms.

The following descriptions include the specific signs and symptoms of how each Influence manifests. Both External and Internal aspects are discussed. Three or more signs under a given category need to manifest to indicate the presence of that Influence. When two or more Pernicious Influences appear together, all the Influences involved are treated.

WIND
Wind tends to rise, disperse, move upward and outward, and because of its movement, is considered a Yang evil. Thus, pathogenic Wind usually attacks the upper and outer Yang parts of the body first, such as the head and face, and the skin and muscle, resulting in such symptoms as headache, dizziness, spasms, rigidity of the muscles and deviation of the eye and mouth. It also brings on sudden colds with headache, stuffy nose, chills and fever. At other times it causes a stiff or rigid neck and shoulders. Often people will remember being exposed to a draft before these symtoms began.

The essence of Wind is movement and change. It tends to migrate to various parts of the body, come and go, change direction and location, alternate in intensity of symptoms or periodically disappear altogether. Diseases of Wind usually occur rapidly and are capricious, variable and tend to wander. Symptoms of pathogenic Internal Wind are characterized by vibration and involuntary movement, such as tremors, convulsions and vertigo. These signs can be observed in nature by watching the wind in trees and leaves, on water or with clouds.

Wind, a mechanism that involves a complex neurological reaction and the proliferation of Pathogenic Influences, is the most commonly involved of the Six Influences. As such, it combines readily with other Influences to form combinations such as Wind-Cold, Wind-Heat, Wind-Dryness and Wind-Damp. While it is associated with the season of spring, Wind can occur during any season. External Wind symptoms occur as a result of the Excess of pathogenic Wind. The resulting chills and fever reflect the conflict between External Influences and the body's innate integrity, or what is called **Righteous Qi**. Exposure to high winds, living in windy environments and insufficient clothing are precipitating causes for an External Wind Influence.

Internal Wind is usually caused by a functional derangement of the Liver, yet it can arise from a Deficiency of Blood or Liver or Kidney Yin, or from a persistently high fever which consumes Body Fluids. In fact, any Deficiency can injure the nervous system and give rise to Interior Wind. It can also be caused by excessive eating of hot-natured, spicy, greasy, fatty and fried foods, excessive activity, "burning the candle at both ends", insufficient rest and stress.

Qualities of Wind:
comes and goes, quickly and abruptly
signs change locations
various signs appear in succession
tendency toward movement and change
itching
spasms
moving pains
twitching
skin eruptions that change locations; urticaria
Pulse: External: floating; Internal: bowstring, tense
Tongue: External: thin white coat, may appear normal
Internal: trembles, deviated to the side, can appear normal

External Wind: Wind-Cold Symptoms
slight fever
aversion to wind and cold
body aches

headache
stronger chills
cough, stuffed nose
sudden onset
itchy or slight sore throat
Pulse: floating and tense
Tongue: thin, white coating

Formula
Schizonepeta and Ledebouriella Combination (Jing fang bai du san)
Actions:
a) Warming Diaphoretic, clears Wind Cold
b) Antipyretic, anti-inflammatory, lowers fevers and clears Heat
c) Diuretic, clears Dampness

External Wind: Wind-Heat Symptoms:
high fever, sudden onset
slight chills
headache
slight aversion to cold
fear of wind
sweating
swollen sore throat
cough with yellow sputum
stuffed nose
Pulse: floating and rapid
Tongue: pale red tongue tip; white or yellow tinged coating

Formulas
1. **Lonicera and Forsythia Combination** (Yin qiao san)
Actions:
a) Diaphoretic, disperses External Wind-Heat
b) Alterative, antibiotic and antiviral, clears Internal Heat and relieves toxicity

2. **Morus and Chrysanthemum Combination** (Sang ju yin)
Actions:
a) Cooling diaphoretic
b) Dispels Wind Heat
c) Antitussive, relieves cough

Internal Wind Symptoms:
convulsions
upward turning of eyeballs
rigidity and pain of neck and head
numbness of limbs
paralysis

dizziness
tremors
apoplexy
vertigo
hemiplegia
tetany
muscle spasms, twitching
deviation of eyes and mouth
urticaria, itching skin eruptions that change locations
Pulse: bowstring, tense
Tongue: trembles, deviated to side, can appear normal

Formulas

1. **Bupleurum Formula** (Yi gan san)
Actions:
a) Antispasmodic, Calms Liver Wind
b) Tonifies Liver Blood and Qi

2. **Gastrodia and Uncaria Combination**
(Tian ma gou teng yin)
Actions:
a) anti-hypertensive
b) clears Heat

3. **Antelope Horn and Uncaria Combination** (Ling yang gou teng tang)
Actions: a) antispasmodic and anti-hypertensive, calms endogenous Liver Wind.
b) eliminates Heat

COLD

Cold, a Yin phenomenon, causes feelings of coldness and a slowing of circulation and all metabolic functions. There is a tendency towards cold extremities, to wear more clothes regardless of the weather, and in general, to contract and hunch over to minimize body surface and maintain inner warmth. Upon examination, the body, or parts of it, feel cold to the touch and have a generally pale appearance, which in some cases can also be an indication of Deficient Blood. Any bodily secretions are clear or white in color, such as clear or white mucus, sputum, vomit, urine, diarrhea or vaginal discharges. Cold is aggravated during colder climates and the season of Winter. It can, however, become an issue any time of year with exposure to Cold.

Just as water turns to ice when exposed to coldness, Cold in the body constricts, contracts and congeals. This causes physical obstructions, blocking the flow of Qi and Blood in the body and often causing various kinds of pain, contraction, spasm, cramps and stiffness. Usually when symptoms favorably respond to the application of Heat, the cause of the symptom is Cold. When Cold stays in the skin and muscles, it contracts the pores and stagnates the immune system's defensive energy (Wei Qi). When this occurs, External Cold invades, resulting in fever, strong chills, a lack of sweating, body aches and an aversion to cold. If Cold remains in the muscles and channels, numbness, rigidity and coldness can occur.

Being Yin in nature, Cold in excess can injure the body's Yang Qi and cause symptoms of Deficient Yang. External Cold comes on quickly and impairs the defensive Yang of the body, for which teas and formulas containing warm spicy herbs such as cinnamon twigs (Ramulus cinnamomi) fresh ginger and black or red peppers are specifically indicated. When this occurs, chills are more pronounced than fever and there is little, if any, sweating. Cold Evil can also invade and injure the Yang-function of the Organs. For example, Cold Evil can attack the Intestines and Stomach, causing a stomach ache and watery diarrhea containing undigested food or vomiting of water.

Cold can also arise Internally from an overall lowering of metabolism or insufficiency of Yang. Internal Cold is usually chronic and is characterized by coldness, slowness and hypo-activity of the Organs and metabolism. Yang then may be unable to warm and nourish the limbs, digest food or assimilate and transport Fluids and nutrients. Internal Cold is most often related to the Kidney/Adrenals since they are the root of the body's Yin and Yang, and the throne of the Life Gate Fire (*Ming Men*). If there is Internal Coldness, the body becomes more susceptible to External Cold invading the body.

Causes of Cold include improper dressing for the season or environment, including seasonal changes; living in cold places; excess eating of foods and drinks with a cold temperature, cold energy or eliminating nature, such as raw foods, fruits, juices, ice cream, popsicles and iced drinks; inactivity; and lack of exercise.

Qualities of Cold:
feeling of coldness
fear of cold
pale, frigid appearance
desire for more clothes, warm foods, drinks and climate
hypo-functioning of organs and slowed metabolism
tendency toward stagnation and contraction
clear or white discharges and secretions
sleeps curled up, hunched body posture
lack of circulation of Qi and Blood

listlessness, slowness
little odor of body or discharges
Pulse: slow, deep
Tongue: pale, moist

External Cold Symptoms:
slight or low grade fever
strong chills
lack of sweating
no thirst
headache
sudden onset
fear of cold and feeling of coldness
body aches
desire for lots of clothes or covers
nasal obstruction
Pulse: floating and tense
Tongue: white coating

Formulas
1. **EPHEDRA DECOCTION** (Ma huang tang)
Actions:
a) Warm stimulating diaphoretic
b) Dispels External Wind Cold
c) Anti-asthmatic
d) For a strong body type

2. **CINNAMON COMBINATION** (Gui zhi tang)
Actions:
a) Warming diaphoretic
b) Tonic, regulating the constructive or nutrient energy
(Ying) and the Wei (immune system)
c) For a weaker body type

3. **PUERARIA COMBINATION** (Ge gen tang)
Actions:
a) Diaphoretic, treats External Wind, Cold and Dampness
b) Antispasmodic, relieves stiffness and pain of the shoulders
and neck
c) For an average body type

Internal Cold Symptoms:
feeling of coldness
aversion to cold
cold limbs
listlessness
sleeps alot

underactivity
frigid appearance
watery stools or stools containing undigested food
craving warm food and drinks
desire for more clothes and covers
pale complexion
pain in the joints and flesh
lack of circulation of Qi and Blood
clear or white discharges (urine, vaginal, mucus, sputum)
Pulse: slow (slower than 60 BPM), deep
Tongue: pale, wet; white creamy coating

Formulas
1. **Aconite, Ginger and Licorice Combination** (Si ni tang)
Actions:
a) Internal warming Yang stimulant

2. **Ephedra and Asarum Combination** (Ma huang fu zi xi xin tang)
Actions:
a) Stimulating and warming diaphoretic; warms and disperses the surface.
b) Internally warming

HEAT (OR FIRE)

Heat and Fire are Yang phenomena, and differ only according to degree, with Fire being the more severe. Furthermore, Heat refers to an External Pernicious Influence while Fire designates an Internal Pernicious Influence. Non-pathogenic heat emanates from the Life Gate (*Ming Men*) of the Kidney-Adrenals, and when in its proper place, it is regarded as the "Clear Yang," which is the normal Yang energy that imbues all Internal Organs with vital warmth, Qi and movement. It is also a part of the External immune system or Wei Qi. Its nature is to rise and circulate, imparting immunological and digestive function, vital warmth and movement throughout the body. The innate vitality and warmth of each Organ is designated as "Ministerial Fire".

Internal Heat as part of Yang Qi is not to be confused with the Pernicious Influence that occurs as a result of External Heat strongly reacting with our innate Yang. Thus, Heat is aggravated in hot or warm climates and during summer, though it appears year round. Being Yang, its qualities are hot, reactive and associated with stagnation. In this way, stagnation caused by Coldness can change to Heat, but when the body's resources are vanquished, it can change back to Coldness again.

The Heat Pernicious Influence causes a person to feel hot, to wear fewer clothes and covers, to crave cold foods and drinks and to be restless and re-active, even to the point of aggressiveness. There is usually thirst, possible burning sensations, strong odors, and sticky or thick excretions and secretions that are yellow, red or blood-tinged. Heat can dry out Bodily Fluids over time and cause Dryness, such as unusual thirst, dry stools, dryness of the throat and mouth or scanty urination. Heat tends to burn and scorch, causing symptoms such as high fever, flushed face and constipation. Just as a physical fire flares up and rises, so does Heat in the body. With the ascension of toxic, Unclear Yang, Heat symptoms often appear on the head and face, resulting in painful, swollen and bleeding gums, swollen, red and painful eyes and a red neck and face. Fire also tends to cause boils, sores and red skin eruptions with local redness, swelling, heat, pain and even suppuration and ulceration. In general, Heat signs are often associated with inflammation or fever.

Pathogenic Heat may accelerate the flow of blood and force it to go astray, causing various bleeding symptoms such as nosebleed, hemorrhage, ecchymosis, and blood in the urine, stool, vomit or mucus from the lungs. Fire can also stir up Liver Wind, causing a reckless movement in the Blood that can affect the Spirit, or Shen. This results in emotional upset and insomnia in mild cases or mania and restlessness, unconsciousness, confused speech or delirium in severe cases.

External Heat invades directly, or is the product of any of the other invading Pernicious Influences transforming into Heat. Internal Fire arises from dysfunction of the Internal Organs, an Excess of Yang or Deficiency of Yin in the body, or from extreme emotional swings. It usually appears as Liver, Stomach or Heart Fire. Over a long time Heat can consume the Body Fluids, or Yin, and cause Deficiency Heat signs such as night sweats, insomnia, malar flush and a burning sensation in the palms, soles and over the heart. Heat can be caused by overactivity, living in or being exposed to hot environments, fried foods, alcohol, coffee, and hot-natured foods such as red meats, and many recreational drugs.

Qualities of Heat:
dislike or fear of heat
ruddy, hot appearance
thirst
craves cold
fast active
irritability
restlessness

prefers cool climate
blood in any discharges
strong body odors
tendency to rise, expand
desire for fewer clothes, covers
yellow, red excretions and secretions that are sticky and hot feeling
Pulse: rapid
Tongue: red

External Heat Symptoms:
sudden onset, acute
sweating
high fever
slight chills
flushed red face
red eyes
headache
dark or red urine
sore, swollen throat
desire for cold
irritability
red skin eruptions, rashes
aversion to heat
nervous, fidgeting or restless
dry mouth
scanty urination
cough with yellow mucus
wants few clothes, covers
few body aches
great thirst with a desire for cold drinks
boils, carbuncles
constipation or diarrhea with foul-smelling yellow stools
Pulse: rapid, full, floating
Tongue: red; dry or sticky yellow coating

In severe cases there may be:
loss of consciousness
delirium
reckless behavior
epistaxis
hematemesis
confused speech
hematuria
coma

Formula
Lonicera and Forsythia Combination (Yin qiao san)
Actions:
a) Diaphoretic, disperses External Wind-Heat
b) Alterative, antibiotic and antiviral, clears internal heat and
relieves toxicity

Internal Heat Symptoms:
quick, agitated movement
delirium
red eyes and face
irritability
thirst
talkative, extroverted manner
hot body or limbs
desire for cold foods and drinks
constipation
dark urine; can be scanty
Pulse: rapid
Tongue: red; yellow coat

Formulas

1. **Coptis and Scutellaria Combination** (Huang lian jie du tang)
Actions:
a) Detoxifies, anti-inflammatory, alterative, antibiotic

2. **Coptis, Scute and Pueraria Combination** (Ge gen huang qin huang lian tang)
Actions:
a) Clears both External and Internal acute inflammations
b) Relieves muscle aches of the neck

3. **White Tiger Decoction** (Bai hu tang)
Actions:
a) To eliminate Heat in the Qi (secondary defense) system and the Yang Ming channel
b) To promote the secretion of Body Fluids

Deficiency Heat Symptoms:
superficial flushed cheeks, nose
insomnia
night sweats
irritability
sore or dry throat (not extreme pain)
low grade fever
fidgeting, restlessness
dry cough with a little sputum
scanty, reddish urine
feverish sensation in the palms, soles and heart area
Pulse: thready, rapid
Tongue: red; denuded or with little coating

Formula

**Anemarrhena, Phellodendron and Rehmannia
Combination (Zhi bai di huang wan): Rehmannia Six
Combination**(Liu wei di huang wan) with 6-9 grams each of
Anemarrhena (Zhi Mu) and Phellodendron (Huang Bai).

Action:
a) Tonify Yin and clear Deficiency Heat
Liver Fire Symptoms:
headache, migraine
red eyes
bitter taste in the mouth
burning pain in the costal region
yellow urine
flushed face
irritability
dry throat
constipation
restlessness
Pulse: rapid
Tongue: red; sides may be redder, yellow coat

Formula

Dang Gui, Gentiana and Aloe (Dang gui long hui wan)
Action:
a) Purges Fire from the Liver and Gallbladder
Stomach Fire Symptoms:
burning epigastric pain
acid regurgitation
foul breath
ulcers
constipation
stomach distress
painful or bleeding gums
thirst with desire for cold drinks
hunger not alleviated by eating large amounts of food
Pulse: rapid, slippery
Tongue: red; creamy, yellow coat, especially in central region

Formula

Clear the Stomach Powder (Qing wei san)
Action:
a) Clears Heat from the Stomach.
Heart Fire Symptoms:
tongue and mouth ulcers
insomnia
painful, burning urination
fidgeting
thirst

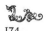

restlessness
Pulse: rapid
Tongue: red tip; yellow coating

Formula
Coptis and Rhubarb Combination (San huang xie xin tang)
Actions:
a) Clears Heart Fire
b) Allays nervousness

DRYNESS

Since Autumn is characterized by low humidity, diseases aggravated by the Dry Pernicious Influence can occur. External Dryness characterized by dehydration can be caused by either Heat or internally by Deficiency of Blood or Yin. Dryness caused by dehydration and Heat causes hot feelings and a flushed, red appearance. Warm-Dryness usually occurs in the heat of late summer and early Autumn. Cool-Dryness usually occurs during late Autumn with the onset of pathogenic Cold of approaching Winter. Dryness is a Yang phenomenon.

Dryness usually invades through the mouth and nose, afflicting the Defensive Qi and the Lungs. If the Lungs, considered a sensitive organ, are lacking sufficient Yin moisture, they become vulnerable to the attack of Dryness. When this occurs there may be dryness of the mouth, nose and throat, dry cough with little phlegm, asthma and chest discomfort. When Dryness invades it impairs body fluids, causing dryness in the mouth, nose and throat with thirst, dry skin and constipation.

Dryness can also arise internally. This is usually caused by a Deficiency of Blood or Yin, the exhaustion of Essence, a loss of blood, excessive vomiting, diarrhea or bleeding, chronic diseases or those with a long disease course, or the consumption of body fluid from febrile diseases. Excessive consumption of spicy, hot-natured foods, over-exposure to dry weather, and not drinking enough fluid can also lead to Dryness.

Qualities of Dryness:
dry, rough, chapped or cracked skin
dry throat, nose, mouth, lips
dry cough with little phlegm
dry, lifeless hair
unusual thirst, dehydration
dry stools
Pulse: thready, hesitant
Tongue: dry with no saliva

External Dryness: Cold-Dryness Symptoms:
fever
headache
aversion to cold
dry skin
no sweating
dry mouth and throat
cough with scanty or no sputum
Pulse: thready, hesitant
Tongue: dry with a white, thin and dry coat

Formula
Apricot Seed and Perilla Formula (Xing su san)
Actions:
a) Diaphoretic
b) Clears Wind-Cold
c) Soothes the Lung and relieves cough

External Dryness: Heat-Dryness Symptoms:
fever
mild chills
headache
thirst
anxiety
a decreased amount of sweat
sore, swollen throat
dry skin, nose and throat
dry cough or cough with scanty, sticky bloody sputum
Pulse: thin (Dryness from Blood or Yin Deficiency), or minute, choppy-
  rapid (Dryness caused by Heat)
Tongue: red tipped or red-edged

Formula
Eriobotrya and Ophiopogon Combination (Qing zao jiu
fei tang)
Actions:
a) Moistens the Lung and treats Dryness
b) Tonifies Qi
c) Lubricates, cools and nourishes Essence of the Lung

Internal Dryness Symptoms:
excessive thirst
dry, rough skin
constipation
dry, lifeless hair
Pulse: thready, hesitant
Tongue: dry with no saliva

Formula
Ophiopogon and Trichosanthes Combination
(Mai men dong yin si)
Actions:
a) Expectorant
b) Tonifies the Yin of the Lung

DAMPNESS

Dampness, a Yin phenomenon, is like heavy rains, snow or a large body of water. It is wet, heavy and slow and causes a sinking sensation with bodily heaviness. Therefore, people with Dampness usually feel sluggish, heavy, dull and stagnant. As a result, they have an expressed dislike for damp environments and seasons. Symptoms of Cold Dampness are aggravated in the colder climates and seasons such as winter, while Hot Dampness (usually termed Damp Heat) is aggravated in seasons and climates associated with high levels of humidity. Similar to the previous Pernicious Influences that are aggravated by exposure, Dampness can show an aggravation with any inordinate exposure to damp conditions during any season or climate or in any environment.

In the body, Dampness appears with excretions and secretions that are turbid, sluggish, sinking, viscous and stagnant as well as copious, slimy, cloudy or sticky. These may be found as eye secretions, diarrhea or mucus in the stool with pus and blood, turbid urine, excessive leukorrhea and oozing, purulent skin eruptions. As Dampness sinks, its symptoms are often found in the lower part of the body. Its heaviness is often felt as lassitude, a sluggish, stuffy and heavy sensation of the body, or a heavy head, as if a tight band surrounds it.

There can also be edema, abdominal distention and chest fullness which, if unattended, can lead to congestive heart failure and symptoms that obstruct the flow of Qi such as nausea, vomiting and/or palpitations. If there is Dampness in the joints, they feel heavy, ache, are stiff or continually painful or sore, as in arthralgia or arthritis. Damp conditions require time and patience to treat as well as a corresponding Dampness-removing diet in order to have any lasting effect. This necessitates the elimination of 'sodden' foods such as high fat, oils, sugar, dairy and flour products, and a simple diet is recommended based on low or non-fat foods including whole grains, beans and vegetables.

The Damp Pernicious Influence obstructs the activities of Qi and impairs Yang. When pathogenic Dampness attacks, it leads to an imbalance of the transforming, ascending and descending functions of Yin and Yang. For examples: retention of Dampness in the epigastrium can lead to distress in the chest; Dampness blocking the Spleen and Stomach can cause anorexia, epigastric distress, nausea, vomiting and loose stool; Spleen Yang may be disturbed resulting in retention of Dampness in the body evidenced by diarrhea, edema and difficult urination.

Besides External Dampness, Internal Dampness is also a possibility. This is caused by a dysfunction of the Spleen's transporting and transforming functions, with impairment of Fluid metabolism and resultant fluid retention. Both External and Internal Dampness can influence each other and are interdependent. External Dampness is more immediately the result of environmental and dietary stresses, but can become chronic and eventually develop into Internal Dampness. Either of them frequently appear with Cold or Heat, which is differentiated as Damp Cold or Damp Heat.

External Damp Evil is aggravated by exposure to damp weather and damp environments. As stated, Internal Dampness is aggravated by the excess use of sodden foods such as dairy, flour products, pasta, oils, fruits, raw foods, juices, tofu, soy milk, cold foods and drinks, dairy, greasy foods, coffee, alcohol and sugar.

Over time, Internal Dampness can collect and stagnate, condensing into Phlegm. This can stress the Yang functions of the Spleen and Kidneys and accumulate in the mucus membranes of the body, causing diseases associated with Damp congestion in the Lungs and reproductive organs as a result of impaired movement of Water and Fluids (lymph) throughout the body.

Phlegm, being heavier than common metabolic Dampness, is less Fluidic and easily causes obstruction in the form of lumps, nodules, cysts or tumors. Obstruction of Phlegm in the Lungs results in chronic cough with heavy expectoration; in the Heart it results in disturbed Spirit (Shen) with muddled thoughts, stupor, coma, erratic behavior or madness. Phlegm obstruction in the Meridians causes numbness, paralysis as well as soft mobile nodules, cysts and tumors.

There are still further complications that can arise as a result of Dampness. It is usually associated with Deficient Spleen Yang and eventually Deficient Kidney Yang. If Dampness overwhelms the Spleen's transporting and transforming power, the original nutritive Qi of the Spleen becomes weakened, and it blocks the ascendancy of the Clear Yang of the Kidney. Then turbid Dampness accumulates in the Lower Warmer and changes to Heat, which eventually burns out and depletes the Yin.

External Cold Damp diseases with mucus can be treated with warm spicy acrid herbs such as fresh ginger, cinnamon twigs and various peppers. External Hot Damp conditions are treated with cool spicy herbs such as mint, basil, coriander and chrysanthemum flowers. Internal Cold Damp conditions are treated with Warm or Hot Internal spicy substances such as cinnamon bark, prepared aconite, cloves and dried ginger. Internal Warm Dampness conditions are treated with herbs that relieve Damp Heat and generally have cholagogue properties, such as gentian root, Chinese scutellaria root, coptis or Western herbs such as barberry root and golden seal.

In general, chronic diseases caused by Dampness are among the most difficult diseases to cure because of their stubborn congested nature.

Qualities of Dampness:
wet
viscous
turbid
heaviness
sluggish
lingering
pus
oozing
tends to sink, obstruct
sweetish taste in mouth
turbid urine
damp, oozing skin eruptions
aching in the limbs or entire body
loose stool or stool with mucus, pus and blood
copious discharges which are cloudy, turbid or sticky
no desire to drink, even if there is thirst
Pulse: slippery
Tongue: wet, slimy, greasy coating

External Dampness Symptoms:
fever not relieved by sweating
heavy vaginal discharge
cloudy urine
constricted feeling in the chest
aversion to cold
oozing skin eruptions
heavy diarrhea
no desire to drink
fullness of chest or abdomen
dribbling or incomplete urination or defecation
heaviness and soreness of body and head
excretions and secretions that are copious, turbid, cloudy or sticky
Pulse: soft, floating
Tongue: slippery coating

Formula
Magnolia and Hoelen Combination (Wei ling tang)
Actions:
a) Eliminates Dampness of the Spleen (relieves bloating)
b) Carminative; restores the function of the Stomach and assists digestion.

Dampness in the Joints (Bi Syndrome) Symptoms:
arthralgia or arthritis with fixed pain
heaviness or achiness in the joints or limbs
numbness of the muscles and skin

Formula
Clematis and Stephania Combination (Shu jing huo xue tang) (Decoction to Dredge the Meridians & Vitalize Blood)
Actions:
a) Opens circulation of the channels and collaterals, stimulates blood circulation, removes Blood stagnation.
b) Antirheumatic, removes Damp stagnation.

Internal Dampness Symptoms:
heavy-headedness
poor appetite
diarrhea or loose stool
abdominal edema
abdominal distention
lassitude
turbid urine
nausea
indigestion
edema
vomiting
heavy vaginal discharge
feeling of oppression in the chest
Pulse: soft, thready; can be slippery
Tongue: creamy coating

Formula
Citrus and Pinellia Combination (Er chen tang)
Actions:
a) Removes Dampness, resolves Phlegm
b) Regulates Spleen and Stomach

Phlegm Symptoms:
lumps
nodules
tumors
delirium

numbness in limbs
thick greasy secretions
tremors
tends to obstruct
Pulse: slippery
Tongue: greasy, thick coating

Phlegm in Lungs Symptoms:
asthma
cough with heavy expectoration of mucus

Formula
Minor Blue Dragon Combination (Xiao qing long tang)
Actions:
a) Dries Damp and dispels Phlegm
b) Regulates Qi and harmonizes the middle warmer
(Stomach and Spleen).

Phlegm in Heart Symptoms:
chaotic or erratic behavior
rattle in throat
muddled thought
madness
stupor
coma

Formula
Bamboo and Poria Combination (Wen dan tang)
(Gall Bladder Warming Decoction)
Actions:
a) It is expectorant; eliminates white, frothy mucus
b) Sedative for restlessness, insomnia, anxiety and nausea

Phlegm in Meridians Symptoms:
numbness
paralysis
soft, mobile tumors, nodules or swellings

Formula
Cinnamon and Poria Combination (Gui zhi fu ling wan)
Actions:
a) Promotes Blood and lymphatic circulation, thus removing
stagnant Blood.
b) Softens and resolves hard lumps such as cysts and fibroids.

SUMMER HEAT

Summer heat is another form of Fire, but is more extreme and occurs in the summer. It is purely an External Pernicious Influence and results from exposure to extreme Heat. In the West it is known as heat stroke. Summer Heat is Yang in nature and is scorching hot. It is acute and tends to rise and disperse. As heat stroke it causes high fever, dizziness and nausea. With overexposure to Summer Heat, it causes profuse perspiration and then exhausts Qi and Body Fluids. It is usually accompanied by Dampness since it can be caused by hot-humid climates or Heat reacting to the body's Damp-Heat environment. In this case, both the Heat and Dampness must be treated.

Summer Heat Symptoms:
dizziness
nausea
extreme thirst
lassitude
sudden fainting
heavy sweating
exhaustion
coma
sudden, very high fever
upset, flushed face
shortness of breath
loss of consciousness
delirium
depletion of fluids
Pulse: full and rapid, or weak and rapid
Tongue: thin, white and creamy coating

Formula
Lotus Stem and Ginseng Combination (Qing shu yi qi tang)
Actions:
a) Clears Summer-Heat and nourishes the Qi
b) Demulcent and cooling; replenishes Body Fluids

Summer Heat With Dampness Symptoms:
lassitude of the limbs
chest distress
poor appetite
feeling of suffocation
low-grade fever rising in the afternoon
nausea, vomiting
sticky, loose stool
general lassitude
Pulse: thready
Tongue: creamy coating

Formula
Agastache Formula (Huo xiang zheng qi san)
Actions:
a) Diuretic, carminative, clears Damp turbidity from the
Spleen and Stomach; for Summer Heat with Dampness
b) Diaphoretic for External conditions

THE SEVEN EMOTIONS

In contrast to contemporary Western scientific medicine, Traditional
Chinese Medicine has for millennia recognized an implicit link between
the emotions and physical health. Besides generally affecting hormonal
secretions, the emotions can promote or impair the secretion of various
neural-transmitter hormones. These include acetylcholine which regulates
brain functions like memory and intellectual abilities; catecholamines
which are involved with mood, attention ability and the control of
bodily movements; and serotonin which is produced from tryptophan
and helps to regulate mood, carbohydrate metabolism, hypothalmic
releasing hormones, (implicated in alcoholism and obsessive-compulsive
disorders), and endorphins that regulate our susceptibility and response
to pain and pleasure.

Through a variety of psychological therapeutic modalities, some
people have experienced complete remission from life-threatening chronic
diseases such as AIDS, cancer and various other autoimmune diseases.
More is being learned regarding the relationship of various nutrients to
the emotions. One example is how a deficiency of niacin (vitamin B3)
can be coincidental with chronic violent behavior and schizophrenia.

Increasingly, anti-depressant drugs are prescribed for chronic
depression and other psychological disorders. The problem is that seldom
is the underlying physiological or psychological cause adequately
addressed, and there may be long term side effects that have not as yet
been recognized.

Be that as it may, emotional stress continues to be the primary
cause of disease, and true healing can only occur when the individual is
guided to make those changes necessary to achieve body-mind wholeness.
This is a place where philosophy plays an important role, since the lack
of inherent values is often at the root of many personal problems.

An essential aspect of a healer's work is to assist their patients
through various life and emotional changes. This can include offering
guidance and direction to terminate an unsatisfying job, changing a
stressful relationship that may be abusive and psychologically harmful,
encouraging appropriate self-assertion of true inner needs that will assist

further emotional growth, and reminding the patient to make time for inspiration and spiritual achievements. There may be an underlying problem of lack of direction, not living a life of personal fulfillment and allowing outside influences to hinder people from their true goals. Patients need to learn safe methods to release their frustrations and anger, to process grief or loss, to achieve a balance of work and play and to value their inner guidance and intuition.

Antidepressants can help some of us move from being dysfunctional to functional humans by chemically lessening the intensity of our feelings. They can also inhibit us from processing the underlying emotional cause, which may be both nutritional as well as emotional, and there is a danger that imbalances will be suppressed to a deeper stage of disharmony.

Through the various theoretical systems, Traditional Chinese Medicine is able to offer nutritional, herbal and physio-therapeutic methods such as 'tui-na' massage and acupuncture as well as psycho-spiritual counseling to assist in the healing process. Specifically, since ancient times, there has been a correlation of interactive effects between the Seven Emotions, the Five Elements and the twelve corresponding Zang Fu (Yin-Yang) organs.

Each Organ has its corresponding emotion. For instance, the Chinese "Heart" corresponds to the physiological heart anatomically, including its relation to the blood and vessels. At the same time, TCM describes the Heart as the 'house of the Spirit' and relates it to the body-mind, thoughts and dreams, as well as the emotions of joy and sadness. From this perspective many colloquial phrases such as "broken heartedness" demonstrate the relationship of the Heart with joy or the lack of it. Similarly, other common sayings such as "having a lot of gall", "unable to stomach a situation", "red with anger" "liverish", "sickeningly sweet" and so forth, demonstrate renewed mind-body validity.

Emotions in and of themselves are not negative; in fact, emotions are a necessary response to life. It is when a feeling is either suppressed or inappropriately indulged or vented that it becomes potentially injurious to its corresponding Organ. When this happens, immunity is lowered and disease, degeneration and general debility occur. As an example, individuals who succumb to prolonged grief after the death of someone to whom they had close emotional ties often become more susceptible to pneumonia, asthma, heart disease and other debilitating or fatal ailments.

On the other hand, when an Organ is out of balance, there may be a noticeable imbalance in its corresponding emotion. For instance, if the Kidneys are Deficient, fear or paranoia may result, or if the Liver is congested, anger, irritability and frustration can arise. Thus, the Seven Emotions can be both the cause as well as an indication of a specific Organ imbalance.

The Seven Emotions are: joy, anger, sadness, pensiveness, grief, fear and fright (shock). Sometimes sadness is coupled with grief and worry and is then considered one of the Seven Emotions. Others consider worry to be part of pensiveness. Each of these emotions has a particular affect on Qi and the other Substances. They each correspond to a particular Organ as follows:

JOY

Of the Seven Emotions, joy associated as the very essence of a positive state, seems the most quizzical. When one joyfully over-celebrates with the over- indulgence usually associated with that, it can damage the Heart and its vessels. In fact either a complete absence of, or an Excess of joy in the sense of over-celebrating, besides injuring the Heart can cause Spirit or Shen disturbances. This manifests symptoms of insomnia, muddled thinking, inappropriate crying or laughter and in extreme cases, fits, hysteria and insanity. When Heart Qi is imbalanced, one may tend towards inappropriate giddiness, laughter or oversensitivity. Constant mental stimulation or excessive excitement, no matter how wonderful, can excessively stimulate the Heart and, in time, lead to Heart Fire or Deficient Heart Yin.

ANGER

Anger includes resentment, frustration, irritability, rage, indignation, bitterness and animosity. Excess anger injures the Liver. Likewise, a Liver imbalance can cause one to get angry or be prone to irrational outbursts of anger more easily, often without apparent cause or provocation. Anger causes Qi to ascend, resulting in Liver Fire or Yang Rising, Stagnation of Liver Qi or Blood, or Deficient Liver Yin. It then appears in symptoms such as headaches, tinnitus, dizziness, blurred vision, mental confusion, red face, vomiting of blood and diarrhea. Long term repressed anger or resentment eventually causes depression. This in turn suppresses and stagnates Qi and leads to such conditions as hypochondriac pain, a lump or plum-pit feeling in the throat, PMS, tension and irritability, swollen breasts before periods, irregular or painful periods, and digestive upsets such as nausea, poor appetite and epigastric pain.

SADNESS

Sadness affects both the Lungs and the Heart, since they both lie in the Upper Warmer. Sadness depletes Qi, leading to Lung Qi or Heart

Qi Deficiency. This results in symptoms such as breathlessness, depression or crying, amenorrhea, shortness of breath, fatigue, and lowered resistance to colds and flus. In time, Lung or Heart Qi Deficiency can cause Heart Blood or Yin Deficiency or Lung Yin Deficiency with such symptoms as palpitations, dizziness, insomnia, anxiety and night sweats.

PENSIVENESS

Pensiveness refers to excessive thinking, studying or mental work. It is often referred to as concentration. Dwelling too much on a particular topic weakens the Spleen, causing Stagnation of Qi. This disrupts the Spleen's function of transforming and transporting food and fluids, resulting in tiredness, loss of appetite, Dampness, weak digestion, abdominal distension and loose stools. Eventually, immunity and resistance are depressed from the body's lack of physical nourishment. This is frequently seen in students and workaholics, especially if the lifestyle includes irregular meals or eating on the run or while working or studying.

Worry is often attributed to the Spleen, as it also depletes Spleen Qi. Further, it affects Lung Qi, resulting in anxiety, breathlessness and stiffness of the neck and shoulders.

GRIEF

Grief is associated with the Lungs and weakens Lung Qi, leading to shortness of breath, mucus, sweating, tiredness, cough and susceptibility to colds, flu, respiratory allergies, asthma, emphysema and other lung complaints. Individuals who experience difficulty breathing are appropriately predisposed to fits of anxiety. It is not uncommon following the sudden loss of a family member to later develop bronchitis, asthma or pneumonia. Grief can also damage the Heart and Pericardium.

FEAR

Fear depletes Kidney Qi and makes Qi descend (it is not uncommon to feel an uncontrollable urge to void when a fearful situation arises). Bedwetting, frequent urination or urinary incontinence can be the result or symptoms of Kidney Deficiency. Fear can also cause Kidney Yin Deficiency with symptoms of night sweats, palpitations and a dry mouth and throat. Constantly living in a fearful situation eventually weakens the Kidneys, while individuals with weak Kidneys and adrenals tend to feel insecure, paranoid, easily frightened and generally more fearful.

FRIGHT

Fright is different than fear in that it is sudden and unexpected. It is shocking and alarming, causing Qi to scatter. Fright injures the Heart, which deprives the Shen of its residence and produces palpitations, breathlessness and insomnia. It also affects the Kidneys, leading to urinary incontinence, night sweating, dizziness or tinnitus. Extreme shock can leave one with chronic Kidney-Adrenal fatigue.

NEITHER INTERNAL NOR EXTERNAL CAUSES OF DISEASE

Causes of disease which are neither External nor Internal include diet, lifestyle habits, and miscellaneous causes including weak constitution, malnutrition, food poisoning, infected wounds, trauma, bites and stings, parasites and toxins.

DIET

Considered as neither an External nor Internal cause of disease, diet is increasingly significant as a factor in disease. Most of the variety of foods eaten today were not available even a century or two ago. People in China ate a basic diet of grains, legumes, vegetables and a small portion of meat and fruit a few times a week as they were seasonally available. Therefore, foods were locally grown and only available within their season, and diet played a key role in helping to maintain homeostasis according to geographic location, climate and lifestyle.

Today our diets are high in refined and processed foods. Food is brought in from all over the world and available any time of the year. For example, what was once appropriate in hot climates for their cooling moistening energy, bananas are now available year round even in cold and damp northern climates. Over time this aggravates Dampness within the body, especially in damp climatic environments.

Furthermore, today most foods are adulterated with chemicals in the form of preservatives, flavoring, coloring, emulsifiers and so forth. From their being cultivated with the use of artificial fertilizers and chemical insecticides as well as the impact of air and water pollution, there are residual chemicals in the food chain. Additionally, commercial meat contains hormones, and many animals are raised in confined prison-like conditions so that the quality of meat is less than optimum. Finally, with the pollution of coastal seas, fish harvested from them show dangerously high levels of heavy metals. As a result of all of this occurring over such a short time span, animal and human evolution is unable to catch up, and many are suffering from acute and chronic immune deficiency disorders.

Every time we eat we are creating, and contributing to, an energy in our bodies. According to TCM these energies can be delineated as cooling, warming, moistening, drying, eliminating, building, Yin or Yang. These energies appear in combinations with each other in the body, even when they seem contradictory, such as Dampness and Dryness co-existing in a situation of edema with dry skin. However, over time a predominance of one or two of these energies appears in the body and creates conditions associated with that energy. For instance, Heat building up in the body over time results in Heat signs such as strong body odors, yellow or red tinged discharges, irritability, restlessness, thirst and so on.

When we eat a predominance of foods which have a heating energy, this contributes to preexisting Heat in the body and can cause an imbalance that eventually gives rise to disease. The same would be true of an imbalance of cold or dry foods and so on (see the chapter on Whole Nutrition). Ideally we should eat a diet comprised of all the energies in balance with each other, and when we do this our desires and cravings are more in accord with our true needs.

For instance, If we have a constitutional predisposition to Dampness we would naturally crave more drying foods; a Hot or high metabolic constitution would naturally be attracted to more cooling foods; and a Cold constitution would naturally want more warming foods. We see this in small children whose innate warmer metabolism necessitates a need for more cooling fruits. An imbalanced diet, therefore, creates extreme cravings which lead to disease.

Excessive consumption of foods which are cooling and/or moistening, such as juices, fruit, salads, cold or iced drinks, raw and cold foods, tofu, soy milk, ice cream, frozen yogurt and popsicles, for instance, create Cold and Dampness in the body and injure Spleen Yang. While raw foods and juices are considered the epitome of healthy food by many, they cause Coldness and Dampness in the Spleen, weaken the digestive process and eventually cause poor appetite, mucus, loose stools, diarrhea, low energy, amenorrhea and a runny nose leading to frequent colds.

Excessive intake of sweets and sugar causes over-stimulation and empty Heat in the Stomach with symptoms of poor focus and general anxiety. Eating lots of flour products creates Dampness and congestion. Both block the Spleen function and injure its ability to transform Fluids. This results in mucus in the lungs or stools, vaginal discharge and abdominal distention and fullness, for example.

Excessive intake of fried or greasy foods such as deep-fried foods, milk, cheese, butter, avocados, nuts and nut butter, chips and fried foods produce Dampness and obstruct the Spleen function. This leads to Phlegm, which causes symptoms such as sinusitis, nasal discharge, heavy and fuzzy feeling in the head, dull headaches and so forth. Excessive consumption of hot, spicy and oily foods such as nuts and nut butters, avocados, cheese, chips, fried foods, curry, alcohol, beef, lamb or hot spices, causes Heat signs, especially in the Liver and Stomach. Excessive intake of caffeinated foods and drinks, including coffee, black tea, cocoa, colas and chocolate, causes Damp Heat in the Liver, depletes the Kidneys and forms acids (another form of Heat) which collect in many places in the body such as the joints, as in arthritis. Smoking tobacco is drying and causes Deficient Lung Yin with initial symptoms of cough and eventually other more serious Lung diseases such as cancer.

Not only what we eat, but how we eat can cause imbalances. Over-eating causes a blockage which obstructs the Spleen and Stomach functions and leads to congestion and Stagnation of Qi. Under-eating leads to Deficient Qi and Blood. Furthermore, eating quickly, distractedly or when in an emotionally distraught state or while reading, studying or working can impair the digestion and eventually cause Qi Stagnation or Spleen Qi Deficiency.

LIFESTYLE

There are many lifestyle habits which can cause disease. These can be generally grouped under either sexual or physical causes.

Sexual Activity

Known as the 'affairs of the bedroom' to the Chinese, sexual activity in excess is deleterious to health because it causes a depletion of Kidney Jing and/or Pre-Heaven Essence. This is especially true if one is already depleted in Jing Essence or as one ages. Depletion of Essence causes symptoms of Kidney Yin and Yang Deficiency (*Ming Men* or Life Gate Fire). The result is low back pain, dizziness, low energy, premature aging signs, teeth problems, tinnitus or loss of hearing and eyesight.

Such excessive sexual activity specifically refers to ejaculation and orgasm, so that any reasonable sexual stimulation without ejaculation actually promotes youthful vigor. Because of this, there are a number of ancient treatises on the practice of Taoist sexual yoga for health and longevity.

Lack of sexual desire, on the other hand, is a sign of Deficient Kidney Yang. This includes symptoms of impotence, premature ejaculation and frigidity. An excessive sexual drive can indicate either Excess Yang or Deficient Kidney Yin. If Kidney Yin is severely Deficient with Empty Fire, it is possible to have vivid sexual dreams with nocturnal emissions in men and orgasms in women.

Physical Activity
Physical activity encompasses both inactivity and excessive activity.

Inactivity
Before the advent of motor vehicles, walking was inseparably integrated into daily life. For most people, day to day life encompassed a healthy amount of exercise just accomplishing routine affairs and chores. Today with motor vehicles, elevators, escalators, electric machines, elaborate communication systems and conveniences of all types and forms, our daily routine movement is minimized, often to the point of severe underactivity. Aerobic exercise in moderation is beneficial, but an excess can further contribute to the frantic mood of modern lifestyles.

Inactivity causes Qi and Blood to stagnate and leads to a degeneration of Yang Qi with the accumulation of Dampness. It can also be a diagnostic sign of Deficient Qi or Deficient Yang.

Various postures and movements can benefit or injure specific internal organs. Sitting is associated with the Spleen and in moderation is beneficial, while excessive sitting is deleterious (often causing enlarged hips due to lymph congestion from Deficient Spleen Qi). The same goes for standing, which in Excess can injure the Kidneys (which is why people with Deficient Kidney Qi often experience lower back ache when they stand for a prolonged period). Walking in moderation, especially out of doors, helps the Liver to spread and harmonize, while excessive walking for a person's ability can deplete the Liver.

Over-activity
Overactivity has taken on new meaning in our fast-paced information-seeking global society. What would have taken years previously, we can now accomplish in days or even hours. While there are many benefits, it also creates "burn-out", or Yin Deficiency. Stress from over-exertion is recognized as a major cause of hypertension, heart disease and other debilitating ailments.

Under normal circumstances the Qi used up in daily activities is easily replenished by proper diet and rest. Even when working hard for a week, such as a student studying for exams or a consultant preparing for a special presentation at work, depleted Qi can be restored within a few days. However, if this intense activity is continued, working long and hard for hours, months or even years without adequate rest, it will result in the body's inability to sufficiently replenish Qi, and it is forced to then draw on its Essence reserves. This ultimately creates Yin Deficiency. Over-exertion can occur in three ways: mental, physical and through over-exercising. Mental over-work includes working long hours, often in a confined space, with unreasonable deadlines under conditions of stress. Furthermore, this often results in skipped, late or irregular meals which further contributes to Qi and Yin Deficiency. Physical over-exertion causes depletion of energy which leads to Blood and Yin Deficiency. Over-exercising depletes Qi, Blood and Yin and ultimately Jing.

Among the most beneficial forms of exercise are Taoist Qi Gong, Tai Qi or Yoga, which combine slower meditative stretching movements with the breath.

OTHER LIFESTYLE HABITS

There are other lifestyle habits which can adversely affect the body. Frequently staying up too late and getting insufficient sleep leads to chronic Qi and Yin Deficiency. The body conforms to a specific cycle of biorhythm which makes certain activities optimal for the different cycles of each day. Following is the Chinese biorhythm chart with corresponding appropriate activities:

Time	Organ
11 AM to 1 PM	Heart
1 PM to 3 PM	Small Intestine
3 PM to 5 PM	Bladder
5 PM to 7 PM	Kidney-Adrenals
7 PM to 9 PM	Pericardium
9 PM to 11 PM	Triple Warmer
11 PM to 1 AM	Gall Bladder
1 AM to 3 AM	Liver
3 AM to 5 AM	Lungs
5 AM to 7 AM	Large Intestine
7 AM to 9 AM	Stomach
9 AM to 11 AM	Spleen-Pancreas

According to this biorhythm chart there are certain activities that are appropriate for different periods throughout each day. For example, defecation naturally occurs during Large Intestine time in the early morning hours between 5AM and 7AM. Eating a nutritious breakfast during Stomach-Spleen time between 7AM and 11AM in the morning is best for digestion. Going to bed by 11PM creates the most regenerative sleep since it is during Wood time, 11-3 AM, that the Liver cleans and replenishes the Blood.

Similarly, organic imbalances and weaknesses are likely to appear at certain times, making the above chart useful as a diagnostic tool. For instance, it is common for people with Deficient Kidney Qi to get tired in the late afternoon, 3 - 7 PM, during Water time. Further, people with lung ailments often wake up between 3 - 5 AM and have breathing difficulties or can't go back to sleep.

As another example of lifestyle issues, childbirth and the responsibilities that follow can be very depleting of a woman's Essence and Kidney Qi. This is why taking tonic herbs such as ginseng and Dang Gui can be very beneficial after childbirth.

MISCELLANEOUS CAUSES

Malnutrition

Malnutrition is an obvious cause of disease. It exists not only in Third World countries, but in slums, ghettoes and impoverished areas of wealthy countries as well. It also occurs in those who think they are supposedly eating adequately, since so many foods such as desserts, sodas, chips, white bread and flour products, canned foods, and refined and processed foods, are full of empty calories and lack adequate nutrition. Others, attracted to an overly rigid diet, often in their quest for superior health, can also develop insidious nutritional deficiencies that often do not appear until years later, at which time the injury to the metabolism is too severe to completely restore. Similarly, women who display anorexic or bulimic tendencies in their quest to remain physically thin and attractive are at high risk for injuring their digestive and immune systems.

Weak Constitution

Each person is born with unique constitutional needs, strengths and deficiencies. This is determined by our ancestors, especially our parents' health at the time of birth. If the parents' health is poor, if the mother drinks alcohol or smokes during pregnancy, or if the mother conceives when she is too old, the child is at risk of being born with a poor constitution. This inherited constitution accounts for the relevant tolerance to dietary and emotional stress of certain individuals while others who, despite a careful diet and lifestyle, seem to be plagued with frail health. Genetic ancestry is probably important for many considerations, especially for some with certain dietary requirements. It is known that many of African and Southeastern Asian ancestry may lack an essential enzyme for the digestion of milk and dairy products. Dairy, on the other hand, has been an important article of diet for those with a Northern European background, and while too much is not necessarily advised, a little will do no harm whatsoever.

Similarly, it may be that certain dietary regimes such as strict vegetarianism may be inappropriate for some individuals while for others it might be beneficial. Ultimately, one must judge for one's self which diet is best, but be wary of fanatical, moralistic rigidity that ultimately does violence and harm to ourselves by keeping us away from the essential foods and nutrients our individual body requires.

Other Causes

Other causes of illness include burns, traumas, parasites, poisons, bites and stings. These are sudden and are usually easily identifiable conditions. They are treated within the context of TCM Organ patterns. Some examples include various parasites and intestinal worms which are typically prevalent in tropical, humid climates. The excessive consumption of greasy and sweet foods causes Dampness which can make one more prone to all parasites, so that it may be necessary to take measures to alleviate the Internal Dampness.

Traumas not only have an immediate effect on the body, but can become the cause of later disease. For instance, previous sports injuries that were mistreated, perhaps with the application of ice, elbow pain from excessive playing of tennis, or a previous fall or injury can, upon exposure to a Cold Damp climate, cause Cold and Damp obstruction. The injured area, with its resulting pain and contraction of movement, can then generate a predisposition to rheumatic pains.

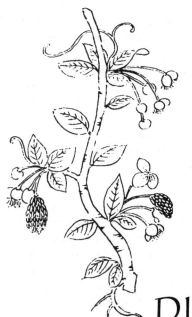

銳州五味子

DIAGNOSIS

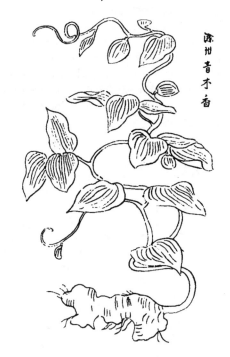

深州青木香

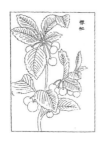

NINE

THE FOUR METHODS OF DIAGNOSIS

Traditional Chinese Medicine outlines four methods of diagnosis: interrogation, observation, audition and palpation. Only after evaluating these various essential parameters is a tentative diagnosis made. Scudder, the great Western Eclectic physician, once said, "Diagnosis means cure". This idea is particularly applicable in the Four Methods of Diagnosis since the purpose is not only to identify the disease itself, but also its mechanism and causes – whether the disease is External acute or Internal chronic, Hot or Cold, Excess (sthenic) or Deficient (asthenic) and Dry or Damp, all of which is encompassed by Yin and Yang (these are all discussed in detail in Chapter 4). Even the reaction to the first herbal treatment is also considered an important and often essential diagnostic parameter.

Contrast this with current Western allopathic diagnosis that seems content with identifying by name a particular pathological condition such as a staphylococcus infection. While it may suggest the use of a particular antibiotic, it does not indicate either the underlying cause of the disease or its relationship to other predisposing imbalances, and it most certainly does not offer a clue as to a treatment that will ultimately heal and restore balance. By first identifying such an infection as Heat in TCM, the traditional practitioner immediately knows to prescribe cool natured herbs and substances to counter it.

The location, along with other aspects concerning the nature of the particular Heat pattern, is also considered. In general, though not always, if it is on the skin, it is an acute External Heat manifestation; if the overall appearance seems robust or strong it would be Excess Heat; or if the patient appears frail with a history of recurring symptoms it would be considered Deficient Heat, requiring an altogether different approach to treatment.

INTERROGATION

Interrogation includes the patient's description of his primary complaint and any other secondary complaints. It also includes specific areas of inquiry by the doctor. Since the Ming Dynasty, it has been customary to follow the method of ten questions when making a diagnosis. This includes: 1. chills and fever; 2. perspiration; 3. headache, chest, abdominal or other pains anywhere in the body; 4. urination and defecation; 5. appetite; 6. mental state; 7. hearing; 8 thirst; 9. history of old diseases and causes of the new illness; 10. if a woman, menstruation, leukorrhea, number of children, childbirth, miscarriages and abortions.

Chills and fever
Chills and fever help determine whether it is an acute External symptom pattern or chronic Internal one. External complexes are always accompanied by chills, while with an Internal condition the patient may be prone to general coldness but not chills.

Colds, influenza, headache, stiff neck, body aches, fevers with chills and an aversion to Cold and Wind are all External symptoms. These need to be further understood as being either of the Wind-Cold or Wind-Heat type. With Wind-Cold the chills are more severe than the fever and there are other indications of Coldness such as pale appearance and a slower pulse (60 or less beats per minute). With Wind-Heat chills are milder while the fever is stronger, and there are other strong indications of Heat such as a flushed appearance and a rapid pulse (closer to 80 or more beats per minute). The Wind-Cold and Wind-Heat diseases are divided into six stages, each having several formulas appropriate for its treatment. These are detailed in chapter 6.

Perspiration
Spontaneous perspiration is generally an indication of a Deficient condition. Fever with perspiration is a sign of either External Wind-Heat or Heat invading the Qi level.
Wind Heat: use **Lonicera and Forsythia Combination** (Yin qiao san)
Wind Cold: use **Cinnamon Combination** (Gui zhi tang)
Qi level fever: use **White Tiger Decoction** (Bai hu tang)

Perspiration accompanying an Internal symptom complex could represent Yang Deficiency when one perspires upon awakening or spontaneously, or Yin Deficiency if perspiration occurs during sleep. Cold extremities, small pulse and a pale complexion with incessant predisposition to sweating can be a sign of exhaustion.

Yang Deficiency: Tonify Yang with **Rehmannia Eight Formula** (Ba wei di huang wan).

Yin Deficiency: Tonify Yin with **Rehmannia Six Formula** (Liu wei di huang wan).

Perspiration Caused by Exhaustion: Use a ginseng or Qi tonic formula such as **Ginseng and Ginger Combination** (Li zhong wan) or **Four Major Herbs** (Si jun zi tang).

Headaches, Chest, Abdominal or Other Aches and Pains

Headaches

External Cold: Incessant headaches with fever and cold, use **Cinnamon Combination** (Gui zhi tang).

Blood Deficiency: Headaches that come and go with dizziness indicates **Dang Gui Four Combination** (Si wu tang).

Greater Yang (Tai Yang) type: Headaches that occur at the neck and the back of the head is treated wth **Ephedra Combination** (Ma huang tang).

Lesser Yang (Shao Yang) type: Bilious headaches located at the temples or sides of the head are treated with **Bupleurum and Cinnamon Combination** (Chai hu gui zhi tang) or **Bupleurum and Dang Gui Formula** (Xiao yao san or Rambling Powder).

Sunlight Yang (Yang Ming) type: Headaches that are located at the forehead to the eyebrow ridge are caused by the Stomach and are treated with **Minor Rhubarb Combination** (Xiao cheng qi tang).

Lesser Yin (Shao Yin) type: Headaches acompanied with vomiting, cold extremities and a deep pulse are treated with **Evodia Combination** (Wu zhu yu tang).

Deficient Qi: Severely painful headaches which occur in the morning, late afternoon or come and go are caused by weakness and are treated with tonics such as **Ginseng and Dang Gui Ten Combination** (Shi chuan da bu wan).

Excess Heat: A severe, continuous headache may be caused by toxic accumulation and is treated with detoxifying herbal formulas such as **Coptis and Scutellaria Combination** (Huang lian jie du tang) or **Major Bupleurum Combination** (Da chai hu tang).

Chest discomfort and pains

Excess: For a feeling of fullness in the chest with labored breathing use **Five Peels Decoction** (Wu pi san).

Deficient Qi: For a feeling of emptiness with shallow breathing use **Rehmannia Eight Combination** (Ba wei di huang wan).

Blood Stagnation: Sharp chest pains are treated with **Decoction for Removing Blood Stasis in the Chest** (Xue fu zhu yu tang).

Asthma or emphysema: For a stuffy feeling in the chest with pain and shortness of breath one can consider **Ephedra and Ginkgo Combination** (Ding chuan tang).

Abdominal Pains

Excess: For abdominal pains with tenderness upon palpation one can consider **Major Bupleurum Combination** (Da chai hu tang); for abdominal pains accompanied with constipation, a hard, distended abdomen and an aversion to warm weather use **Major Rhubarb Combination** (Da cheng qi tang), **Minor Rhubarb Combination** (Xiao cheng qi tang), **Rhubarb and Moutan Combination** (Da huang mu dan pi tang) or **Major Bupleurum Combination** (Da chai hu tang).

Deficiency: For abdominal pains alleviated with pressure and warmth one can use **Ginseng and Ginger Combination** (Li zhong wan); for abdominal pains associated with malnourishment use **Minor Cinnamon and Paeonia Combination** (Xiao jian zhong tang), or **Ginseng and Ginger Combination** (Li zhong tang) when there is Qi Deficiency and weakness.

Stagnation of Blood, Dampness or Qi: For masses or lumps in the abdomen use **Cinnamon Twig and Poria Combination** (Gui zhi fu ling tang).

General Pain

In general, pains that move or come and go are caused by Wind, intractable pains are caused by Damp stagnation, while Deficiency pains are dull and aching.

Wind-Damp-Cold: For pains especially in the lower back and legs use **Du huo and Loranthes Combination** (Du huo ji sheng tang) or for generalized pains use **Clematis and Stephania Combination** (Shu jing huo xue tang).

Wind-Damp-Heat: For rheumatic pains in the bodily extremities use **White Tiger and Cinnamon Twig Decoction** (Bai hu jia gui zhi tang).

Blood Stagnation: Sharp, stabbing pains use **Du Huo and Loranthes Combination** (Du huo ji sheng tang) and add persica seed (Tao Ren), carthamus (Hong Hua) and cyperus (Xiang Fu) to this formula.

Shoulder and neck stiffness and pain

For those with a stronger conformation, **Pueraria Combination** (Ge gen tang) is generally effective.

Joint and lower back pain

Kidney Deficiency: Joint and lower back pains with aching weakness and fatigue is treated with **Du huo and Loranthes Combination** (Du huo ji sheng tang) and/or **Rehmannia Eight Combination** (Ba wei di huang wan).

<u>Stagnant Blood</u>: Joint and lower back pains that are sharp and fixed are treated with **Fantastically Effective Pill to Invigorate the Collaterals** (Huo luo xia ling dan) or **Cinnamon Twig and Poria Combination** (Gui zhi ful ling wan).

<u>Arthritic and Rheumatic Pains</u>: May be treated with **Dang Gui, Dipsacus and Tienchi Combination** (Shu jin san) or **Clematis and Stephania Combination** (Shu jing huo xue tang).

A single herb that is often taken by the elderly for aching lower back pains, hypertension and heart disease and to strengthen the bones and sinews is Loranthus parasiticus (Sang Ji Sheng) or Mulberry mistletoe. It works for diseases associated with aging by replenishing the Liver and Kidney Qi.

Defecation

<u>Yang Stagnation and Excess</u>: Constipation in one with a normal appetite or a feeling of abdominal fullness with discomfort and pain indicates **Major Rhubarb Combination** (Da cheng qi tang) or **Minor Rhubarb Combination** (Xiao cheng qi tang).

<u>Deficiency</u>: A thinner patient with less appetite and constipation without either abdominal fullness or pain indicates **Blood Replenishing Decoction** (Ji chuan jian).

<u>Dryness of Blood and Internal Heat</u>: Chronic constipation in older individuals indicates **Blood Replenishing Decoction** (Ji chuan jian) with the addition of Scutellaria and cannabis seed (or flax seed).

<u>Spleen Qi or Yang Deficiency with Dampness</u>: Loose bowels indicates the use of a ginseng tonic formula such as **Four Major Herbs** (Si jun zi tang) or **Ginseng and Ginger Combination** (Li zhong wan).

<u>Indigestion and improper diet</u>: Diarrhea with abdominal pain and strong smelling stools may indicate the use of a carminative Qi regulating formula or a formula to remove food stagnation such as **Citrus and Crataegus Combination** (Bao he wan).

<u>Dysentery</u>: For tenesmus, an urgent need to defecate but often with no result, one might consider **Spleen Warming Decoction** (Wen pi tang).

<u>Internal Cold</u>: Persistent watery diarrhea may indicate a formula such as **Ginger, Licorice and Aconite Combination** (Si ni tang).

<u>Gastroenteritis or cholera</u>: persistent diarrhea with nausea and vomiting can indicate **Mume formula** (Wu mei wan) or **Citrus and Crataegus Combination** (Bao he wan).

Urination

Urination six times daily is average; more is a sign of Deficiency while less is a sign of Excess. The darker the urine the more concentrated it is, which indicates a Heat condition.

Deficiency of Kidney Yang: Pale or light urine is an indication of a Cold condition and one would consider **Rehmannia Eight Combination** (Ba wei di huang wan).

Diabetes: Frequent urination with thirst are signs of diabetes. One might consider **Rehmannia Six Combination** (Liu wei di huang wan).

Deficiency of either Yin Essence, Yang or Qi: For incontinence of urine, in older individuals, or enuresis (night time urination) in adults or children use **Mantis Egg-case Powder** (Sang piao xiao san), one of the primary formulas to consider for urinary frequency associated with Deficiency.

Cystitis (bladder infection), nephritis (kidney infection) or urinary stones: Dark yellow urine with hematuresis (blood) and pain during urination is a sign of serious urinary disturbance and one should consider either **Gentiana Combination** (Long dan xie gan tang) or **Polyporus Combination** (Zhu ling tang).

Appetite

More superficial digestive or appetite problems relate to the Stomach symptom complex while deeper, chronic problems with metabolism and assimilation relate to the Spleen complex. Excessive appetite is an indication of excessive Stomach Heat while lack of appetite with digestive weakness is a sign of a Deficient Spleen or Cold Stomach. Stomach Heat is caused by overeating fatty, spicy and hot foods. There may also be symptoms of thirst, foul breath, preference for cold drinks and foods and in extreme cases, nausea.

Qi Deficiency: Lack of appetite is treated with **Six Major Herb Formula** (Liu jun zi tang).

Cold Stomach: This is caused by a Deficiency of Yang possibly as a result of overeating cold, raw foods. Cold Stomach pains are usually relieved by the application of warmth or ginger tea. Treatment for Cold Stomach is **Ginseng and Ginger Combination** (Li zhong wan) or **Cinnamon, Ginseng and Ginger Combination** (Gui zhi li zhong wan).

Morning sickness: Nausea and vomiting during the early stages of pregnancy is an indication of morning sickness. It can be treated with **Saussurea and Cardamon Combination with Six Noble Ingredients** (Xiang sha liu jun zi tang).

Hearing
Sudden hearing loss is an Excess condition, while gradual diminution of hearing is a sign of Deficiency.

Tinnitus (ear ringing): That sounds like blowing or wind indicates a Wind Heat condition. Consider using **Magnetite and Cinnabar Sedative** (Ci zhu wan). Tinnitus that is more like a humming or cicada sound indicates Liver or Kidney imbalance. Use a variation of **Magnetite and Cinnabar Sedative** (Ci zhu wan) that adds lycii berries, ligustrum, cuscuta and prepared rehmannia.

Ear ache: Possibly with pus is an indication of Damp Heat. One might use **Gentiana Combination** (Long dan xie gan tang).

Thirst
Thirst with a desire to drink cold fluids is a sign of Internal Heat. Thirst with a desire for Warm drinks is a sign of Internal Cold. Excessive thirst is a sign of Yin Deficiency. Thirst with no desire to drink is a sign of Damp Heat. Excessive thirst with normal urination, an individual who urinates twice as much as is the fluid that is taken in, or a person who urinates as much as is taken represent three different types of diabetes.

Thirst with Internal Heat: Consider **White Tiger Decoction** (Bai hu tang).

Thirst with Internal Cold: Consider **Rehmannia Eight Combination** (Ba wei di huang wan).

Thirst caused by Yin Deficiency: One can consider **Anemarrhena, Phellodendron with Rehmannia Combination** (Zhi bai di huang wan) or **Rehmannia Six Combination** (Liu wei di huang wan).

Mental condition
For depression and moodiness: Use **Bupleurum and Peony Combination** (Jia wei xiao yao wan) or **Cinnabar Combination** (Zhu sha an shen wan).

For Heart and Kidneys or Yin Deficiency: For insomnia, forgetfulness and mental exhaustion consider **Ginseng and Zizyphus Combination** (Tian wang bu xin tang - This is sometimes called the "scholar's formula") or **Mantis Egg-case Powder** (Sang piao xiao san) with zizyphus seeds and schizandra.

For anemia with Spleen Deficiency: Consider **Ginseng and Longan Combination** (Gui pi tang).

For mental off-centeredness and forgetfulness associated with hypoglycemia: Consider **Minor Cinnamon and Paeonia Combination** (Xiao jian zhong tang).

For insomnia with a tendency to awaken early or in the middle of the night: Consider **Zizyphus Combination** (Suan zao ren tang).

<u>For insomnia with extreme nervousness and emotional instability</u>:
Use **Bupleurum and Dragon Bone Combination** (Chai hu jia long
gu mu li tang).

Menstruation

The amount and color of the menstrual blood as well as its regularity or irregularity is indicative of the condition and treatment. Pains that occur during ovulation represent stagnation and are treated with emmenagogue herbs such as Dang Gui (Angelica sinensis), lovage (ligusticum species), motherwort (Leonurus cardiaca), Chinese red sage root (Salvia milthiorrhiza), red peony root (Paeonia rubra), safflower (Carthamus tinctorii) and calendula (Calendula officinalis) flowers.

<u>Hot Blood</u>: Women with frequent periods and extreme blood flow can be treated with **Gentiana Combination** (Long dan xie gan tang).

<u>Blood Deficiency</u>: Women with scanty menstruation and irregular or missed menstruation can be treated with **Dang Gui Four** (Si wu tang).

<u>Blood Stagnation</u>: Women who exhibit a lot of clots are treated with **Cinnamon Twig and Poria Combination** (Gui zhi fu ling wan).

OBSERVATION

A skilled TCM doctor is often able to diagnose a patient as soon as they walk into their presence. This is not so difficult to understand since our imbalances reflect themselves in every aspect of our expression and manner.

We can presume an underlying Deficiency when an individual presents themselves as soft spoken, shy or somewhat timorous with a greater tendency towards negative states and a generally lifeless manner, which is especially noticed in their eyes. A pale complexion is usually an indication of Blood Deficiency; it may also indicate Qi Deficiency if there are complaints or indications of Deficient Qi as well. In Chinese medicine, Deficiency issues of men usually, but not always, involve Qi, while with women, because of menstruation and childbirth, Blood Deficiency is more likely. Since, according to the classics, Blood is the mother of Qi and Qi the commander of Blood, it is not uncommon for both Blood and Qi to be simultaneously Deficient.

Yang Deficiency will have a similar presentation, but the individual may be more densely clothed, suggesting Coldness. Upon interrogation, they would also express a lack of motivation and drive and lack of libido. Yin Deficiency manifests similarly to Excess Yang but arises more out of an overall Deficient state. Yin Deficient individuals tend to be

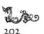

thinner, the complexion may be red but more in blotches on the surface of the skin, especially the nose and face, the voice may be loud but hollow sounding and while they may issue forth with a burst of enthusiasm, they have a tendency to not complete what they begin and therefore drift about as if somewhat lost, making them appear to be unfocused. As a contrast, Excess individuals are generally of a stocky build, not at all shy in manner or speech, more strongly opinionated with a cheerful disposition, a deeper ruddy complexion, and bright clear and lively eyes. We would not consider this individual to be either Excess Qi or Blood, because any imbalance other than Deficiency of these two paradigms would be described as Stagnation with specific corresponding symptoms.

An individual could, however, present as Excess Yin or Yang. Excess Yin is characterized by edema, or a more phlegmatic appearance, while with Excess Yang there is more of an aggressive manner and a certain overbearing aspect to their presentation. While there is often a combination of both Yin and Yang Excess together in the same individual, Yin Excess tends to a somewhat paler complexion, while Yang is definitely of a more ruddy complexion.

Qi Stagnation is often accompanied by a moody or depressed attitude with a tendency towards fullness and pains in the chest, and gas and bloating after meals. Blood Stagnation on the other hand presents with a more deeply scarlet or purplish appearance and fixed, stabbing pains.

When treating any Deficiency, we must use tonification therapy. It there is Qi Deficiency, integrate herbs such as ginseng, astragalus, jujube dates and honey-baked licorice in the preparations. Sugar is also a Qi tonic and preparations made with whole, unrefined cane sugar, maple syrup, blackstrap molasses, barley malt and rice syrup would give Qi tonic properties.

For Blood Deficiency use herbs such as Dang Gui (Angelica sinensis), lycii berries (Gou Qi Zi), prepared Rehmannia glutinosa (Shu Di Huang) or Polygonum multiflorum (He Shou Wou) and Blood nourishing herbs and iron-rich foods such as various dark colored berries, grapes and red meat.

For Yang Deficiency, use Internal warming stimulants such as cinnamon bark (Rou gui) and/or prepared aconite root (Fu Zi), and other spicy acrid herbs including cloves and peppers. For Yin Deficiency, we use Yin tonics which may include a number of Blood tonics (because of the close relationship of Blood and Yin), such as prepared rehmannia (Shu Di Huang) and lycii berries (Gou Qi Zi) along with Yin tonics such as ophiopogon (Mai Men Dong), American ginseng (Panax quinquefolium), tortoise shell (Bie Jia), black donkey skin gelatin (E jiao), demulcent herbs such as marshmallow root (Althea officinalis), comfrey root (Symphytum officinale), slippery elm bark (Ulmus fulva), Iceland moss (Cetraria islandica) and Irish moss (Chondrus crispus), and foods such as okra, pork and turtle soup.

When treating Excess, use more therapeutically active herbs and formulas with reducing or detoxifying therapies. These may include purgatives, cholagogues (herbs that stimulate the liver to discharge bile), alteratives (Heat clearing herbs), diuretics or diaphoretics.

In general, often behind every Excess there is a latent Deficiency and behind every Deficiency there may be a latent Excess. Always treat what is most apparent first. Following the principle of treating the branch symptoms before the root will allow us to eventually access any latent imbalances as they may appear.

Skin: A puffy appearance of the skin indicates edema and Dampness. Dry or rough skin can indicate Blood Deficiency and is treated with Blood tonics such as Polygonum multiflorum (He Shou Wou) in the compound called "Shou Wou Chih" sold in most Chinese pharmacies. Skin that feels moist to the touch is an indication of Dampness.

Hair: Dry, lusterless hair that breaks easily represents a general Deficiency, especially of Blood and Yin.

Mucus secretions: The Chinese mother formula for all types of Excess mucus is the formula **Two Cured Decoction** (Er chen tang - also found in pill form), which can be appropriately modified for Cold or Hot conditions. Thick yellow or greenish phlegm indicates Heat and is treated with cooling, alterative herbs such as echinacea (Echinacea spp.), golden seal (Hydrastis canadensis), chaparral (Larrea divaricata), coptis (Huang Lian), honeysuckle (Jin Yin Hua), forsythia fruit (Lian Qiao), gentian (Long Dan Cao) and poke (Phytolacca spp.).

Thin, clear mucus secretions usually indicates Coldness, Dampness and Deficiency and is treated with Internal warming herbs and formulas such as garlic, cayenne pepper and raw ginger or the Ayurvedic Trikatu formula. This consists of equal parts pippali long pepper, black pepper and ginger powders mixed with honey. One half to one teaspoon is taken as a single dose. Two parts anise seed powder could be substituted for pippali to make it milder for children.

A large amount of mucus secretion is described as Excess Dampness if it is purulent white. Yellowish or blood tinged exudate is classified as Damp Heat, for which one would use **Gentiana Combination** (Long dan xie gan tang) or formulas containing cholagogue herbs such as dandelion root (Taraxacum officinale), barberry (Berberis vulgaris) or oregon grape (Mahonia repens), golden seal (Hydrastis canadensis), fringetree bark (Chionanthus virginicus), gentian root (Long dan cao), yellow dock root (Rumex crispus), as is found in the Planetary formula, HerbaDerm Complex. Dry phlegm that is difficult to expectorate requires expectorants such as platycodon (Jie Geng), ophiopogon (Mai Men Dong), yerba santa (Eriodictyon spp.) and balm of gilead (Grindelia spp.).

Blood (coughing, vomiting, menses): Thin, light colored-blood indicates Deficiency while dark red, clotted blood is Excess. Blood Stagnation manifests in women as more pain and clots immediately before and during menstruation. Pain that occurs more after menstruation indicates a Deficiency.

Stool: Loose stools represent Dampness and Spleen Deficiency. Hard, constipated stools represent Heat.

Urine: Cloudy urine represents Dampness and possibly Heat. Dark yellow, concentrated urine, possibly with blood, indicates Heat. Clear urine may indicate Qi and Yang Deficiency with Coldness and weakness. Brown-colored urine can indicate a chronic condition such as diabetes. An excessive volume of urine also can indicate diabetes while a small volume can be edema.

Herbs used to clear Excess Heat and Dampness include cooling or neutral diuretics such as cleavers (Galium aparine), uva ursi (Arctostaphylos uva urse) and horsetail (Equisetum spp.) in Western herbalism. Chinese formulas include the mushrooms poria (Fu Ling) and polyporus (Zhu Ling) and dianthus (Qu Mai) herb. Herbs that clear Damp Heat are cholagogues such as gentian root (Long Dan Cao), barberry (Berberis vulgaris), oregon grape (Mahonia repens), and golden seal (Hydrastis canadensis). Chinese formulas to consider for Damp Heat conditions include **Gentiana Combination** (Long dan xie gan tang) and **Dianthus Combination** (Ba zheng san).

TONGUE DIAGNOSIS

This is one of the most important methods of diagnosis and, along with pulse diagnosis, warrants a more extensive presentation.

History

The earliest record of tongue diagnosis is found on inscriptions of bones and tortoise shells unearthed from the ruins of the Yuan dynasty, the first dynasty of the Bronze Age. A thousand years later, around 400 to 300 B.C., descriptions of tongue diagnosis were recorded in the Yellow Emperor's Classic of Internal Medicine (*Huang Ti Nei Jing*). Tongue diagnosis evolved further from the Han to the Tang millennia (200 BC to 907 BC) and continues to evolve with extensive research during the present day in China.

Not too long ago, one of the first Western medical diagnostic procedures was when the doctor asked us to open the mouth so he could examine the tongue. Thus, tongue diagnosis represents an effective and low-tech method of diagnosis when combined with other diagnostic parameters of observation. It is unfortunate that for many simple, non-life-threatening conditions, such an economic and artful procedure is seldom utilized in contemporary Western clinics.

Following is a table that compares traditional TCM diagnosis of the tongue with that of contemporary Western medicine. (Note that a normal tongue appears as pink, slightly moist, neither too thick or thin and with a slight white coat.)

Table 1. Comparative Clinical Significance of Tongue Appearances in TCM and Western Medicine [1]

Tongue Feature	In TCM	In Western Medicine
COLOR **Pale**	Deficiency of Qi and Blood	Anemia, malnutrition
Red	Heat evil invades Ying level [2] ; Heat in the Pericardium meridian, Zang Fu or the extremities.	Toxemia/pyemia caused by infection; acute or suppurative infectious disease; high fever; severe pneumonia; hyperemia; tongue vessel dilation.
Cardinal red	Heat evil invades Ying and Blood levels; Heat affecting Pericardium; Heat Fire flushing up.	High fever; septicemia and other serious disease conditions.
Purplish	Extreme Heat; Stagnant Blood; Heat in Heart Meridian; insidious pathogenic factors in Lung; Heat phlegm in Upper Warmer; Excess Heat both Interior and Exterior.	Severe infection; respiratory/ circulatory disorder; thrombosis or microcirculatory bleeding; sublingual vein stasis; pigmentation disease.

Tongue Feature	In TCM	In Western Medicine
Bluish	Internal accumulation of Damp-Phlegm; Heat in Blood level; Cold Liver and Kidney.	Respiratory/circulatory failure; anoxia; cyanotic Heart disease.

BODY

Contracted	Heart-Blood Deficiency; Internal Heat consuming the muscles.	Tongue atrophy; severe infection; late stage disease; extreme weakness and emaciation.
Swollen	Cold Dampness; Heat Dampness; Phlegm overflow; Heart Fire.	Edema; lingual inflammation and congestion; macroglossia.
Stiff/swollen	Excessive Heart Fire; Heat in Heart and Spleen.	Tongue severely swollen.
Double Tongue (rare)	Phlegm-Wind, Phlegm-Fire in the Heart and Spleen.	Tumor; sublingual gland cyst or inflammation.
Protruding	Phlegm-Heat in the Heart; epidemic Toxin attacking the Heart; Deficiency of Original Qi.	Down's syndrome; toxemia; high fever.
With Thorns (Strawberry)	Heat-Toxin; Excess symptom complex; Blood Stagnation.	High or scarlet fever; severe pneumonia.
Fissured	Heat damage to Stomach Fluid; Yin and Blood Deficiency.	High fever; dehydration; malnutrition; tongue inflammation.
Smooth	Over-sweating or overuse of purgatives; consumption of Yin; Stomach Qi exhaustion.	Malnutrition, macrocytic anemia; atrophy of filiform and fungiform papillae.
Ulcerated	Heat in the upper warmer	Stomatitis; ulcerative stomatitis
Denuded	Yin Deficiency.	Malnutrition; geographic tongue, allergic or exudative constitution. Some filiform papillae atrophy, some proliferate.
Crooked	Liver Wind.	Stroke; similar injury to, or stimulation of, nerves of the tongue.
Trembling	Internal movement of Liver Wind.	Can be a sign of either weakness or Excess, depending on the other signs. It is often associated with hyperthyroidism, general poor health and neurosis.
Flaccid	Blood Deficiency or Yin damage.	Weakness, fatigue, low thyroid, hypoglycemia, etc.
Hyperactive	Excess or Weakness; Heat in the Spleen and Heart.	Depending on other signs it can indicate anemia and exhaustion, or the aftermath of cerebral vascular accidents or stroke.

TONGUE COATING
COLOR

White	Normal or Exterior symptom-complex; febrile diseases, Cold Evil in the Tai Yang Stage[3] or Heat Evil in Wei level. (In Deficiency, Cold	Normal. Initial stage of febrile disease; chronic mild disease, or convalescence.

⤸

207

	and Interior symptoms complex can also be seen.)	
Yellow	Interior, Excess, and Heat symptom-complex, Excess Heat diseases; Excess Heat affecting the gastro-intestinal tract or Stomach (Bright Yang level); Heat Evil between Ying and Wei levels.	Bacterial infectious disorder; constipation.
Gray	Interior symptom-complex; febrile disease in three Yin Stages; (Cold, or with a pseudo-Heat appearance); Heat Evil invading Blood level; epidemic disease (Excess Heat).	Severe disease; long term digestive disorder; dehydration; acidosis; or result of smoking.
Black	Interior symptom-complex; Heat Evil invading Blood level.	Disease conditions more severe than in gray coating; fungal infections.
CHARACTER		
Thin	Normal or Exterior symptom-complex in febrile disease.	Mild pathogenic factors.
Thick	Interior symptom-complex; Excess Evil such as Heat, Cold, or Phlegm.	Stronger pathogenic factors, influencing digestive or respiratory tract; filiform papillae proliferation.
Moist	Normal, or mild disease that has not injured Body Fluid.	Normal saliva secretion.
Dry	Heat Evil consuming Body Fluid.	High fever; dehydration; open-mouth breathing; decreased saliva secretion.
Creamy/Greasy	Dampness and Turbid Qi in Stomach, Spleen or Lung.	Poor digestion; poor oral cleaning ability or habit.

In TCM tongue and pulse diagnosis, there are always signs of primary consideration and signs which are only considered when there is a corresponding indication in a designated area. What is of primary consideration involves the overall description of the shape, tongue body and coat of the tongue. Further, if specific signs or indications are particularly noticeable at certain areas, these may be correlated with specific internal viscera.

While there is some disagreement concerning the significance of signs observed on certain tongue areas, there is enough empirically based agreement that most TCM physicians place considerable importance on them. In general the tongue tip corresponds to the Heart; the intermediate horizontal zone between the middle and the tip represents the Lungs; the root or back of the tongue to the Kidney; the center of the tongue indicates the Spleen and Stomach; while the side edges correspond to the Liver and Gall Bladder. Following another TCM model, the front of the tongue corresponds to the Organs of the Upper Warmer, the middle area to the Middle Warmer Organs and the root or back of the tongue to the Lower Warmer Organs.

Tongue Inspection

We divide our inspection of the tongue into three main areas: appearance of the tongue, the tongue body and the coat. From the appearance and body of the tongue we learn of the relative state of Yin, Yang, Xu (Depletion or Deficiency) or Shi (Repletion or Excess). Overall the tongue is under the domain of the Heart because it reflects the overall circulatory condition. However, the tissue of the tongue is comprised of the same continuous tissue of the stomach so that the tongue also indicates the condition of the Stomach. The coat on the tongue represents the vaporized waste of the Stomach Qi.

Since the condition of the coat is more transient depending on the External Influences (Wind, Cold, Damp, Heat, Dryness, Summer Heat) and on food, it is only of secondary importance, while the tongue body which reflects the underlying state of vitality is of primary importance. As a result, no matter what the condition of the coat, the disease is relatively easy to cure if the tongue body appears healthy. However, since the tongue body reflects a deeper imbalance, if it appears imbalanced treatment will be longer and more difficult.

Tongue Appearance
1. **Thin and shriveled** – This generally indicates Deficiency. If it is pale then there is poor circulation with weakness of the Heart and Spleen. If it is dry, then it is Yin Deficient and is difficult to treat.
2. **Swollen** – The tongue may be enlarged or have noticeable scallops on its edges outlining tooth indentations. This indicates Dampness and edema caused by Excess Yin or Deficient Spleen.
3. **Stiff tongue** – This may be deflected to one side of the mouth or the other. This indicates apoplexy (stroke) and Internal Wind.
4. **Protruding** – A tendency to frequently extrude the tongue from the mouth indicates Internal Heat affecting the Heart and Spleen Organ meridians.
5. **Trembling** – If the tongue is trembling excessively, this is an indication of Internal Liver Wind, possibly associated with epilepsy or Parkinson's disease. If there is an associated tendency to refrain from speech, this can be a symptom of Heart and Spleen Qi Deficiency.

Inspecting the Tongue Body: Color of the tongue
A normal, healthy tongue is pinkish and moist. If it is lighter than

normal it is considered a pale tongue, darker than normal is a red tongue. A more intensely dark red tongue is called a cardinal red tongue and is an indication of fire. A bluish-purple tongue is an indication of stagnation of either Cold or Heat.

A. The pale tongue

A plump and tender pale tongue is most commonly seen and indicates Cold-Dampness with Deficient Yang (poor circulation and low metabolism). A thin and small bodied pale tongue indicates a Deficiency of Qi and Blood.

These indications are further elucidated in terms of its overall appearance or character. A so called "withered" pale, white tongue indicates that the visceral Qi and Blood are not adequately supplying the tongue with nourishment. Usually this is accompanied with colorless lips and gums. A withered, white and moist tongue is an indication of anemia, physical weakness or Deficiency of Yang with stagnated Cold-Dampness.

Tooth prints, or scalloped edges, on the tongue are generally considered to be an indication of edema caused by Deficient Spleen Qi and accumulated Dampness. It is a hypotensive state and is treated with Fluid-dispersing diuretics and warming Spleen and Kidney Yang Qi tonics.

B. Red and Cardinal Red Tongues

Pink is the normal color of the tongue. A tongue that is red progressing to deep cardinal red is an indication of pathological Heat and febrile disease. There are two types:

1. **Excess Heat Type**

There may be a high fever, even delirium, but the Heat has not accumulated to the degree that it has injured the normal Qi. One may perceive that in this type the tongue substance appears relatively fresh. Sometimes there are red thorns which can increase in size and protrude. The surface of the tongue is dry and fissured, the tongue coating may be white and dry, coarse yellow or charred black, indicating that Evil Heat has penetrated between the Qi and Ying level or has already entered the nutritive Ying level. This is an Excess Evil where, even though the Yin essence has sustained injury, it is not of primary concern. At this stage, one should use anti-inflammatory, Heat clearing herbs that also cool the Ying.

2. **Yin Deficient Type**

This type is seen in chronic wasting conditions or the late stages of acute febrile diseases. At this stage, the Qi has become Deficient and the

Evil is also somewhat weak. Tidal fever occurs with an elevation of temperature in the afternoon. The complexion is red with a sensation of Heat in the chest, palms and soles. The tongue body is cardinal red but relatively dark, not fresh. There is little or no coating and the tongue surface is dry and lacking moisture. Sometimes only the sides of the tongue and tip are cardinal red. This is an indication of Yin Deficiency, and Yin nourishing herbs should be used to control the exuberant Yang.

A more advanced situation is when the Stomach and Kidney Yin dry up. Here the Fluids are severely injured and the tongue surface is dark red, not fresh, and is shiny, like a mirror. It is usually thin, withered and shriveled. This can be seen in patients with diagnosed TB, advanced stages of AIDS or any autoconsumptive condition.

C. Cyanic or Purple Tongue body

There are two types of cyanic or purplish tongues. While both are an indication of stagnation of Blood and Qi, the blue color is more a sign of Cold stagnation while the purplish color is a sign of Heat stagnation. In view of the fact that TCM theory describes how a stagnation of Cold can change into Heat and vice versa, we see a close relationship between the blue and purplish colors on the tongue.

Tongue Coat

A. The White Tongue Coat

The white tongue coat can be differentiated into four types:

1. External Cold Type

This is seen in early-stage Wind-Cold disease. The coat is white, thin and moist and the tongue body is paler than normal. This is an indication of Cold invading and the patient should be given warming diaphoretic therapy.

2. External Heat Type

In early stage Wind-Heat disease the coating can also be white but somewhat thinner, dry and smooth. The tongue substance is red, indicating a not so serious invasion causing a Heat reaction. The patient is treated with cooling diaphoretics.

3. Stagnant Cold-Dampness type

The white coat is thick and filthy. It cannot be scraped off and its surface is Damp and smooth with a lot of saliva on it. This usually indicates Cold, Dampness with phlegm and food stagnation. Warming therapy is used to dry the Dampness and to help expectorate the Phlegm.

4. Excess Heat Type

The white coating is dry and fissured. It appears like white powder spread out over the entire tongue surface. It indicates the penetration of Evil Heat. It is a Yang Ming stage Heat where there is Dampness and Heat together. The patient should be given Heat clearing herbs, Damp dispelling diuretics and laxatives if there is constipation.

Individuals with a thin emaciated appearance, constipation, a thin rapid pulse and only a faint thin whitish-yellow coating would manifest Heat from the perspective of Yin Deficiency.

B. The Yellow Tongue Coat

A yellow coat indicates Heat, be it from Interior, Exterior, or Excess conditions. It can also represent Heat in the gastrointestinal tract or Stomach (Bright Yang level), or Heat Evil between Ying and Wei levels.

1. Exterior Type:

A pale yellow coating that is thin and white on the central surface of the tongue signifies that the disease is about to turn from Cold to Hot and from the Exterior to the Interior.

2. Damp Heat in the Middle Burner with stagnation of Qi:

The tongue coating is light yellow but thick and indicates Damp Heat and Qi stagnation in the Middle Warmer.

3. Damp Heat type:

The coating looks creamy, yellow and sticky with saliva. It may also appear dirty yellow, indicating long-standing retention of Damp Heat, usually in the Stomach and Intestines. Herbs which clear Dampness and Heat are used.

4. Heat injuring Fluids:

If the coating is dry and yellow, it reflects the presence of Heat which has injured the Body Fluids. Herbs which clear Heat and moisten Fluids are used.

C. Black Tongue Coat

A grayish or grayish-black coating represents a potentially serious disease. There are three basic types of black tongue coats:

1. High Fever, Yin-Wasting type

A Cold or Warm disease that is prolonged can penetrate to the Interior of the body where it transforms into Fire. The coat may first turn from white to yellow and finally to black. As the fever progresses it can look thorny, charred and cracked (fissured).

2. Deficient Yang and Cold Yin Type
The tongue substance is pale and the coating is thin, black and moist. It is not as black as the one with extreme fever. The tongue itself looks tender, slippery and moist. It represents Deficient Yang with extreme Cold.

3. Renal Depletion Type
The tongue coat is black and dry but not charred. The tongue body is relatively emaciated. It indicates an exhausted Kidney but without fever, and hence termed a Deficient Yin/insufficient Kidney Water type of person.

AUDITION AND SMELLING
The fourth method of diagnosis involves listening to the sounds and smelling the odors of the patient's body. This includes the voice, breathing, coughing, sighing, vomiting, hiccups and rumbling abdominal sounds. It also includes an awareness of general body odor, mouth and breath odors and any malodorous smell of various bodily discharges and excretions.

Voice: A strong, clear voice indicates a more Yang condition while a soft low voice is Yin. If the voice is loud and hollow sounding it indicates External Excess with Internal Deficiency. If it has a sing-song quality with noticeable rising and lowering of pitch it indicates Spleen imbalance. If it has a groaning or gravely quality it indicates depletion of the Kidney-adrenals. An overbearing or shouting sound indicates Liver Yang Excess. A weepy, sighing quality is Lung imbalance. An individual whose speech appears as if they are laughing indicates a Heart imbalance.

Breath: Loud, rapid, deep breathing indicates Excess or Yang. Soft, shallow breath suggests Deficiency or Yin. Breathing with the sound of mucus or Phlegm indicates upper respiratory congestion, possibly bronchitis or asthma.

Cough: One may have a dry or non-productive cough or a wet-productive cough.
1) **Wet cough**: This indicates External Damp Wind and is treated with **Minor Blue Dragon Combination** (Xiao qing long tang) if the mucus is thinner. If it is thicker then use **Minor Bupleurum Combination** (Xiao chai hu tang) for more Deficient type individuals,

or **Major Bupleurum Combination** (Da chai hu tang) for more Excess types.

An Ayurvedic formula for the whitish or thin mucus type is called Sito Paladi Churna. Western herbs include warming expectorants such as angelica root (Angelica archangelica) or lovage root (Ligusticum levisticum), osha (Ligusticum porteri), ginger root (Zingiber offincinale), hyssop (Hyssopus officinalis), wild ginger (Asarum canadensis), yerba santa (Eriodictyon spp.) and elecampane (Inula helinium). The same type of Western herbs are also used for wet cough with Deficiency, especially elecampane root. For accompanying Excess conditions, especially of Heat, one would use coltsfoot (Tussilago farfara) leaves and pleurisy root (Asclepias tuberosa). Lobelia (Lobelia inflata) is indicated for all types because it possesses expectorant, antispasmodic and stimulant properties.

2) **Dry cough**: This indicates Lung Yin Deficiency and is treated with **Ophiopogon Decoction** (Mai men dong tang).

Western herbalism would employ demulcent expectorants such as mullein leaf (Verbascum thapsus), chickweed (Stellaria media), American ginseng (Panax quinquefolium), marshmallow root (Althea officinalis), slippery elm (Ulmus fulva) and comfrey leaf or root (Symphytum officinalis). Herbs that specifically help to inhibit the cough reflex include apricot seed (Xing Ren), wild cherry bark (Prunus virginiana) and loquat leaves (Eriobotrya japonica).

3) **Yang cough**: Individuals who have a cough with a more Yang constitution would use **Minor Blue Dragon** (Xiao qing long tang) or **Minor Bupleurum Combination** (Xiao chai hu tang). Western herbs include Western coltsfoot (Tussilago farfara), pleurisy root (Asclepias tuberosa), marshmallow root (Althea officinalis), mullein leaf (Verbascum thapsus), comfrey leaf (Symphytum officinalis), wild cherry bark (Prunus virginiana) and slippery elm (Ulmus fulva).

4) **Yin cough**: Individuals who have a cough with a more Yin constitution would use **Ephedra and Asarum Combination** (Ma huang fu zi xi xin tang). Western herbs would contain a combination of ephedra (Ephedra species), wild ginger (Asarum canadensis), elecampane root (Inula helinium), fresh ginger (Zingiber officinale), honey and wild cherry bark (Prunus virginiana).

Vomiting: Loud vomiting represents an Excess, Yang conformation while weak vomiting is a more Yin conformation.

Abdominal rumbling sounds: Rumbling sounds in the abdomen indicates Coldness and Fluid in the gastrointestinal tract.

Body odors: A fragrant body odor suggests Spleen imbalance; a scorched or burnt odor is Heart; a rancid odor is Liver; a putrid (stale water) odor is the Kidneys; and a metallic odor is Lungs. All of these correspond to the Five Elements. In general a strong body or breath odor is Excess while a faint or unnoticeable odor is more Deficient.

PALPATION

Palpation is a diagnostic method used by the physician involving palpating or touching specific areas. The most important method included is pulse diagnosis, along with back and abdominal palpation of specific areas.

Pulse diagnosis

In ancient times, the pulse was taken at nine different areas on or near seven major arteries. The three acupuncture points on the head at the level of *Heaven* were Extra-point Taiyang and Triple warmer 21 on the temporal artery corresponding to the sides of the head, the ears and eyes respectively, and one on the facial artery, Stomach 3, corresponding to the teeth and mouth. The three at the wrist corresponding to the level of *Human* are Lung 9 on the radial artery corresponding to the Lungs, and Large Intestine 4, posteriorly between the index finger and thumb. The third corresponding to the chest was on Heart 7 located on the ulnar artery corresponding to the Heart. The three at the *Earth* level are pulses on Liver 3 and Liver 10 on the Dorsal artery corresponding to the Liver; pulses on Stomach 42 and Spleen 11 also on the Dorsal artery corresponding to the Spleen, and pulse on Kidney 3 on the Tibial artery corresponding to the Kidneys.

Sometime around the 6th century AD it became improper to touch women on various parts of the body. For this reason, the *Nan Jing* (Classic of Difficulties) first described studying the entire body with all the 12 major organs by solely reading the pulse of the radial artery of the wrist. Since that time, the pulse has been regarded as the most definitive indication of one's state of health and a directly palpable manifestation of a person's energy, capable of revealing past, present and future conditions as well as internal psycho-physiological states. Unlike other diagnostic criteria, the pulse is very reactive and reflects the most current state of the individual. As such, its use in traditional diagnosis is synonymous with the high degree of skill and sensitivity required to be a traditional physician.

For the Chinese people, pulse taking is so ingrained amongst the people that upon first contact with a physician, the patient automatically holds out his/her arm for a pulse reading. It is expected that a qualified physician, without any further questioning, would be able to tell the patient something that is relevant to their condition. Failing to do this, patients would have no faith in the doctor's qualifications. Nevertheless, despite its high regard in traditional cultures, in modern TCM the pulse is taken as being of secondary importance, with interrogation being primary.

An old common saying concerning the difficulty of learning pulse diagnosis is: "In the mind quite certain, under the finger unsure". The idea is to unite the knowledge of pulse taking with the actual process of feeling. It may be of some consolation to most beginners or less experienced practitioners that despite the fact that pulse diagnosis is such a distinctive aspect of TCM diagnosis, it is generally considered to be only about 40% reliable as a sole diagnostic method by most TCM practitioners. It is the experienced masters who are able to offer physiological and lifestyle guidance based strictly on their pulse reading. Then, of course, inadvertent observation of the patient's complexion, voice, manner, degree of warmth or coldness of the hand may also provide a great deal of information that is used to corroborate the findings on the pulse.

As mentioned in the section on tongue diagnosis, pulse diagnosis provides areas of primary consideration based on the overall quality of the pulse and secondary consideration based on specific qualities that may be noticeable in specific areas.

The Triple Warmer is still the model for corroborating Internal Organs to various locations on the wrist. The Upper Warmer with all its corresponding Organs includes the Heart and Lungs and is located on the radial artery pulses at the base of the wrist. The Middle Warmer corresponds to the Spleen, Stomach, Liver and Gall Bladder and is directly over the thenar prominence of the wrist in the middle position. The Lower Warmer Organs include the Kidneys, Bladder, Pericardium, Triple Warmer or Colon depending upon which system one uses, and is further up the wrist proximally behind the thenar prominence.

Method of pulse taking:

Three fingers are placed on three different positions called *cun, guan* and *chi*, respectively. At the base of the wrist with the index finger closest to the hand in the *cun* position, is the Upper Warmer, including the Heart on the left and the Lungs on the right wrist. The middle fingers over the thenar prominence in the *guan* position is the Middle Warmer with the Liver-Gall Bladder on the left and the Spleen-Stomach on the right wrist. The ring finger higher and just proximal to the thenar prominence is the *chi* position, and is the Lower Warmer with the Kidney-

Bladder on the left and the Triple Warmer-Pericardium on the right wrist. This last *chi* position on both wrists is usually interpreted as Kidney Yin on the left and Kidney Yang on the right.

Ideally the pulses are studied in the early morning. The practitioner should take about 15 minutes to study each wrist. The patient's wrist should be at a horizontal level to the heart. The breath of the practitioner and the patient should be as still as possible.

This latter recommendation has two functions. Traditionally, without a second hand on a watch, the speed of the pulse could only be measured by counting the number of beats per normal respiration of the patient. Less than four beats per complete respiration indicates a slow pulse, while more than five indicates a fast pulse. Another reason for stilling the mind is that pulse diagnosis is a subtle intuitive art requiring an empty, open and receptive mental state. The fact is that the best pulse diagnosticians combine a balance of rational observation with intuitive thought processes.

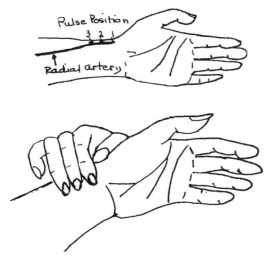

Most individuals are able to discern six relatively easily verifiable qualities which form the basis for pulse study. Following are the six basic pulse qualities:

1. **Weak or empty pulse:** An empty pulse may feel rather big but soft or empty upon slightly stronger pressure. This type of pulse signifies Deficient Qi. A weak pulse can also feel thin or thready which signifies Deficient Blood.

2. **Full pulse:** This pulse feels full, big, rather hard and long. If the pulse

is full and rapid, it represent Excess Heat, if it is full and slow, it indicates Excess Cold.

3. Slow=cold: Less than four beats per complete respiration of the patient or less than 60 beats a minute, a slow and empty pulse indicates Empty-Cold from Deficient Yang, while a slow and full pulse indicates Full-Cold from Excess Yin.

4. Fast=Heat: More than 5 beats per respiration of the patient or 80 or more beats per minute, surface or floating indicates Exterior or acute disease or in rarer cases, it will appear as floating for Internal Deficient conditions such as anemia, cancer or Yin-wasting diseases. This pulse is felt with a light pressure of the fingers, just resting on the artery.

5. Deep pulse: This pulse requires a deeper pressure to discern. It must be felt with a heavy pressure of the fingers close to the bone. A deep and weak pulse indicates Deficiency of Qi and Yang; a deep and full pulse indicates stagnation of Qi or Blood in the Interior, or Internal Cold or Heat.

6. Floating or superficial pulse: This is opposite of the one previous. The pulse is felt with a light pressure of the fingers just resting on the artery. A floating pulse indicates a surface condition or in chronic disease, an exhaustion of the Internal (Yin) Organs. A floating and fast pulse indicates surface Heat while a floating, slow pulse indicates surface Cold. Most often a floating pulse indicates a superficial acute condition such as a cold, cough or flu.

Treatment: If the pulse feels weak and Deficient, one would not use eliminative or strong Heat clearing herbs but rather, would emphasize the use of tonics. If it feels strong and full, one would prescribe some type of clearing or eliminative strategy. If it feels slow which signifies Cold, one would prescribe warming and stimulating herbs; if fast, cooling and sedating remedies. If it is floating, one would use some type of surface-relieving diaphoretic herbs. If the pulse feels floating and slow one would prescribe warming and stimulating diaphoretics such as cayenne pepper or ginger, for instance. If it is floating and fast, one might give relaxing diaphoretics such as lemon balm or catnip to relieve the External condition. If it is floating at the superficial level but empty at the deep level, it indicates Yin Deficiency and would require Yin-nutritive tonics. If the pulse is deep, one would treat Internal Organ conditions. If deep and weak, it is a Deficiency of Qi and Yang and would require tonics. If it is deep and full, it indicates stagnation of Qi and Blood, and one would use emmenagogue herbs and foods that would promote Blood circulation, or carminative herbs to promote Qi circulation.

Summary of the various pulse qualities

The 6 categories of pulse types can be further subdivided into specific quality types comprising 28 different pulse types altogether:

Floating pulse category

Floating – Is felt on the surface of the body. It is felt by slightly pressing down, and the pulse disappears when pressed deeper. It is an indication of an External condition. Learn this pulse by studying the pulse of an individual with a cold or flu.

Flooding – Floating with great strength on the surface. It enters strongly and exits gradually. It indicates acute hypertension. Learn to recognize this pulse by studying the pulse of an individual with acute hypertension or anger.

Big pulse – A large pulse without the excessive force of the flooding pulse. It can represent either Excess Heat or extreme Deficiency (especially in the aged).

Leekstalk – Floating and big on the surface but hollow upon depression. This indicates blood loss and Spleen Yang Deficiency. Learn this pulse by studying someone who has experienced recent acute blood loss.

Soft – The pulse feels floating, soft and thready and indicates Deficiency and weakness.

Leathery – The pulse feels like striking a stick against a soft drum head. It represents chronic loss of blood and sperm. Feel this pulse in a woman who has recently experienced excessive and prolonged bleeding either from menorrhagia or childbirth.

Bowstring pulse – This pulse is in the category of External or floating and feels tense and taut like the string of a guitar. It is associated with nervous tension, Liver Wind and depression. The best way to learn this pulse is to find someone who is extremely nervous and agitated and feel the pulse at the middle position of their left wrist.

Deep pulse category
Sinking – This pulse is only felt by heavy palpation. It represents an Internal Yin condition or Qi stagnation.

Deep pulse – One must depress deeper than average to find the pulse, nearly to the bone. It represents Coldness. Feel this pulse on a thin, timid, cold and pale individual. It will be very similar to the following latent pulse but easier to find.

Latent or hidden pulse – The pulse is difficult to find. One must push aside the ligaments and reach to the bone. This represents Internal collapse or extreme pain.

Prison or taut pulse – It feels deep, full, big and long. It represents Excess Yin with severe Fluid accumulation. Feel this pulse on an edemic, obese individual.

Slow pulse category
Slow pulse – The pulse is 60 beats or less per minute, or only 3 beats for one complete respiration of the patient. It represents Yang Deficiency with Internal Coldness.

Leisurely or relaxed pulse – The pulse is close to 60 beats per minute, or 4 beats for one complete respiration of the patient. It is mostly a quality of slowness. It may be normal, or it could also indicate Dampness depending on other qualities.

Choppy or astringent pulse – This is in the category of a slow, small pulse. It feels rough and astringent. It is described like a knife scraping against bamboo. It indicates blood loss, Deficient Qi or stagnant Qi and Blood. Learn to differentiate this pulse by feeling someone's pulse who has recently experienced traumatic blood loss.

Knotted pulse – The pulse is slow with occasional interruption. It indicates Blood, Qi or Fluid Stagnation. Learn to differentiate this pulse between the uneven or replacement pulse with regular interruptions and the accelerated pulse that is rapid with irregular stops.

Uneven or replacement pulse – This is a slower pulse with regular interruptions. It indicates more serious degeneration or feebleness.

Rapid pulse category

Fast pulse – 80 beats or more per minute, or 6 beats or more for each complete respiration of the patient. It represents Heat, fever and/or inflammation. Learn to recognize this pulse by studying the pulse of an individual who has a high fever.

Agitated pulse – This pulse is faster than the previous, faster than 80 beats per minute, or 7-8 beats for each complete respiration of the patient. This is a condition of Yang and Yin collapse.

Accelerated pulse – This is a rapid pulse with occasional irregular interruptions. It represents Yang Stagnation with Stagnation of Qi, Blood, Phlegm or Food.

Tight pulse – The pulse feels tense, like a rope. The difference between this and the Bowstring pulse is that the Tight pulse can move from left to right while the bowstring pulse can't. It indicates Coldness and severe pain. Learn to recognize this pulse by studying the pulse of an individual who is experiencing severe pain.

Deficient pulse category

Deficient pulse – Weak and Deficient at both the superficial and the deep levels. It is difficult to find. It indicates Deficiency of Qi, Blood or Yang.

Scattered pulse – The pulse feels confused and floating, lacking a clear point of entry or exit and easily disappearing under palpation. It is an indication of dissolving of Original Qi. It is associated with an individual who is near death.

Diminutive or feeble pulse – The diameter of the artery is extremely thin and thready. It is differentiated from the thready pulse in that it is nearly imperceptible. It indicates a serious Yang, Qi and Blood Deficiency.

Weak pulse – This pulse is small, deep and weak. It represents prolonged illness causing Qi, Blood and Yang Deficiency. Feel this pulse on an individual who is thin, highly sensitive, has multiple allergies and easily gets sick.

Thready or small pulse – Extremely thin and thready, like a silk thread. It represents Blood and Qi Deficiency with frequent urination. Feel this pulse on an individual who is pale, hypersensitive, shy, and soft spoken with chronic fatigue.

Excess pulse category
Short pulse – The pulse feels strong in the middle position and weaker, if it can be felt at all, in the first and third positions. It represents an Excess condition. Feel this pulse in a forceful, heavy set and aggressive individual.

Long pulse – This pulse is so strong that it extends beyond the three positions. It indicates severe Excess Heat. Feel this pulse in a strong, heavy set, loud voiced, constipated individual.

Slippery or Damp pulse – This pulse feels smooth and gliding. The Chinese liken it to feeling pearls in a porcelain basin. It is an important pulse for diagnosing Dampness, mucus and edema. The best way to learn to recognize this pulse is to find someone who obviously has edema, a lot of mucus or a pregnant woman. Especially notice this pulse in the deeper middle position of the right wrist.

Ayurvedic Pulse Diagnosis
Ayurvedic medicine correlates the pulse with Tridosha, or the Three Humours. The pulse on the wrist closest to the hand, taken by the index finger of the physician, corresponds to the Vata-air, or nerve oriented humour; the middle position is taken with the middle finger and corresponds to the Pitta-fire, or digestive and circulatory humour; while the third position, taken with the ring finger, corresponds to the Kapha-fluid or bodily substance humour.

The individual qualities of the pulse are described as different animals. A Vata, or air predominant pulse, is compared with the movement of a snake or leech. Usually this pulse feels faster and indicates indigestion, nervous problems, and fever, for instance. In Chinese medicine it might be classified as Yin Deficient. A Pitta, or fire predominant pulse, is described as resembling the jerky movement of a frog, sparrow or crow. Since these represent a jerky or jumpy movement, it can indicate insomnia, diarrhea, vertigo, hypertension, Heat of the skin, palms, soles and burning eyes. A Kapha, or water predominant pulse, is described as the movement of a swan, cock or peacock. This is generally a slow pulse and indicates the presence of phlegm coughs, a melancholic disposition and other Damp conditions.

Western Pulse Diagnosis:
Western medical diagnosis also recognizes various pulse indications that correlate with disease factors. For instance, a fast pulse indicates fever or inflammation; a slow pulse indicates inaction or a weak digestion; and a small or weak pulse indicates general debility and possible anemia. There are literally dozens of other pulse indications that once were part of the medical doctor's training and are seldom used today in modern clinical practice, except for the speed of the pulse.

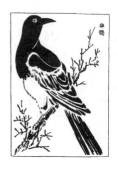

TEN

PATTERNS OF
DISHARMONY

QI, BLOOD, FLUIDS, ESSENCE, YIN AND YANG

When determining how to treat illnesses in TCM, the practitioner looks at all the signs and symptoms experienced by the person and then identifies their corresponding patterns. The patterns are then treated rather than the disease itself, using acupuncture, herbs and other therapies. These patterns may or may not correspond to specific Western diseases. For example, a stuffy nose, sneezing, coughing, fever and chills fits the Western definition of a cold. However, in TCM, this same illness can be identified by different patterns, depending on the specific traits of each symptom. For instance, if the coughing involves yellow mucus, the fever is high and chills slight, the resulting pattern is Invasion of the Lungs by Wind Heat. If the coughing involves clear watery mucus, the fever is slight but the chills are pronounced, then the pattern is Invasion of the Lungs by Wind Cold. The acupuncture and herbal treatment for each condition is thus different. Therefore, rather than treating diseases per se, TCM further refines the symptoms being presented to identify a specific pattern, so more accurate treatment can then be given.

For example, a patient presenting with recurring headaches may think nothing of their experience of stomach upset. The stomach discomfort comes and goes, but the headaches are more bothersome, and so this is what she wants corrected. In TCM, the symptoms of headache and stomach upset are connected and form a pattern that, when treated, eliminates the stomach problem along with the headaches.

Another person might complain of headaches, yet when questioned reveal he is also periodically dizzy, has frequent low back pain and sometimes sweats at night. Again, all symptoms taken together form a pattern, and in this case, it is a different one from the first type of headache. A different approach is then taken with this type of headache than with the first, and the symptoms experienced other than the headache clear up with the appropriate treatment.

The patterns of disharmony are determined by matching the signs and symptoms presented with those of the Pernicious Influences, Qi, Blood, Yin, Yang and the Organs. Each of these has its own particular qualities which define it according to its functions. Perhaps the easiest way to learn these patterns is to first learn the individual functions of each of these aspects in the body. Then it is possible to "overlay" or combine them in all the various ways possible. Breaking it down into the various components and their functions makes it much easier to understand and recognize how they all inter-relate and combine together.

Let's look at a few examples. Weakness and tiredness indicate a Deficiency of Qi, while frequent copious urination and low back pain indicate the Kidneys are involved. Put together, it forms the pattern of Deficient Kidney Qi. As another example, a sensation of heaviness in the body, sluggishness and a discharge which is copious and cloudy indicate the presence of Dampness. Frequently feeling cold, copious discharge and loose stools signal there is also Cold in the body. These two categories combined with the further symptoms of lack of appetite, sweetish taste in the mouth, stuffiness in the chest and epigastrium, all aspects signaling the involvement of the Spleen. This defines the pattern of Cold-Damp invading the Spleen.

When determining which categories are involved in a given condition, there need to be three or more symptoms from a category for it to be indicated. Several symptoms appear in more than one category, so more signs need to be present from that same category to signal its involvement. For instance, a headache is one sign of an External Pernicious Influence pattern and one sign of the Excess Liver Yang pattern. If it is an External Pernicious Influence invading, there will also be chills and fever, sudden onset and a floating pulse. If it is Excess Liver Yang, there will also be signs of dizziness, red face and eyes, thirst, dream-disturbed sleep and/or a full, wiry and rapid pulse.

The following patterns are first described individually according to Pernicious Influences, Qi, Blood, Yin, Yang, and Organs, and are then combined to form the traditional patterns of disharmony, described in the next chapter, Differential Diagnosis. The herb formulas listed are not the only possibilities, but represent the most common ones used.

QI DISHARMONIES

Several pathologies of Qi exist and involve either insufficient Qi (Deficiency conditions) or stagnant Qi (Excess conditions), in which Qi is either flowing improperly or is impeded. Qi may be Deficient or

Stagnant throughout the body, but usually is associated with specific organs. While we may speak of Qi as being in Excess or Deficiency, this is only apparent as a result of its inability to transform or evolve through a given circumstance. Thus, excess Qi is really a manifestation of Stagnation, while Deficient Qi represents an inability to adequately respond to specific conditions.

Qi changes form according to its locality and its function. A derangement of Qi will thus appear differently according to where it is found and what its function is. However, the overall characteristics of Qi remain the same. The following are the various pathologies of Qi found in the body.

Deficient Qi

When Qi is Deficient, it generally appears as tiredness or weakness in the body. Because Qi is lacking, it is unable to perform any of its functions. This may apply to any of the different types of Qi, including that of the Organs. For instance, if defensive Qi is insufficient, the person may be prone to frequent colds and flu and spontaneous sweating. If Spleen Qi is Deficient, the uterus or bladder may prolapse or the appetite may be poor and digestion sluggish. A Deficiency of the Qi of the Kidneys may cause them to be unable to regulate water, causing edema, frequent urination or resulting in incontinence.

The following signs of Qi Deficiency include several of the possible ways in which this may manifest. Some of these signs may be from different causes; for example, loose stools can be from Dampness. The overall differentiating symptoms for Qi Deficiency, however, is that there will be accompanying tiredness and weakness as well.

Symptoms:
general weakness, lethargy
low, soft voice
tiredness, listlessness
dislike of talking or speaking
spontaneous sweating
frequent colds and flu
daytime sweating
frequent urination
shallow respiration
palpitations
pale bright face that is puffy or bloated
weak cough
prolonged menses with a very light flow
weakness of limbs
amenorrhea
excessive bleeding with light blood

dislike of movement
shortness of breath
spermatorrhea
loose stools
Pulse: empty, frail, weak
Tongue: pale body

Herbal Categories and Formulas: Tonify Qi herbs
Four Major Herbs Decoction (Si jun zi tang)
Six Major Herbs (Liu jun zi tang)

Sinking or Collapsed Qi

Another form of Qi Deficiency, the weakened Qi in this case is unable to perform its holding function, resulting in a prolapse of the organs. This function mostly applies to the Qi of the Spleen.

Symptoms:
prolapse of uterus, bladder, stomach, kidneys, anus
bearing down sensation in abdomen
piles or certain types of hemorrhoids
extreme chronic diarrhea
urinary frequency, urgency or incontinence

Herbal Categories and Formulas: Tonify Qi and regulate Qi herbs
Ginseng and Astragalus Combination (Bu zhong yi qi tang)

Stagnant Qi

If the flow of Qi is impeded in any way, it becomes stuck or stagnant. This can be likened to a traffic jam on the freeway. In this case, Qi does not flow smoothly or evenly. It can then lead to impairment of any of the Organs. When Qi is stagnant in the limbs or in the meridians of the body, aches and pains may result. Tonification is contra-indicated in this case; it would be adding more cars to the traffic jam. Instead, Qi moving or regulating therapy is required.

Stagnant Qi is an Excess condition. When Qi is Stagnant it can lead to other types of Stagnation such as Blood, Fluids or food Stagnation. Likewise, poor circulation can result in Qi condensing and stagnating, resulting in lumps, physical masses or tumors. In a Qi Stagnation condition, the person is usually not tired as in Qi Deficiency, but may be "stuck", frustrated or easily irritated.

Symptoms:
distention in the ribs and abdomen
fluctuating emotions or mental state; depression; moodiness

distention, soreness and pain which change in severity and
location
soft palpable lumps
frequent sighing
a sensation of tightness around ribs or chest
lump in the throat
irregular menses
swelling of breasts during menses
Pulse: wiry or tight
Tongue: dark, or purplish tinge to tongue body

Herbal Categories and Formulas: Regulate Qi herbs
Bupleurum and Peony Combination (Xiao yao wan)
Disperse Vital Energy in the Liver Powder (Chai hu su gan san)

Rebellious Qi

An Excess condition, rebellious Qi is another form of Qi Stagnation.
In this case, Qi flows in the wrong direction. For instance, if the normal
downward flow of Stomach Qi is disrupted and it goes upward instead,
nausea, vomiting, belching or hiccuping may result. The following signs
may indicate rebellious Qi; however, some may be from other causes.
For instance, nausea may also be due to food Stagnation or Damp
Stagnation in the epigastrium. If so, other signs of food Stagnation or
Dampness will be present.

> **Symptoms:**
> hiccuping
> belching
> nausea
> vomiting
> some forms of coughing
> some forms of asthma

Herbal Categories and Formulas: Regulate Qi Herbs
Inula Flower and Hematite Decoction (Xuan fu dai zhe tang)

BLOOD DISHARMONIES

There are three basic categories of Blood pathologies. These are
Blood Deficiency, Blood Heat and Blood Stagnation. In the first, there
is insufficient Blood to nourish and moisten the body. This usually
occurs with the Organs with which it has special relationships and
includes, among many other things, anemia and circulatory problems.
In the second, too much Heat in the body, usually in the Liver, causes
Heat in the Blood and pushes it out of the vessels. Varicose veins or
hemorrhage can result. Extravasated blood with congealment in the
capillaries, abdomen or pelvis can cause a variety of symptoms including

edema, obesity, menstrual pains and bluish or purplish discoloration on the surface of the skin or tongue. Stagnation occurs from Blood moving improperly due to Coldness, Heat or Stagnation of Qi. Circulatory problems, pelvic pains and menstrual problems can occur. Blood tonic herbs are used to treat Deficient Blood and anemic syndromes. Usually these also have some Blood invigorating properties as well. For Heat in the Blood, herbs that clear Heat out of the Blood, hemostatic herbs, or herbs that stop bleeding are given. When there is Blood Stagnation, Blood moving, Blood invigorating or Blood tonic herbs are used. Blood moving herbs and formulas can be either warm or cool and are classified as emmenagogues (any substance that specifically is used to promote menstruation) in Western herbalism. More broadly useful, Chinese herbalism classifies these emmenagogue herbs as "herbs that invigorate or regulate Blood".

Deficient Blood
A Deficiency of Blood occurs when the entire body or a particular Organ or other body part is insufficiently nourished by Blood. This can be caused by a loss of blood, insufficient Spleen Qi to produce Blood, or congealed Blood which prevents new Blood from forming. Since Blood is part of Yin, a long term Deficiency of Blood gives rise to dryness, causing dry skin and hair. The Organs most likely to be affected by Deficient Blood include the Heart, Spleen and Liver.

Symptoms:
dizziness
scanty menses or amenorrhea
thin, emaciated body
spots in the visual field; impaired vision
numb limbs
weak tremors in the limbs
dry skin, hair or eyes
lusterless, pale face and lips
depression
tiredness
poor memory
insomnia
Pulse: thin, fine or choppy
Tongue: pale, thin body

Herbal Categories and Formulas: Tonify Blood herbs
Dang Gui Four (Si wu tang)

Blood Stagnation

Blood Stagnation is one of the most important diagnostic conditions in Chinese Medicine because it is frequently the cause of intractable pain syndromes anywhere in the body. Stagnant Blood results in a fixed stabbing pain, whereas stagnant Qi tends to move and change locations and intensity of sensation. Blood invigorating or Qi regulating herbs are used separately or together for these conditions. Other symptoms of Blood Stagnation can include traumatic swelling, difficult pregnancy and impairment of ovarian function. Patients may have a ruddy complexion, blotchy skin, increase in skin capillaries, coarseness of the skin and peri-oral and/or peri-orbital bluish discoloration.

The causes for Stagnant Blood conditions can include:

1) heredity
2) childbirth, abortion, miscarriage and menopause
3) gynecological diseases
4) fevers
5) injuries
6) circulatory disorders (stagnant Qi)
7) Liver disorders (Liver stores the Blood)
8) Spleen disorders (Spleen maintains Blood in the vessels)
9) chronic inflammation and infections
10) excessive lipids
11) hormone imbalance
12) trauma or injuries such as bruises, sprains and swelling
13) Deficiency of Qi
14) Heat in the Blood
15) Internal Coldness
16) Blood Deficiency

Blood Stagnation is a condition of toxicity which can include lower abdominal pains as well as itchy scalp, shoulder stiffness, dizziness, feelings of chills in the waist, numbness, and dry mouth. There may be a feeling of abdominal fullness, even when there isn't any, especially in women before menses. Portions of the body can feel feverish, an outbreak of goose bumps, dryness, red spots and varicosities appear on the skin; the tongue may exhibit a purplish cast especially noticeable on the sides, and there may be a tendency to bleed.

Acute lower abdominal pain is a primary symptom of Blood Stagnation. To determine this, have the patient lie on his or her back with legs flexed, then rather gently at first, palpate the lower abdomen below the umbilicus, especially the left and right sides (over the ovaries in women). If there is severe Blood Stagnation, the patient will usually feel pain upon palpation. Milder Stagnation may result in lumps or swelling in the area.

Two rhubarb-containing formulas (rhubarb is a laxative-astringent) are frequently indicated for Blood Stagnation and are of particular interest because their indications are predominantly for either right or left sided pelvic pains. Symptoms of Blood Stagnation that occur at the lower left quadrant of the pelvis could represent intestinal blockage, fibroids or cysts for which **Persica and Rhubarb Combination** (Tao he cheng qi tang) is used. Similar conditions involving ileocaecal valve, appendicitis, and cysts and fibroids respond better to **Rhubarb and Moutan Combination** (Da huang mu dan pi tang). Both formulas are commonly indicated and quite often are effective for endometriosis, regardless of whether or not there is normal or loose bowels.

> **Symptoms:**
> fixed, stabbing or boring pain
> lumps
> hard, relatively immobile masses
> recurring, frequent hemorrhages
> clots of a dark, purple tinge
> dark colored blood
> a dark complexion
> purple lips, nails
> tremors
> swelling of the Organs
> **Pulse**: choppy, wiry or firm
> **Tongue**: dark purple tongue material with red spots

Herbal Categories and Herbs: Regulate and vitalize Blood herbs
Persica and Rhubarb Combination (Tao he cheng qi tang)
Rhubarb and Moutan Combination (Da huang mu dan pi tang)
Cinnamon and Poria Combination (Gui zhi fu ling wan)

Heat in the Blood
Heat in the Blood may be from Excess or Deficiency. If Excess, it is often caused by a Heat Pernicious Influence that has invaded deep inside the body and agitated the Blood, making it "reckless". Too much Heat in the Blood pushes it out of its pathways and causes bleeding, somewhat like a boiling volcano erupting. Thus its major symptom is bleeding. The blood will be fresh red or dark colored, with a heavy loss of blood. Stagnation of Blood can also cause Heat in the Blood and consequent bleeding. The Blood in this case will be very dark colored with clots.

Another cause of Heat in the Blood may be from Yin Deficiency, in which case the bleeding is scanty and bright-red in color. Note that bleeding can also be caused by the Qi unable to hold the Blood in its pathways. This is not caused by Heat in the Blood, but because the Qi is weak and cannot perform its holding function. The blood will be pale in this case, with prolonged bleeding and heavy loss of blood.

Symptoms:
blood in the sputum, stools, urine, or vomiting of blood
coughing up blood
bloody nose
excessive menses
red skin eruptions
Pulse: rapid
Tongue: scarlet red
Note: Other Heat signs may be present such as thirst, irritability, feeling of heat, dry mouth and, in extreme cases, delirium

Herbal Categories and Formulas: Clear heat from the Blood herbs **Rhinoceros and Rehmannia Combination** (Xi jiao di huang tang)

FLUID DISHARMONIES

The categories of Fluid imbalances include Deficiency of Fluids, Edema, and the Phlegm patterns. A Deficiency of Fluids can cause Yin Deficiency, and Yin Deficiency can cause a lack of Fluids. It may also be caused by heavy or prolonged diarrhea, vomiting, sweating and bleeding. A Fluid Deficiency mostly affects the Lungs, Stomach, Kidneys and Large Intestine.

Edema is caused by Spleen Qi Deficiency and may also involve Lung or Kidney Qi deficiency, since all three are involved in the transformation, transportation and excretion of Fluids. Edema from Lung Qi Deficiency mostly appears in the Upper Warmer, while that from the Spleen occurs in the Middle Warmer and from the Kidneys in the Lower Warmer.

Substantial Phlegm occurs mainly in the Lungs. Non-substantial Phlegm can appear in the channels, joints and under the skin, causing lumps, nodules, numbness and bone deformities. It can also appear in the head, Stomach or Lungs, or obstruct certain Organs, such as the orifices of the Heart, the Kidneys or Gall-Bladder where it forms stones. It can also appear with Wind, Heat, Cold Damp and Qi Stagnation.

Deficiency of Fluids Symptoms:
dry, rough, chapped or cracked skin
dry throat, nose, mouth, lips

dry cough with little phlegm
dry stools
dehydration
unusual thirst
Pulse: thready, hesitant
Tongue: dry with no saliva

Herbal Categories and Formulas: Moisten Dryness, Blood and
Yin tonic herbs and formulas, some herbs that clear Heat from the
Blood, demulcents, emollients
Apricot Seed and Perilla Formula (Xing su san)
Lily Bulb Decoction to Consolidate the Lungs (Bai he gu jin
tang)
Ophiopogon and Trichosanthes Combination
(Mai men dong yin si)
Scrophularia and Ophiopogon Combination (Zeng ye tang)

> **Edema Symptoms:**
> edema of hands and face (usually from Lung Qi Deficiency)
> edema of the abdomen (usually from Spleen Qi Deficiency)
> edema of the legs and ankles (usually from Kidney Qi
> Deficiency)

> **Phlegm Symptoms:**
> Phlegm
> lumps
> nodules
> thick greasy secretions
> tumors
> delirium
> numbness in limbs
> **Pulse:** slippery
> **Tongue:** greasy, thick coating

> **Phlegm in Lungs Symptoms:**
> asthma
> cough with heavy expectoration of mucus

> **Phlegm Misting the Heart Symptoms:**
> chaotic or erratic behavior
> madness
> muddled thought
> stupor
> coma
> rattle in throat
> schizophrenia
> manic-depression
> epilepsy

Phlegm in Kidneys or Gall-Bladder Symptoms:
stones in Kidneys or Gall-Bladder

Phlegm in Meridians Symptoms:
numbness
paralysis
soft, mobile tumors, nodules or swellings

Phlegm Under the Skin Symptoms:
lumps under the skin
nerve-ganglia swellings
lymph node swelling
swollen thyroid
some fibroids and lipomas

Phlegm in the Joints Symptoms:
bone deformities with arthritis and rheumatoid arthritis
heaviness or achiness in the joints or limbs
numbness of the muscles and skin

Wind-Phlegm Symptoms:
dizziness
nausea
vomiting
aphasia
coughing of phlegm
rattling sound in throat
numbness of limbs

Phlegm-Heat Symptoms:
red face
restlessness
yellow-sticky phlegm
dry mouth and lips
Pulse: rapid and slippery
Tongue: red body with sticky-yellow coat

Phlegm-Cold Symptoms:
white-watery phlegm
nausea
cold feeling in limbs and back
Pulse: deep, slippery, slow
Tongue: pale body, white-wet coat

Qi Phlegm Symptoms:
(often called "plum-stone" or "plum-pit" syndrome)
stuffiness of chest and diaphragm
difficulty in swallowing
feeling of a lump in the throat which comes and goes, especially
with emotional swings

Phlegm-Fluids Symptoms:

This is very similar to Dampness and is very watery and thin. It can be heard splashing in the body, found usually in the Stomach, Intestines, hypochondrium, limbs or above the diaphragm.

Phlegm-Fluids In Stomach and Intestines Symptoms:
abdominal fullness and distention
vomiting of watery fluids
no desire to drink
splashing sound in the stomach
feeling of fullness of the chest
loose stools
loss of weight
Pulse: deep, slippery
Tongue: swollen with sticky coating

Phlegm-Fluids in Hypochondrium Symptoms:
hypochondriac pain, worse when coughing and breathing
feeling of distention of hypochondrium
shortness of breath
Pulse: deep, wiry
Tongue: sticky coating

Phlegm-Fluids in the Limbs Symptoms:
heaviness of the body
pain in the muscles
no sweating
no desire to drink
cough with abundant-white sputum
Pulse: wiry or tight
Tongue: sticky, white coat

Phlegm-Fluids above Diaphragm Symptoms:
cough
asthma
edema
dizziness
copious white sputum
Pulse: wiry
Tongue: thick, white coat

Herbal Categories and Formulas: Herbs that remove Dampness, diuretics, warming stimulants for Cold Dampness, Qi and Yang tonics for Dampness caused by Deficiency, herbs that remove Damp Heat for Hot Dampness are employed.

Citrus and Pinellia Combination (Er chen tang) and variations
Bamboo and Poria Combination (Wen dan tang)
Poria Five Herbs (Wu ling san)

ESSENCE DISHARMONIES

Pathologies of Essence result from either injured Pre-Heaven Essence resulting in a weak inherited constitution, or from damaged Post-Heaven Essence occurring from improper diet or lifestyle activities. The natural decline of old age also shows signs of Essence Deficiency. The inherited Pre-Heaven Essence problems represent inherited deficiencies and tendencies that can, at best, only be managed. However, we can greatly influence what happens to our Post-Heaven Essence.

The injury of Post-Heaven Essence may begin during fetal growth or afterwards if impure air, food or water combines with overly stressful, imbalanced living to injure the depth of our being. Problems that result from fetal injury may be caused by impure foods, alcohol, tobacco, recreational drugs and certain prescription drugs taken by the mother during gestation. Consider the health effects on babies who are born addicted to drugs, such as heroin or cocaine, or the significantly higher cancer risks we have seen in women whose mothers took the prescription drug thalidomide, widely prescribed by medical doctors during the sixties. Are we to assume that the only damage caused by these drugs taken during fetal development is the increased risk of birth defects, or might we also suspect a correlation with the many individuals who suffer a lifetime with a compromised immune system, battling fatigue and multiple susceptibilities to environmental and food allergies?

Essence can also be depleted by an improper diet, excessive abuse of alcohol, tobacco, sugar and other drugs, excessive sex, "burning the candle at both ends", overwork, stress and insufficient rest or sleep. These injuries from longer, more protracted abuse and stress may, with great persistence and difficulty, improve over time. However, they necessitate changes in diet and lifestyle and, in such instances, herbal and other natural therapies may offer a safer, less invasive means of management, avoiding the long term risks and side effects caused by most synthetic drugs.

Another option is to use herbs to optimize and minimize drugs, such as using herbs to increase blood circulation to optimize the effects of chemotherapy, or Fu Zheng employing immune-potentiating herbs to protect the immune system to minimize the negative effects of drug treatment. This approach offers the potential to greatly decrease risks, especially if the use of the herbs can bring about an ultimate reduction in the required drug dosage.

Because Essence is a part of Yin and Yang, symptoms of Essence Deficiency often present with a Deficiency of Kidney Yin and/or Kidney Yang. If there is a lack of Kidney Yin, there also may be premature ejaculation, insufficient vaginal secretions, tinnitus, dizziness or other Kidney Yin Deficiency signs, since the Yin is not holding the Yang. If there is an accompanying Deficiency of Kidney Yang, there may be impotence, coldness or other Kidney Yang Deficiency signs, since the Yang is not holding the Yin.

Essence Deficiency - in Children - Symptoms:
improper or poor bone development
late or incomplete fontanel closure
mental dullness or retardation
premature aging
slow physical development

Essence Deficiency - in Adults - Symptoms:
premature aging
senility
bad or loose teeth
poor memory or concentration
brittle or softening of bones
weakness of knees and legs
falling of hair
premature graying of hair
low libido or impotence
habitual miscarriage or infertility
constantly prone to colds, flu or other External diseases
wasting of flesh
Pulse: floating and empty; sometimes deep and nearly non-existent in the rear position
Tongue: red and peeled

Herbal Categories and Formulas: Qi, Blood and Yin tonics
Minor Cinnamon and Paeonia Combination (Xiao jian zhong tang)
Achyranthes and Rehmannia Combination (Restore the Left Pill - Zuo gui wan)

YIN DISHARMONIES

The two major Yin disharmonies are Excess Yin and Deficient Yin, with a rarely seen pattern of collapse of Yin. Yin includes all the substance and Fluids in the body. It cools, moistens, nourishes and gives form to all the bodily processes. Excess Yin occurs when too much Coldness and Dampness collect in the body, while Deficiency arises from a lack of cooling moisture, giving rise to superficial Heat signs.

Excess Yin

Excess Yin is a Full Yin state. Its signs are similar to those of the Cold and Damp Heat Pernicious Influences. When Yin becomes Excess, there is a condition of surplus Fluids that have built up in the body. They may collect throughout the body, giving a general appearance of swelling and heaviness, or they may accumulate in a particular area of the body, as in the abdomen causing nausea and vomiting, or the Lungs, resulting in cough with copious mucus. Because Yin is cooling in nature, and since the excessive occurrence of Yin causes the Yang fires to be extinguished, an Excess of Yin frequently gives rise to Cold symptoms similar to Yang Deficiency.

Yin Excess arises from over-exposure to cold or hot damp environments and climates, the Stagnation and obstruction of pathogenic Cold inside so that Yang is unable to balance Yin, Dampness stagnating and turning to Heat, and underactivity. It especially occurs with over-eating, and the excessive consumption of cold, damp foods, such as salads, fruits, juices, raw foods, iced drinks and frozen items such as ice cream and frozen yogurt, refined foods, flour products, and hot greasy foods such as fried red meats.

Symptoms:
lack of thirst
forceful but slow movements
dampness
epigastric pain aggravated with pressure
loose stools
clear or turbid and abundant urination
feelings of heaviness, pressure or oppression
abdominal distention
nausea
edema
heavy vaginal discharge
poor appetite
pain is worse with pressure, but relieved by warmth
Pulse: full, slippery, tight or wiry, but strong
Tongue: Pale with white, wet and/or creamy thick coat

Herbal Categories and Formulas: Dampness removing herbs (diuretics)
Poria Five Herb Combination (Wu ling san)
Five Peel Powder (Wu pi yin)

Deficient Yin
When Yin is Deficient the cooling, moistening and nurturing aspects of the body are lacking. This gives rise to Dryness and Heat accompanied by weakness and lack of strength and resistance. Because Yin is lacking, it cannot control Yang, so the Heat of the Yang becomes more apparent. Water cannot control Fire so it gets out of hand. Heat signs arising from

this are called empty-Heat, or false Heat, because they are not from a true Excess Yang condition. The result is signs of Heat, but without the strength of Yang.

For instance, there may be fever, but it would only appear in the afternoon; the sensation of Heat in the body only occurs in the palms and soles and chest region; the person may talk rapidly, but cannot sustain it, or the Heat spurts come and go, with an apparent underlying weakness and Deficiency. Because Yin is abundant at night, signs of Yin Deficiency especially appear then, such as night sweats, dry throat and insomnia, or at its opposite time of greatest decrease, the afternoon, such as low-grade afternoon fever.

While there are general symptoms categorizing Deficient Yin, the symptoms change according to the Organs involved, such as the Kidneys, Heart, Liver and Lungs. Because the Kidneys are the root of Yin and Yang in the body, anything that depletes the Kidneys can cause their Yin to be Deficient, and then the Yin throughout the rest of the body tends to become Deficient. When Kidney Yin is depleted, low grade sore throats, dizziness, night sweating or poor memory might occur. When the Heart Yin is Deficient, insomnia and mental agitation or restlessness result. Liver Yin Deficiency creates irritability and headaches. A Deficiency of Lung Yin produces dry cough and malar flush.

Yin can become Deficient by "burning the candle at both ends", over-working, lack of sleep, over-exercising, overindulgence in sex, Yang becoming so excessive it consumes the Yin, long-term chronic diseases, internal injury due to the seven emotions, and the over-eating of dry and hot-natured foods. Yin is strengthened primarily by rest and Yin tonic herbs.

Symptoms:
night sweats
burning, feverish or hot sensation in the palms, soles and chest
fever or feeling of heat, especially in the afternoon
malar flush
superficially red or flushed nose
emaciation
dry or chronically sore throat, especially at night
thirst
weakness and fragility, but fast movements
agitated manner; jumpy; anxious
mental restlessness
scanty dark urine
dry cough
dry stools
dry mouth at night
nocturnal emissions

pain relieved by pressure and cold
Pulse: thready, thin and rapid, or floating-empty and rapid
Tongue: red with no coat, or a thin shiny tongue body (called a mirror or peeled tongue)

Herbal Categories and Formulas: Tonify Yin herbs
Rehmannia Six Formula (Liu wei di huang wan)
Achyranthes and Rehmannia Combination (Restore the Left Pill - Zuo gui wan)

Collapse of Yin

When Yin becomes extremely depleted, it collapses. At its extreme, death can occur because the Yin at that point cannot control the Yang and they separate. This is seen only in extreme cases.

Symptoms:
abundant sweating
hot limbs
dry mouth with desire for cold liquids in small amounts
constipation
retention of urine
skin hot to the touch
Pulse: rapid, floating and empty
Tongue: red, dry and peeled (no coat)

Herbal Categories and Formulas: Yin tonics, lubricating herbs, Heat clearing herbs
Big Pearl for Internal Wind (Da ding feng zhu)
Sweet Wormwood and Tortoise Shell Formula (Qing hao bie jia tang)
Anemarrhena, Phellodendron and Rehmannia Combination

(Zhi bai di huang wan)
Rhinoceros and Rehmannia Combination (Xi jiao di huang tang)

YANG DISHARMONIES

There are two basic Yang disharmonies: an Excess of Yang and a Deficiency of Yang. The condition of false Yang is not a Yang disharmony, but arises from a Yin Deficiency, and so is included under Deficiency of Yin. Because Yang is Heat and activity, an excess of Yang is characterized by excessive Heat signs and hyperactivity, and a Deficiency of Yang is distinguished by a lack of Heat, or Coldness, and hypoactivity. A third disharmony of Yang, Collapse of Yang, is rarely seen. This occurs from an extreme depletion of Yang to the point where it collapses.

Excess Yang

Excess Yang is a Full Yang state, and its signs are similar to those of the Heat Pernicious Influence. Because Yang is associated with Heat, activity and dryness, the symptoms are exemplified by any of these qualities. There are general symptoms which designate Excess Yang, yet they become more specific depending on the Organ involved. For instance, migraines often arise from Excess Liver Yang, or manic behavior and extreme restlessness result from Excess Heart Yang. When there is Excess Yang, the body is in a hyperfunctional state. Over time the presence of excessive Yang "burns off" the Fluids in the body, resulting in a condition of Deficient Yin.

Excess Yang is most often due to the Heat Pernicious Influence, either External or Internal. It can also be caused by internal damage from the Seven Emotions, the Stagnation of Qi or Blood, over-exposure to hot climates or environments, indigestion, and the overconsumption of hot-natured and fried greasy foods, coffee, alcohol and red meat.

Symptoms:
high fever
thirst
red face
aversion to heat
restlessness
delirium
burning sensations
constipation
red eyes
scanty dark urine
large loss of blood which is bright-red
irritability
yellow discharges
sticky, thick and hot-feeling excretions
pain which is intensified by pressure and relieved by cold
Pulse: rapid, full and strong
Tongue: red with dry, rough and yellowish thick tongue fur

Herbal Categories and Formulas: Clear Heat Herbs
Major Rhubarb Combination (Da cheng qi tang)

Deficient Yang

Deficiency of Yang is an Empty-Cold condition marked by Deficiency and Coldness. In this case the Yang energy is insufficient to warm the body or internal organs, or lacks activity to function normally in the organism. When Yang is insufficient, Fluids collect and congest, resulting in edema and puffiness; Qi and Blood tend to stagnate; and a general hypoactivity of the organic processes occurs. This pattern differs from Excess Yin in that Deficient Yang also includes signs of Coldness. A Deficiency of Yang is mostly related to Spleen-Yang, Kidney-Yang, Heart-Yang or Lung-Qi. The root of Yin and Yang in the body "resides" in the Kidneys, so if they become weakened from excessive standing, sex, activity or overwork, the depleted Kidney-Yang affects the Yang of the rest of the body, creating Deficient Spleen or Heart Yang, for instance. When Spleen Yang is Deficient, it fails to warm the muscles and to properly metabolize food, resulting in Coldness and Deficient Qi and Blood.

Yang Deficiency can occur from congenital defects of improper care after birth. Yet, it becomes Deficient from lack of activity or exercise, excessive sex, over-exposure to cold environments and climates, and excessive consumption of cold, raw foods and juices, sweets, alcohol, coffee, iced drinks and frozen foods such as ice cream and frozen yogurt.

Symptoms:
pale, frigid appearance
fear of cold
chilliness
cold limbs
lassitude with no desire to move
frail, weak and slow pulse
fatigue
edema in various parts of the body
abdominal pain relieved by warmth and pressure
loose stools
copious or scanty, frequent and clear urination
night time urination
clear to white colored discharges and excretions
faint odors, if any at all
infertility
impotence or frigidity
premature ejaculation
watery stools with undigested food
pain relieved by pressure and warmth
Pulse: slow, deep, feeble, weak, empty
Tongue: pale, swollen, moist; possibly white or wet tongue
coating

Herbal Categories and Formulas: Tonify Yang herbs
Rehmannia Eight Combination (Ba wei di huang wan)
Replenishing the Right (You gui wan)

Collapse of Yang

When Yang becomes extremely depleted, it collapses. At its extreme, death can occur because the Yang at that point cannot control the Yin and they separate. This is seen only in extreme cases.

Symptoms:
chilliness
cold limbs
no thirst
loose stools or incontinence
profuse and frequent urination or incontinence
weak breathing
profuse sweating with an oily sweat
Pulse: deep, minute
Tongue: pale, wet and swollen

Herbal Categories and Formulas: Internal Warming Stimulants, Qi and Yang tonics
Aconite, Ginger and Licorice Combination (Si ni tang)

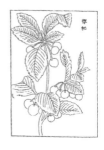

ELEVEN

DIFFERENTIAL DIAGNOSIS

THE ORGANS
ZANG FU SYMPTOM SIGN DIAGNOSIS

The Patterns of Organ Disharmonies are the next step in Differential Diagnosis. The most important Yin Organ systems are called the "Zang" and the lesser important Yang Organ systems are the "Fu". Especially useful for chronic disease, Zang-Fu symptom sign diagnosis is the most important diagnostic method of evaluating disease imbalance in clinical practice because it gives detailed information for treatment. For instance, diagnosing a general Deficient Yang condition is not specific enough to render adequate treatment without further knowing if it is Deficient Yang of the Kidneys, Spleen or Heart.

In many cases there is a correspondence between Western medical diagnosis and TCM. Because, however, the correspondence between TCM Organ patterns and organ diseases of Western medicine is more functional than organ specific, a condition of Stagnant Liver Qi in TCM symptom-sign diagnosis for example, may not test positive in a standard Western medical blood test. The opposite is true, however, in that a specific disease will appear as some pattern of imbalance in TCM. Therefore, these patterns may present specific diseases as we know them in the West, but are regarded and treated as imbalances. This enables the practitioner and patient to consider other possibilities so that even so-called "incurable" diseases can be treated.

The best way to identify a pattern is to also understand how it arises and develops. This can vary individually, as can the number and type of symptoms that occur. The more severe an Organ imbalance, the more and greater severity of signs and symptoms. On the other hand, one may only need two to three symptoms to signal a particular Organ involvement, and these may be milder in manifestation. Whether few or many, the signs that arise distinguish the Organ or Organs involved and these are subsequently treated.

The Patterns of Organ Disharmonies can be best understood by overlapping the signs of the Eight Principles - External, Internal, Hot, Cold, Excess, Deficiency and Yin and Yang - with those of the Pernicious Influences, Qi, Blood, Fluids and Essence and the functions of the Organs to form the various patterns found in TCM. These encompass those found in clinical practice throughout centuries of experience and observation. Certain Organs are more prone to particular patterns than others, and therefore specific combinations, such as Excess Spleen Yang, are not described as such but are seen as Excess Stomach Heat instead. Further, patterns frequently appear together, often from cause and effect relationships. For instance, a Deficiency of Kidney Yin can lead to Deficient Lung Yin concurrently, or Excess Liver Yang can cause Excess Heart Yang at the same time.

Many factors contribute to the development of Organ disharmonies, encompassing dietary, environmental, lifestyle, emotional, mental and hereditary issues. These are discussed in detail in the chapter on Causes of Disease. In describing these, along with the individual and combined patterns, the most common ones seen in clinic practice are the ones included. The key symptoms of each Organ disharmony are in bold type.

Note that only the major formula used for each category is given. Usually several formulas are appropriate and useful for each pattern, however, and these can be determined in Volume II. Further, each of the formulas listed below, a full description of the formula and a listing of the herbs of which it is comprised are also given in Volume II.

Under each pattern, therapies are mentioned which are useful for healing that pattern. Several of the therapies are detailed in the appendix Accessory Healing Therapies for the Herbalist, such as harimaki[1], cupping, moxibustion and nasal wash. Refer there for complete details and instructions to perform them. Note: the major symptoms in each category are in bold.

YIN ORGANS

HEART

The primary functions of the Heart are to control Blood and blood vessels and to rule the Mind (Shen). Therefore, most Heart disharmonies involve these aspects. The different categories for Heart Patterns include Deficiency of Heart Blood, Yin, Qi or Yang, Heart Fire, Congealed Heart Blood and Mucus obstructing the Heart Orifices. Climatic influences which cause Heart imbalances are Fire and Heat, although these do not invade the Heart directly, but instead affect the Pericardium.

Emotions such as sadness, anger or excessive joy can cause Heart Qi Deficiency and Heart Fire.

Causes for Heart Disharmonies

Pathogenic Influences: Heat is the main Pernicious Influence which can invade the Heart, and even then, not directly. Strictly speaking, Exterior pathogens do not attack the Heart itself, rather they invade the Pericardium instead. The Pericardium acts as a protector for the Heart and thus is the one assaulted. This pattern is called Invasion of the Pericardium by Heat and is characterized by acute and rapid invasion of External Heat at the Nutritive Qi level with symptoms of extreme temperature, delirium and, in severe cases coma.

Emotions: The Heart is especially affected by the emotions of joy, sadness and anger. When a person is excessively excited or frequently laughs inappropriately, it is described as excessive joy. Over time, such excesses can create Deficient Heart Qi. Because the Lungs and Heart are in close proximity as part of the "Upper Warmer", they are both affected by sadness, the emotion of the Lungs. This initially causes Deficient Lung Qi, and can eventually lead to Deficient Heart Qi. Prolonged sadness can also cause Qi Stagnation which changes to Heart Fire. Anger causes Liver Fire to rise, which, through the Five Element connection of the Liver as the mother of the Heart, is indirectly transferred to the Heart, causing Heart Fire.

Diet: Fatty, fried and excessively spicy foods cause Stagnation and Heat in the Heart, while excessive consumption of Lamb can cause Heart Fire. On the other hand, someone who has Deficient Heart Blood or Yang would benefit from lamb.

Lifestyle Habits: The Heart represents the inner self. When we are in a state of pure being and inner tranquility, there is a purity and goodness in the Heart. Only when we attempt to extend beyond ourselves, either through excessive desire, ambition or fear, do we threaten the well-being of the Heart.. Therefore, excessive laughter, celebrating, going out, staying up late, reading, and studying injure the Heart. The Heart benefits from rest, aerobic exercise, sufficient sleep, laughter, following one's heart's desires, meditation and contemplation, music, dance and spiritual pursuits.

Heart Blood Deficiency

When Heart Blood is Deficient, the Mind suffers and specifically affects thought, memory and sleep. Further, Heart Qi becomes Deficient, causing palpitations, usually in the evenings and at rest, and with a feeling of anxiety or uneasiness in the chest.

Heart Blood Deficiency arises from Deficient Spleen Qi unable to produce Blood, long-term anxiety and worry which disturb the Mind and suppress the Heart function of governing Blood, a severe loss of blood such as hemorrhaging during childbirth, and excessive long-term studying.

Symptoms:
palpitations
insomnia, with difficulty falling asleep but then sleeping well
forgetfulness and poor memory, especially long term
dizziness
excessive dreaming
dream-disturbed sleep
anxiety
easily startled
dull pale complexion
pale lips
Pulse: fine or choppy
Tongue: pale, thin, slightly dry

Herbal Therapy: Dang Gui Four Combination (Si wu tang) for Heart Blood Deficiency; For Heart Qi and Blood Deficiency use **Ginseng and Longan Combination** (Gui pi tang).

Food Therapy: Eat a balanced diet including lamb, Dang Gui and ginger soup, bone marrow soup, milk, black and aduki beans, congee; eat all cooked foods; do not skip meals.

Other Therapies: Contemplation and meditation, following one's heart's desires, rest, breathing exercises, harimaki and moxibustion over the lower abdomen. Avoid saunas and hot tubs.

Exercise: Light aerobic and stretching exercises including Yoga, Tai Chi and Qi Gong.

Heart Yin Deficiency

Heart Yin Deficiency includes Heart Blood Deficiency. Its signs include those of Heart Blood Deficiency along with empty-Heat signs such as malar flush, mental restlessness and night sweats. Heart Yin Deficiency is caused by or occurs with Kidney Yin Deficiency since Kidney Water cannot then rise to nourish the Heart and prevent the flaring up of empty-Heat. It is more common in middle-aged or old people while Heart Blood Deficiency is more common in young people, especially women.

As with Yin Deficiency in general, doing too much, keeping too busy, staying up too late and getting up early cause Deficient Heart Yin.

It is also caused by excessive study, working, talking, long term anxiety or worry and attack by Exterior Heat consuming Fluids.

Symptoms:
palpitations
mental restlessness
feeling of heat, especially in the evening
malar flush
insomnia with difficulty falling asleep and waking frequently
dream-disturbed sleep
easily startled
forgetfulness and poor memory, especially long term
anxiety
uneasiness, agitation, fidgetness
low-grade fever
night sweating
dry mouth and throat heat in the palms and soles and chest
Pulse: floating, empty and rapid, or thin (fine) and rapid
Tongue: red with no coat; tip redder and swollen with red points; **deep midline crack reaching the tip**

Herbal Therapy: Emperor of Heaven's Tonic Pill for the Mind (Tian wang bu xin dan)

Food Therapy: Avoid spicy and heating foods. If digestion is good, fruit is beneficial, especially berries and purple grapes. If digestion is not good, eat all cooked foods. Sufficient protein at each meal is important. Do not skip meals. Include black and aduki beans, soya, tofu and milk in the diet.

Other Therapies: Oil massage, breathing exercises, rest, cupping over the upper back to relieve Stagnation and Deficient Heat, harimaki; counseling to relieve emotional issues, such as anxiety, worry and lack of joy. Limit mental and sexual activity and reading until the Yin is restored. Being asleep by 9 - 9:30 PM is very beneficial. Avoid saunas and hot tubs.

Exercise: Aerobic exercise is contraindicated. While it is useful for Excess conditions, it will increase Yin Deficiency. Instead one should emphasize more stretching exercise that invites the mind to participate in the circulation of Qi and Blood, such as Yoga, Tai Chi, Qi Gong. Other forms that one can employ are stretching, walking and swimming.

Heart Qi Deficiency

This pattern includes general Qi Deficiency signs along with Heart symptoms. It can be caused by long-term chronic illness, after acute or chronic hemorrhage, and excessive sadness. This pattern often appears with Deficient Lung Qi because the Heart and Lungs are linked in the Upper Warmer and the Sea of Qi in the chest

Symptoms:
palpitations
fatigue
Iethargy shortness of breath on exertion
sweating
pallor
Pulse: empty; in severe cases superficially strong but empty underneath
Tongue: pale, or normal color; midline crack to tip with swelling on each side in more severe cases

Herbal Therapy: Stephania and Ginseng Combination (Mu fang chi tang) and/or **Baked Licorice Combination** (Zhi gan cao tang)

Food Therapy: Eat all cooked foods and warm or room temperature drinks. Whole grains, protein, legumes (especially aduki beans), lots of vegetables and congee are important. Make sure you eat three meals, or more as needed, per day. Avoid raw and cold foods and juices. Do not skip meals.

Other Therapies: Moxibustion, especially on the lower abdomen and on the back over the kidneys; ginger fomentations on both locations; getting plenty of rest, going to bed by 9 - 10 P.M.; not over-extending yourself; journal work to get in touch with the causes of any sadness or lack of joy; breathing exercises; harimaki. Avoid excessive work and sexual activity. Working on and resolving any emotional issues involved is very important. If using saunas or hot tubs, be sure to rinse in cool water afterwards to push the heat back in the body; otherwise it dissipates and can cause Yang Deficiency over time.

Exercise: Exercise is important since it helps give energy; however, do not overdo or push yourself. Do light walking, swimming, dancing, Yoga, Tai Chi, Qi Gong or bicycling.

Deficient Heart Yang

This pattern has similar signs to Deficient Heart Qi, though they are usually more severe and occur with symptoms of Coldness. It is from similar causes to Heart Qi Deficiency, or can be from a Deficiency of Kidney Yang since that is the body's source of Yang. In fact, this imbalance often appears concurrent with Deficient Kidney Yang.

Symptoms:
palpitations

feeling of cold
cold limbs, especially hands
shortness of breath on exertion
tiredness
lethargy
sweating
feeling of stuffiness or discomfort in heart region
bright-pale face
Pulse: deep and weak, or knotted
Tongue: pale, wet, swollen

Herbal Therapy: Cinnamon and Dragon Bone Combination
(Gui zhi long gu mu li tang)

Food Therapy: All cooked foods and warm drinks are essential.
Lamb and beef are beneficial as are spicy foods. Avoid cold,
refrigerated, raw and iced drinks and foods, including salads. Do
not skip meals.

Other Therapies: The same as for Deficient Heart Qi.

Exercise: The same as for Deficient Heart Qi.

Collapse of Heart Yang

Yang can become so Deficient that it suddenly "collapses," causing
profuse sweating, extreme cold in the limbs or entire body, purple lips
and minute or even imperceptible pulse. This is a more extreme form of
Yang Deficiency and could lead to Yin and Yang separating, resulting in
death. The extreme Coldness causes loss of control of sweating and
severe Blood Stagnation.

Coma may occur because the loss of Heart Qi means the Mind has
no "residence". The tongue is short from either the Yang Qi being
unable to move the tongue muscle, or Internal Cold contracting the
tongue muscle. This pattern is caused from long term Heart Yang
Deficiency and collapse of Kidney Yang. This is an acute Heart condition
that results after years of debilitating stressful work and sexual excess. It
can also be precipitated after a chronic, long term illness.

Symptoms:
cold limbs
cyanosis of lips
profuse sweating
shortness of breath
palpitations
weak and shallow breathing

250

coma in severe cases
Pulse: minute, knotted, hidden
Tongue: very pale or bluish-purple; short

Herbal Therapy: **Aconite, Ginger and Licorice Combination** (Si ni tang) or **Restore and Revive the Yang Decoction** (Hui yang jiu ji tang)

Heart Blood Stagnation

This serious condition occurs from other Heart patterns, usually Heart Qi, Yang or Blood Deficiency or from Heart Fire, making it an Excess/Deficiency pattern. If Blood is Deficient, it becomes Stagnant. Likewise, a Deficiency of Qi or Yang also stagnates the Blood. If there is Heart Fire, the Heat congeals the Blood in the chest. This pattern is caused by long term emotional issues such as anxiety, grief, resentment or held-in anger, or from Heart Yang Deficiency.

Symptoms:
pain in the heart region which may radiate to inner aspect of
left arm or shoulder
cyanosis of lips
palpitations
stuffiness, feeling of oppression or constriction in the chest
cyanosis of nails
cold hands
Pulse: knotted
Tongue: purple

Herbal Therapy: Warm and Activate the Circulation of the Heart Pills (Guan xin su he wan)

Food Therapy: Same as for Deficient Heart Blood

Other Therapies: Same as for Deficient Heart Blood

Exercise: Only gentle movement, such as walking

Heart Fire

An Excess pattern, it is different than Heart Yin Deficiency, as it manifests true Heat signs such as thirst, dark urine and full rapid pulse. The bitter taste in the mouth is different from that of Liver Fire in that Heart Fire only appears in the morning and is related to quality of sleep. The tongue ulcers are red with a raised red rim and are painful, whereas ulcers with a white rim can be due to Empty-Heat.

Mental restlessness and agitation are caused by Excess Heat. Dark, condensed urine with or without blood is the result of Heart Fire being transmitted to the Small Intestine and from there to the Bladder (to which the Small Intestine is related in the Greater Yang). Chronic Qi Stagnation with mental depression can cause Heart Fire, as can long term anxiety, constant worrying and Liver-Fire.

> **Symptoms:**
> mouth and tongue ulcers
> thirst
> **palpitations**
> mental restlessness
> feeling agitated
> feelings of heat
> insomnia with feverish sensation
> red or flushed face
> hot, dark urine or blood in urine
> bitter taste in mouth in morning
> **Pulse:** rapid and full or rapid and irregular
> **Tongue: red**, redder tip and swollen with red points, yellow
> coat; there may be a midline crack reaching to the tip

Herbal Therapy: Decoction of the Four Ingredients and Three Yellow Herbs (San huang si wu tang)

Food Therapy: Fasting on fruit or vegetable juices; including fruits (especially watermelon), salads and juices in the diet; limit meat intake to 24 oz. per day maximum, although it's better to avoid meat altogether, especially red, for several weeks. Use legumes instead for protein, including tofu and mung beans. Include plenty of fresh vegetables and greens in the diet. Avoid iced or refrigerated drinks as they can perpetuate the problem by aggravating a Heat reaction. Avoid hot and greasy foods, caffeine, alcohol, nuts, avocados and cheese.

Other Therapies: Meditation; breathing exercises; cupping over the upper back.

Exercise: Martial arts are beneficial as they help focus restless and excessive energy.

Cold Mucus Obstructing the Heart Orifices

This is an extreme pattern where the Mind, blocked by Cold Phlegm, causes disharmonies of Shen (Spirit). Because Cold contracts and stagnates, irrational behaviors are more introverted. Autism and retardation in children as well as strokes, paralysis and aphasia in adults can be the result of Cold Mucus Obstructing. Excessive consumption of greasy, cold and raw foods can cause Phlegm to form. This, combined with severe long term emotional problems, produces this pattern. Further, Spleen Qi Deficiency contributes by not transforming Dampness which then accumulates into Phlegm.

Symptoms:
mental confusion
rattling sound in throat
lethargic stupor
abnormal, inward, restrained and foolish behavior
muttering to oneself
staring at walls
vomiting
aphasia
unconsciousness or sudden blackouts
Pulse: slippery, possibly slow
Tongue: thick, sticky, slippery coat; white coating; midline crack reaching to the tip with prickles in it; swollen tongue body

Herbal Therapy: Bamboo and Poria Combination (Wen dan tang)

Food Therapy: Avoid dairy, wheat, flour products, desserts, greasy and fried foods, chocolate, caffeinated foods and drinks, alcohol, processed foods, especially those with additives, sodas, cold and iced drinks and foods, raw foods, fruit and vegetable juices, salads. Eat rice, millet and barley, black bean soup with onions and garlic, protein and vegetables.

Other Therapies: Professional psychotherapy; cupping over the upper back; moxibustion over the lower abdomen and upper and lower back; harimaki; avoid cold damp environments.

Exercise: Whatever can be safely undertaken; movement would be beneficial such as walking, especially in the woods.

Hot Mucus Obstructing the Heart Orifices

When the Mind is blocked by Heated Phlegm, it results in disharmonies of Shen. Because Heat expands and activates, irrational behaviors are more extroverted and violent. It is a combination of Fire, Heart Disharmonies and Deficient Spleen Qi unable to transform Fluids. This pattern is caused by excessive consumption of hot-greasy foods and/or severe emotional problems leading to Qi Stagnation and then Fire. It can also be caused by overexposure to External Heat. It can manifest as symptoms of manic-depression, extreme mental instability, agitation and brain injury.

Symptoms:
mental restlessness
incoherent speech
mental confusion
rash behavior
tendency to hit or scold people
uncontrolled laughter or crying
shouting
muttering to oneself
mental depression and dullness
dream disturbed sleep
palpitations
bitter taste in the mouth in the mornings
insomnia
easily startled
agitation
aphasia in severe cases
coma in severe cases
Pulse: full, rapid and slippery; or full, rapid and wiry
Tongue: red, yellow sticky coat; midline crack with yellow
    prickles in it; tip may be redder and swollen with red points

Herbal Therapy: Bamboo and Poria Combination (Wen dan tang) with **Scutellaria, Coptis and Platycodon** (Variation of Wen dan tang)

Food Therapy: Avoid hot, spicy, greasy and fried foods, meat, processed foods especially with additives in them, alcohol, tobacco, coffee and other caffeinated foods and drinks, sodas and juices. Eat lots of vegetables, tofu, black beans, greens, rice, barley, legumes.

Other Therapies: Psychotherapy; meditation and relaxation techniques; breathing exercises; cupping over the upper back.

Exercise: In Yoga pranayam, various breathing exercises are described as Heating or Cooling and are described in the appendix, Healing Therapies for the Herbalist. Perform Shitali or Sitkari.

Combined Pattern

Heart and Lungs

Both Organs are located in the chest and are part of the Upper Warmer. The Heart controls the circulation of Blood, while the Lungs control the circulation of Qi. They are, therefore, closely inter-dependent because of the close relationship of Qi and Blood. A Deficiency of

Lung Qi can adversely affect Blood circulation, manifesting as shortness of breath, palpitations, a stuffy feeling in the chest, cyanosis of the lips and a purplish tongue; Deficient Heart Qi stagnates Blood and may in turn affect the Lung's dispersing and descending function, also causing shortness of breath with cough, asthmatic breathing, and a stuffy feeling in the chest.

> **Heart and Lung Qi Deficiency Symptoms:**
> shortness of breath
> palpitations
> **stuffy feeling in chest**
> purple lips and tongue
> cough
> tiredness
> sweating
> **Pulse:** empty
> **Tongue:** pale or normal-colored

Herbal Therapy: Stephania and Ginseng Combination (Mu fang chi tang)

Food Therapy: Refer to this category under Heart Qi Deficiency and Lung Qi Deficiency.

Other Therapies: Refer to this category under Heart Qi Deficiency and Lung Qi Deficiency.

Exercise: Four Purifications, Eight Brocades especially number one, two and six.

Heart and Spleen

While the Heart controls Blood circulation, the Spleen is the source of Blood production and keeps it flowing within the vessels. If the Spleen functions properly in providing sufficient nutrients for growth and development, transporting and distributing them properly, then the Blood of the Heart will be plentiful. In turn, Heart Blood circulates and provides the Spleen with nutrients to better help it perform its functions.

In Five Elements, the Heart is the Mother of the Spleen. If there is Deficient Heart Blood or Qi, it will result in mental anxiety causing the transforming and transporting functions of the Spleen to become disrupted. The result will be improper distribution of nutrients for growth and development with an inability of the Spleen to keep the Blood flowing within the vessels. Finally, a combination of Heart and Spleen symptoms and signs such as palpitation, insomnia, anorexia, lassitude and pallor will result in the TCM condition known as Deficiency of Heart Blood and Spleen Qi or Blood. To treat it, formulas to invigorate the Spleen and nourish the Heart are used, such as **Ginseng and Longan Combination** (Gui pi tang).

> **Heart Blood and Spleen Qi or Blood Deficiency Symptoms:**
> palpitations
> insomnia
> anorexia
> **lassitude**
> fatigue
> pale-dull face
> bleeding
> poor memory
> **Pulse**: fine or choppy
> **Tongue**: pale

Herbal Therapy: Ginseng and Longan Combination (Gui pi tang)

Food Therapy: Refer to this category under Heart Blood and Qi Deficiency and Spleen Qi Deficiency.

Other Therapies: Refer to this category under Heart Blood and Qi Deficiency and Spleen Qi Deficiency.

Exercise: Refer to this category under Heart Blood Deficiency, Heart Qi Deficiency and Spleen Qi Deficiency.

Heart and Liver

The Heart controls Blood circulation while the Liver stores the Blood. Only when Heart Blood is plentiful does the Liver have Blood to store. When Liver Blood is Deficient, Heart Blood is certain to be Deficient also. Thus, signs of Heart Blood Deficiency almost always occur along with Liver Blood Deficiency. Herbs such as Dang Gui and white peony are used to nourish the Blood of the Liver and the Heart. Both the Heart and Liver are involved in mental activities and mood: the Heart because it rules the Mind, the Liver because it is in charge of the smooth and regular flow of Qi to all parts of the body. Further, the Liver is the Mother of the Heart. Liver imbalances frequently affect the Heart and vice versa. When there is Heart Yin Deficiency with signs of insomnia, frequent dreaming and anxiety, there are often Liver signs of fidgetiness, restlessness and anger. Likewise, Liver Yang symptoms of dizziness, fidgetiness, irritability and a sensation of distension in the head can lead to Heart signs of palpitation and insomnia.

> **Heart and Liver Blood Deficiency Symptoms:**
> blurred vision
> scanty periods
> poor memory
> dizziness
> palpitations
> **insomnia**
> anxiety
> pale-dull complexion
> pale lips
> **Pulse:** choppy or fine
> **Tongue:** pale

Herbal Therapy: Ginseng and Zizyphus Combination (Emperor of Heaven's Tonic Pill for the Mind) (Tian wang bu xin dan)

Food Therapy: Refer to this category under Heart Blood Deficiency and Liver Blood Deficiency.

Other Therapies: Refer to this category under Heart Blood Deficiency and Liver Blood Deficiency.

Exercise: Refer to this category under Heart Blood Deficiency and Liver Blood Deficiency.

Heart and Kidneys

The Heart and Kidneys have an interdependent and mutually sustaining relationship. One is Fire, the other Water. Kidney Yin ascends to the Heart to nourish its Yin and protect it from the Yang becoming Excessive, while Yang descends into the Kidneys to nourish their Yang. When Heart Yang is Deficient, it can't warm that of the Kidneys, resulting in excessive water which can lead to possible heart attacks, palpitations and edema. This is called Heart trouble caused by retention of water, and occurs from a Deficiency of Heart and Kidney Yang.

> **Heart and Kidney Yang Deficiency Symptoms:**
> palpitations
> feeling of cold
> **cold limbs**, especially hands and knees
> feeling of cold and soreness in the back
> edema, especially of the legs
> shortness of breath on exertion
> tiredness

lethargy
bright-pale face
Pulse: deep and weak, or knotted
Tongue: pale, wet, swollen

Herbal Therapy: Warm and Activate the Circulation of the Heart Pills (Guan xin su he wan)

Food Therapy: Refer to this category under Heart Yang Deficiency and Kidney Yang Deficiency.

Other Therapies: Refer to this category under Heart Yang Deficiency and Kidney Yang Deficiency.

Exercise: Refer to this category under Heart Yang Deficiency and Kidney Yang Deficiency.

Heart and Kidney not Harmonized (Heart and Kidney Yin Deficiency)
When Kidney Yin is Deficient and cannot nourish the Heart, or Deficient Kidney Yang cannot distill the Yin of the Kidney, Heart Yang becomes excessive resulting in mental restlessness, insomnia, dream-disturbed sleep and seminal emission. This incoordination between the Heart and the Kidneys can be caused by prolonged overwork or overactivity, excessive sexual activity, long term chronic illnesses and emotional shocks or protracted emotional problems such as anxiety, sadness, depression or chronic Heart Yin Deficiency.

> **Heart and Kidney not Harmonized Symptoms:**
> palpitations
> insomnia
> night sweating
> poor memory
> dizziness
> tinnitus
> deafness
> soreness of lower back
> nocturnal emission with dreams
> fever or feeling of heat in the afternoon
> scanty-dark urine
> **Pulse:** floating, empty and rapid
> **Tongue: red-peeling with redder tip and midline crack**

Herbal Therapy: **Coptis and Cinnamon Formula** (Jiao tai wan)

Food Therapy: Refer to this category under Heart Yin Deficiency and Kidney Yin Deficiency.

Other Therapies: Refer to this category under Heart Yin Deficiency and Kidney Yin Deficiency.

Exercise: Refer to this category under Heart Yin Deficiency and Kidney Yin Deficiency.

LUNGS

The Lungs rule Qi, have a dispersing and descending function and are directly connected to the exterior environment. This makes them vulnerable to External invasion of Pernicious Influences. Because of this, patterns of Lung disharmony include External as well as Internal conditions.

Causes for Lung Disharmonies

Pathogenic Influences: The Lungs are the only Internal Organ that has direct contact with the outer environment through breathing, controlling the skin and influencing Defensive Qi. Being vulnerable to External Pernicious Influences, they are regarded as the "sensitive", or the "princess", of the Organs. Any of the External Pernicious Influences can invade - Wind, Heat, Summer Heat, Cold, Damp, and Dryness - although Wind[2] generally combines with any of the other factors. Thus, exposure to any of these Influences, or to environments in homes or work places where these are present, can cause any of the external patterns of disharmony.

Emotions: Grief, worry and sadness in excess can have a profoundly debilitating affect on the Lungs, being a precipitating cause of conditions such as asthma, emphysema, bronchitis, frequent colds and flu or pneumonia.

Diet: Diet is very important to Lung health, as it is to all the Organs. Excessive consumption of cold, raw and damp foods, such as salads, fruits, juices, dairy, wheat, iced or refrigerated drinks and foods, causes Dampness[3] in the Spleen which is often "stored" in the Lungs. This is why Lung Dampness, manifested as certain types of bronchitis and asthma, can often be healed by moving to a dry environment, eliminating foods such as dairy and various fruit juices like orange juice from the diet and taking herbs that eliminate Spleen Dampness such as **Citrus and Pinellia Combination** (Er chen tang).

Lifestyle Habits: Exercise stimulates Fire in the body and is essential in moving the lymphatic system and drying Dampness. Those whose work or inclination involves lack of physical activity will be especially susceptible to Damp accumulation caused by injury to the Spleen and Lungs. Coldness ultimately tends to inhibit circulation, which further slows the lymphatic system and leads to Dampness. Sudden exposure to Cold, Heat and Damp may not give the body sufficient time to prepare for the climatic changes and eventually can compromise the immune system. Finally, mucus-forming foods such as dairy and flour products, denatured foods such as white sugar and Damp-natured foods such as citrus and fruit juices can weaken the body and cause External invasion.

External Patterns
Invasion of the Lungs by Wind-Cold
This pattern is one of Wind and Cold Pernicious Influences invading and obstructing the Lungs. The descending function is disrupted, causing cough and a runny or stuffed nose, and the dispersing function is impaired, resulting in sneezing. When Wind-Chill attacks the Defensive Qi, the pores try to stay closed in the "battle" against the attack, resulting in lack of perspiration, fever, chills, body aches and aversion to cold. However, in this case the chills are stronger from the Cold invasion.

This pattern occurs from over-exposure to a cold and possibly windy environment, air conditioning, drafts or refrigerated store-rooms. Further, it can occur if there is a weakness of the Defensive, or "Wei", energy, thus allowing the External Influences to more easily and frequently invade the body. Finally, the nature of External acute conditions is that they can change quickly, and can move back and forth from Wind Heat to Wind Cold, or vice versa.

Symptoms:
aversion to cold
sneezing
slight fever strong chills
body aches
cough with thin, watery sputum
lack of sweating
itchy throat
stuffy or runny nose with clear-watery mucus
occipital headache
Pulse: floating, tight
Tongue: thin white coat

Herbal Therapy: Trikatu[4], ginger tea, garlic, **Nine Herbs with Notopterygii Decoction** (Jiu wei qiang huo tang), **Ephedra Combination** (Ma huang tang) for Excess conformation or when there is no sweating, **Pueraria Combination** (Ge gen tang) for middle strength constitutions or when there is accompanying tight neck and shoulders, **Cinnamon Combination** (Gui zhi tang) for Deficient types or when there is sweating.

Food Therapy: Eat all cooked foods, keeping them simple, such as soups of grains or black beans with garlic and onions, vegetables and a little chicken. Avoid all else until healed.

Other Therapies: Avoid exposure to air conditioning, drafts, cold and windy environments; dress warmly to conserve the body's heat and immune potential. One of the places that is most exposed is the neck and shoulders so that in cold, windy environments, a warm scarf is good protection. Again, to support the immune system which emanates from the power of the Kidneys, a Harimaki will be gratefully appreciated in cold environments. In addition, therapies such as cupping and moxibustion over the upper back, chest, kidneys and lower abdomen is useful; breathing exercises; morning saline nasal wash; ginger fomentation, onion poultice or mustard plaster over the chest are traditional methods that can be employed with great benefit.

Exercise: Bed rest

Invasion of Lungs by Wind-Heat

Similar to invasion of the Lungs by Wind-Chill, in this case the Wind enters with Heat[5], such as high fever, sweating and aversion to heat as part of the symptom complex. It can be caused by exposure to climatic Heat and possibly Wind, overly heated environments in the home and work place, or Wind-Cold conditions changing to Heat.

> **Symptoms:**
> fever
> aversion to cold
> sore throat
> slight chills
> stuffy or runny nose with yellow mucus
> perspiration
> thirst
> constipation
> dark urine
> swollen tonsils
> body aches
> headache
> cough with yellow mucus
> **Pulse:** floating and rapid
> **Tongue:** red on the sides or tip with a white or yellow coat

Herbal Therapy: Lonicera and Forsythia Combination (Yin qiao san)

Food Therapy: Keep the diet simple, perhaps fasting on fruit or vegetable juices or soups, such as rice and black or mung beans. Avoid all else until healed.

Other Therapies: Avoid exposure to overly heated and perhaps windy environments and climates; do cupping over the upper back, breathing exercises as appropriate.

Exercise: Bed rest

Cold Dampness Obstructing the Lungs

This pattern can occur from an External Damp Pernicious Influence attacking the body, or from any External Influence invading and mixing with a preexisting chronic disharmony of Deficient Spleen or Kidney Qi. The result is an accumulation of Dampness, causing Phlegm and obstruction of the Lung functions. In this case, the Dampness is accompanied by Cold and thus, Cold signs. It is caused by lowered immunity, Deficient Spleen Qi or Yang and possibly Deficient Kidney Qi, and a diet high in cold, raw foods and drinks.

> **Symptoms:**
> cough with profuse white sputum
> wheezing or asthma with copious white sputum
> chest and flank stuffiness, distension and soreness
> difficulty in breathing, especially when lying down
> white-pasty complexion
> shortness of breath or breathlessness
> **Pulse:** slippery and weak-floating or fine
> **Tongue:** thick, greasy white coat

Herbal Therapy: Citrus and Pinellia Combination (Er chen tang)

Food Therapy: Only eat and drink cooked warm foods and fluids, keeping them simple, such as soups. Some spicy tasting things can be helpful, such as ginger tea or horseradish. Avoid all else until healed. When over the acute stage, eat a diet of only cooked foods and warm drinks, avoiding cold raw and damp foods, such as dairy and flour products, salads, fruits, fruit and vegetable juices (especially orange[6] juice), refined foods such as white sugar, and refrigerated or iced foods and drinks..

Other Therapies: Onion and/or ginger poultices over the chest; cupping on chest or over upper back; moxibustion in the same areas; nasal wash; keep warmly dressed, with a neck scarf and a harimaki, and avoid exposure to cold, damp and windy environments.

Exercise: Bed rest

Phlegm Heat Obstructing the Lungs

This is similar to Cold Damp Obstructing the Lungs, but it is accompanied by Heat instead. It can be caused by an External Damp or Wind-Heat Pernicious Influence attacking the body and mixing with a preexisting chronic disharmony of Deficient Spleen Qi. It results in an accumulation of Dampness and Heat, causing Phlegm and obstruction of the Lung functions. It is caused by lowered immunity, Deficient Spleen Qi and a diet high in hot, greasy, spicy, fried foods, meat, alcohol and tobacco.

> **Symptoms:**
> **cough with profuse yellow or green sputum**
> **which is foul-smelling**
> shortness of breath
> wheezing or asthma with copious yellow or green sputum
> chest and flank stuffiness, distension and soreness
> difficulty in breathing, especially when lying down
> shortness of breath or breathlessness
> **Pulse: slippery, rapid** or slippery, rapid-floating
> **Tongue: thick, greasy yellow coat**

Herbal Therapy: Ma Huang and Apricot Seed Combination (Ma xing shi gan tang) and **Citrus and Pinellia Combination** (Er chen tang) with scutellaria, gardenia, apricot seed and platycodon.

Food Therapy: Simple soups or vegetable juice fast until healed. When over the acute stage, avoid: alcohol, red meat, tobacco, spicy, greasy and fried foods and dairy.

Other Therapies: Cupping over the chest or upper back; nasal wash; breathing exercises as appropriate.

Exercise: Bed rest

Internal Patterns
Deficient Lung Qi

When Lung Qi is Deficient, there is tiredness, weakness, cough, sweating and a propensity to catching colds and flu, because the Qi cannot adequately perform its protecting, dispersing or descending functions. It occurs from a prolonged External Pernicious Influence remaining in the Lungs and injuring the Qi, excessive use of antibiotics which locks Cold in the Lungs and injures the Qi and its functions, from hereditary weakness, especially if one of the parents or grandparents had tuberculosis, from excessive stooping or leaning over desks and tables to work, or a diet high in cold raw foods and drinks.

Symptoms:
shortness of breath
weak voice
bright-white complexion
cough watery sputum
exhausted appearance and Spirit
low voice and lack of desire to talk
weak respiration
daytime sweats
lowered resistance to colds and flu
tiredness
Pulse: empty
Tongue: pale or normal colored

Herbal Therapy: Four Major ingredients (Si jun zi tang) with astragalus root.

Food Therapy: Eat all cooked foods and warm drinks, plenty of grains, especially rice, sufficient protein at each meal, black bean soup with ginseng, garlic and onions, cooked vegetables and greens; avoid cold, raw foods and drinks, salads, fruit, juices, alcohol, caffeine.

Other Therapies: Avoid excessive stooping or leaning over tables or desks; rest; dress warmly according to the season, especially with a scarf around the neck; avoid over-exertion in work or sexual activity; get plenty of rest, going to bed early such as 9 - 9:30 at night; moxibustion, especially over the lower abdomen; harimaki; breathing exercises; nasal wash; working on emotional issues such as sadness, grief and worry.

Exercise: Light to moderate exercise within the body's limits; do not over exercise or do strong aerobics; walking, swimming, cycling, Yoga, Tai Chi, Qi Gong are beneficial.

Deficient Lung Yin

Fluids can become depleted in the Lungs from invasion of Exterior Heat and Dryness which remains so long that it injures the Yin. Other causes are from Yin Deficiency of the Kidneys or Stomach which affects the Lungs, long-term Lung Qi Deficiency and from excessive and prolonged tobacco smoking. Characteristically, there will be Dry and Empty Heat signs along with Lung symptoms.

> **Symptoms**:
> unproductive dry cough with little or no phlegm,
>   or blood-tinged phlegm
> feeling of heat in the afternoon
> dry mouth and throat
> emaciated appearance
> malar flush
> night sweats
> burning sensation in palms, soles and chest
> insomnia
> **Pulse**: floating, empty and rapid
> **Tongue**: red, peeled, dry; possible cracks in the Lung area

Herbal Therapy: Eriobotrya and Ophiopogon Combination (Qing zao jiu fei tang)

Food Therapy: Avoid hot, spicy, fried and greasy foods. Eat grains, protein, vegetables and greens and, if digestion is good, some fruit (especially pears) and juices. Include asparagus, duck, black beans. and milk in the diet.

Other Therapies: Oil massage; breathing exercises; harimaki; rest; cupping over upper back; breathing exercises; meditation, contemplation and prayer. Limit mental and sexual activity until the Yin is restored. Avoid saunas and hot tubs.

Exercise: Rest is extremely important in replenishing Yin, both during the day and at night; going to bed early, by 9 - 9:30 PM, is very beneficial. Avoid aerobic exercise or any activity causing sweating, but do Yoga, Tai Chi, Qi Gong and other stretches, and light walking and swimming.

Combined Patterns

Lungs and Liver

The Lungs rule Qi while the Liver stores and regulates Blood. The Lungs are dependent on Liver Qi for the smooth movement of Qi, while the Liver relies on Lung Qi to regulate Blood. A dysfunction of the Lungs in dispersing and descending Qi causes Dryness and Heat to go downward, which can stagnate Liver Qi or cause Heat in the Liver. On the other hand, if Liver Qi stagnates in the chest, it can impair the flow of Lung-Qi or turn into fire and burn the Yin of the Lungs.

Lung Qi Deficiency and Liver Qi Stagnation Symptoms:
cough
moving pains
distension and fullness in the sternocostal or hypochondriac regions
dizziness
headache
depression
listlessness
Pulse: empty and tight
Tongue: pale or normal colored

Herbal Therapy: Bupleurum and Dang Gui Formula (Xiao yao san or Rambling Powder) with 9 grams of codonopsis and 6 grams of apricot seed.

Food Therapy: Refer to this category under Lung Qi Deficiency and Liver Qi Stagnation.

Other Therapies: Refer to this category under Lung Qi Deficiency and Liver Qi Stagnation.

Exercise: Four Purifications breathing practices, meditation and Eight Brocades Qi Gong practice.

Liver Qi Stagnation Invading the Lungs Symptoms:
cough
breathlessness or difficulty breathing .
asthma
distension and fullness in the sternocostal region
Pulse: tight, wiry
Tongue: normal colored

Herbal Therapy: Minor Bupleurum Combination (Xiao chai hu tang)

Food Therapy: The same as for Lung Qi Deficiency and Liver Qi Stagnation.

Other Therapies: The same as for Lung Qi Deficiency and Liver Qi Stagnation.

Exercise: The same as for Lung Qi Deficiency and Liver Qi Stagnation.

> **Liver Fire Invading the Lungs Symptoms:**
> breathlessness
> asthma
> stuffiness and pain of hypochondrium and chest
> headache
> irritability
> cough with painful breathing
> coughing up of blood or yellow-tinged sputum
> scanty dark urine .
> constipation
> dizziness
> **Pulse: wiry** and slippery
> **Tongue**: red, especially on sides; swollen in Lung area; yellow coat

Herbal Therapy: Morus and Lycium Formula (Xie bai san) with **Major Bupleurum Combination** (Da chai hu tang)

Food Therapy: Refer to this category under Liver Fire rising and Lung Qi Deficiency.

Other Therapies: Refer to this category under Liver Fire rising and Lung Qi Deficiency.

Exercise: Four Purifications and Shitali Pranayam exercise and the Eight Brocades, especially exercise number 5.

Lungs and Kidneys

The Lungs and Kidneys coordinate to promote movement of respiration. The Lungs rule Qi and respiration, perform the function of respiration and send Qi down to the Kidneys. Kidney Yang holds the Qi down and thus controls and promotes inspiration. Therefore, a Deficiency of Lung Qi causes painful and difficult breathing, while a Deficiency of Kidney Yang causes Lung Qi to not be received and results in difficulty of inhaling.

The Lungs also send Fluids down to the Kidneys, which evaporates some of it and sends that vapor back up to the Lungs to keep them moist. A dysfunction of either Organ can impair Fluid metabolism in the body, leading to either urinary incontinence or retention, or a Deficiency of Lung Yin from lack of moisture returning to the Lungs.

Lung Qi and Kidney Yang Deficiency

This is the same as the pattern of Kidneys Failing to Receive Qi under the Kidneys. Refer to that pattern for more details.

> **Lung and Kidney Yin Deficiency Symptoms:**
> dry cough which is worse in the evening
> feeling of heat in the afternoon
> night sweating
> hoarse voice
> malar flush
> tidal fever
> lassitude of loins and legs
> soreness of lower back
> thin body
> breathlessness on exertion
> nocturnal emissions
> heat in palms, soles and chest
> **Pulse:** empty and floating
> **Tongue: red and peeled** with two transverse cracks in Lung area

Herbal Therapy: Ophiopogon Combination (Mai men dong tang) or **Rehmannia Six Combination** (Liu wei di huang wan) with schizandra, apricot seed and American ginseng.

Food Therapy: Refer to this category under Lung Qi Deficiency and Kidney Yang Deficiency.

Other Therapies: Refer to this category under Lung Qi Deficiency and Kidney Yang Deficiency.

Exercise: Refer to this category under Lung Qi Deficiency and Kidney Yang Deficiency.

Lungs and Spleen

This is described under the Spleen Combined patterns.

SPLEEN

The major functions of the Spleen are to transform food and fluids into Qi and Blood and to rule Blood. Thus, disorders of the Spleen usually involve metabolic conditions such as low energy, digestive disorders, Dampness and menstrual irregularities.

Causes for Spleen Disharmonies:

Pathogenic Influences: The External Pernicious Influence which can invade the Spleen is Dampness. This can occur from excessive exposure to damp, humid and foggy areas and climates, living or working in damp environments, wearing wet clothing, sitting on damp surfaces and being in water for prolonged periods. When it invades, Dampness causes lack of appetite, nausea, abdominal distension. feeling of heaviness. slippery pulse and a thick white tongue coating.

Emotions: Yi, the intellectual function of the psyche, includes the ability to absorb and remember information, focusing, memorization, concentration, studying, thinking and organizing ideas. Thus, excessive thinking, studying, concentrating and memorizing weaken the Spleen. When the Spleen is imbalanced it often appears in our emotions. These include worry, brooding, pensiveness, obsession and nostalgia. Over thinking and obsessively dwelling on certain ideas and thoughts all reflect an imbalanced Yi. Further, being uncentered in ourselves reflects a Spleen disharmony. Being overly emotionally dependent or sympathetically overly sensitive to others are also possible symptoms of Spleen imbalance. All of these tend to weaken the Spleen and affect our digestive function.

Diet: Diet is central to Spleen imbalances since it is the major Organ involved with transforming food and fluids. The Spleen prefers to be warm and dry and loathes being wet and cold. This includes foods and their inherent warming and cooling energies. Thus, foods which are damp and/or cold, such as raw foods, salads, juices, fruits, refrigerated foods and drinks, frozen foods such as ice cream and iced drinks all impair the digestive capacity. Further, the excessive intake of sugar ultimately creates Heat in the Stomach and Depletes Spleen Qi. Warm and/or dry foods, such as whole grains, chicken, lamb, legumes, cooked vegetables, greens, ginger and pepper warm the Spleen and aid the digestive process.

Lifestyle Habits: Eating on the run, while standing up, driving or doing business, mental work or excessive reading all weaken the Spleen and its digestive function. Skipping meals, overeating, undereating and excessive dieting damage the Spleen and can incapacitate the body's ability to digest and extract food essence to build Blood and Qi

Deficient Spleen Qi

This is a very commonly seen pattern of imbalance. Modern diets are rich in sugars, fats, iced drinks, fast foods and cold raw foods. This, along with irregular eating habits such as inconsistent meals, eating standing up or on the run, eating while reading or discussing business over meals, eating too little or too much food, or eating a protein-deficient diet, all contribute to Deficient Spleen Qi. Extensive mental activity in work and study further causes Spleen Qi Deficiency. Excessive exposure to dampness, either in the environment or in one's home or work place, can create Dampness in the Spleen, obstructing its functions. Further, any long-term illness tends to weaken the Spleen, causing Deficient Spleen Qi. When Spleen Qi is Deficient, it cannot transform food and fluids to create Qi and Blood, and this ultimately causes a Deficiency of Blood and Qi in the body.

> **Symptoms:**
> no appetite
> fatigue
> Ioose stools
> slight abdominal pain and distension relieved by pressure
> gas and bloating
> poor digestion
> fatigue and lethargy
> sallow complexion
> weakness of the limbs
> **Pulse:** empty
> **Tongue:** pale or normal-colored with thin white moss; possible swollen sides with tooth marks and transverse cracks

Herbal Therapy: Four Major Herbs (Si jun zi tang); **Six Major Herbs** (Liu jun zi tang)

Food Therapy: Eat only cooked foods, including rice, millet, meat (especially beef), winter squash, vegetables, greens, aduki beans, congee and warm or room temperature drinks such as warm milk with ginger, cinnamon or cardamom and honey. Avoid cold, raw vegetables and fruits, juices, iced drinks, ice cream and frozen yogurt, salads, uncooked foods and the excessive use of sugar and other sweeteners.

Other Therapies: Moxibustion over the lower abdomen and Kidneys; meditation; getting in touch with emotional needs and finding ways other than "pleasure" foods to satisfy them; focusing on the present; rest; breathing exercises.

Exercise: Very light aerobic exercise, Yoga, Tai Chi, Qi Gong, swimming, walking and light Bicycling avoid strenuous exercise.

Deficient Spleen Yang
Deficient Spleen Yang is a more extensive and serious disorder than Spleen Qi Deficiency. Along with signs of Deficiency of Spleen Qi, it includes symptoms of Coldness. In fact, the metabolism can become so cold and slow that undigested food passes into the stools. Further, a Yang Deficiency usually impairs the circulation of Fluids, resulting in such symptoms as edema, leukorrhea and mucus in the lungs. The causes are the same as Spleen Qi Deficiency, along with excessive intake of cold, raw foods and drinks and overexposure to cold damp environments and climates.

Symptoms:
chilliness
cold limbs
fatigue
loose stools
undigested food in the stools
lack of appetite
gas and bloatedness
abdominal pain and distension relieved by pressure and warmth
sallow or bright-white complexion
weakness of the four limbs
edema
Pulse: weak, slow, deep
Tongue: pale, swollen, wet

Herbal Therapy: Vitality Combination (Zhen wu tang)

Food Therapy: Beef, lamb, all cooked foods and absolutely nothing raw or cold in energy or temperature, rice, millet, barley, whole grains, winter squash, cooked vegetables, greens and plenty of protein.

Other Therapies: Moxibustion over the navel, lower abdomen and Kidneys; finding constructive ways to meet one's emotional needs; singing; breathing exercises, rest.

Exercise: Light walking, swimming, bicycling and dancing; Yoga, Tai Chi, Qi Gong, Four Purifications and Ujjayi pranayam. Eight Brocades with special emphasis on exercises numbers 2, 3 and 7.

Sinking Spleen Qi
When Spleen Qi becomes Deficient, it may not be able to perform its function of raising Qi, including holding the Organs in place. It is produced by any of the causes of Spleen Qi Deficiency along with excessive and prolonged standing.

Symptoms:
bearing down sensation
prolapse of stomach, vagina, urinary bladder, uterus, anus
frequency and urgency of urination or urinary incontinence .
hemorrhoids .
hemorrhage
possibly varicose veins
extreme chronic diarrhea
other Spleen Qi Deficiency signs
Pulse: weak
Tongue: pale

Herbal Therapy: Ginseng and Astragalus Combination (Bu zhong yi qi tang)

Food Therapy: Same as Deficient Spleen Qi

Other Therapies: Same as Deficient Spleen Qi

Exercise: Four Purifications plus Ujjayi pranayam, also Eight Brocades with special emphasis on exercises numbers 1, 3, 5 and 7.

Spleen Unable to Control Blood
   In this form of Spleen Qi Deficiency, the Qi is unable to hold the Blood in the vessels. This causes extravasation including bleeding, hemorrhaging and bruising. It is provoked by any of the factors causing Spleen Qi Deficiency.

Symptoms:
bleeding
purpura
subcutaneous hemorrhaging
blood spots under the skin
blood in the urine or stools
bloody nose
excessive menses
uterine bleeding
sallow complexion
shortness of breath
Pulse: fine
Tongue: pale

Herbal Therapy: Ginseng and Longan Combination (Gui pi tang)

Food Therapy: The same as Deficient Spleen Qi.

Other Therapies: The same as Deficient Spleen Qi

Exercise: The same as Deficient Spleen Qi.

Cold Damp Invading the Spleen

The Spleen loathes Dampness. Long term exposure to cold damp environments or climates, or Deficient Spleen Qi or Yang not properly metabolizing Fluids often cause an Excess of Dampness in the Spleen. Thus, this can be an acute pattern from invasion of External Cold and Damp, or a chronic Internal one. If acute it will appear suddenly and possibly with a low fever; if chronic it will develop over a long period of time.

When Dampness obstructs the Spleen, it often collects in the chest and epigastrium, causing a feeling of stuffiness or heaviness there or in the head. Tastes become difficult to distinguish or are flat and sweetish. Further, vaginal discharge becomes excessive, resulting in leukorrhea.

Symptoms:
stuffiness of chest or epigastrium
feeling of heaviness
leukorrhea
lack of appetite
no thirst or desire to drink
lack of sensation of taste, or flat sweetish taste in mouth
skin eruptions containing fluid
watery stools
nausea
Pulse: slippery, slow
Tongue: thick, greasy white coat

Herbal Therapy: Ginseng, Poria and Atractylodes Powder (Shen ling bai zhu san) and **Sausurrea and Cardamon Combination** (Xiang sha liu jun zi tang)

Food Therapy: The same as Deficient Spleen Yang.

Other Therapies: The same as Deficient Spleen Yang.

Exercise: The same as Deficient Spleen Yang.

Damp Heat Invading the Spleen

Dampness can also appear with Heat and invade the Spleen as an External Pernicious Influence, such as inordinate exposure to hot and humid weather. However, prolonged and excessive intake of hot, greasy, fatty, fried or contaminated foods and abundant intake of alcohol can also cause this pattern.

Symptoms:
loose stools with offensive odor

low-grade fever constant throughout the day
stuffiness of epigastrium and lower abdomen with some pain
no appetite
feeling of heaviness
thirst without desire to drink, or desire to drink only in small
sips
nausea
vomiting
abdominal pain
burning sensation of anus
scanty and dark-colored urine
headache
Pulse: slippery, rapid
Tongue: sticky, greasy, yellow coat

Herbal Therapy: Capillaris and Poria Five Herbs Formula (Yin chen wu ling san).

Food Therapy: Avoid greasy, fatty or fried foods and alcohol; eat grains, legumes, vegetables and greens.

Other Therapies: Breathing exercises, especially Shitali or Sitkari pranayam; cupping over the entire back.

Exercise: Bed rest.

Combined Patterns

Spleen and Lungs

The Spleen transforms food and fluids and transports the resulting Grain Qi to the Lungs, where it is combined with Air Qi to form True Qi. Thus, both Organs are crucial to the production of Qi in the body. Furthermore, the Lungs control Qi and have a dispersing and descending function. If impaired, or if there is not enough deep breathing or exercise to bring in sufficient Air Qi, the Spleen is affected and can't function well in transporting, distributing and transforming nutrients or in performing Fluid metabolism.

On the other hand, an impairment of Spleen function or a diet high in cold raw foods leads to Deficient Qi of the Lungs and creates Dampness in the Lungs with symptoms of cough, excessive mucus and asthma. That is why one major way to treat Lung Dampness is to warm, strengthen and dry the Spleen.

Deficient Lung and Spleen Qi Symptoms:
no appetite
fatigue
breathlessness
loose stools

weak voice
bright-white complexion
slight spontaneous sweating
Pulse: empty
Tongue: pale

Herbal Therapy: Six Major Herbs (Liu jun zi tang) with astragalus

Food Therapy: Refer to this category under Deficient Lung Qi and Deficient Spleen Qi.

Other Therapies: Refer to this category under Deficient Lung Qi and Deficient Spleen Qi.

Exercise: Refer to this category under Deficient Lung Qi and Deficient Spleen Qi.

Spleen and Liver

The Spleen metabolizes and distributes nutrients and promotes water metabolism, while the Liver ensures the smooth and regular flow of energy and Blood. When this Liver function is normal, the Spleen can raise Qi in the body and properly send nutrients upward while the Stomach digests and sends food downwards. This ensures a plentiful supply of food essence, which is carried continuously to the Liver.

However, if any of these functions are disrupted, the Liver may affect the functions of the Spleen, resulting in two possible patterns: Spleen Qi Deficiency and Liver Blood Deficiency or Incoordination Between the Liver and the Spleen. In the former, when Spleen Qi is Deficient, it cannot produce Blood and its Deficiency directly affects the Liver's function of storing the Blood, resulting in Deficient Blood signs. In the latter, Dampness obstructs the Spleen, usually from excessive intake of fried, fatty and greasy foods and drinks, which eventually leads to Stagnation of Liver Qi.

> **Spleen Qi Deficiency and Liver Blood Deficiency Symptoms:**
> dizziness
> loose stools
> blurred vision
> numbness or tingling of limbs
> no appetite
> tiredness
> sallow complexion
> **Pulse:** choppy
> **Tongue: pale**, paler on sides; in severe cases sides could have
> slight orange color

Herbal Therapy: **Dang Gui Four** (Si wu tang) with **Four Major Herbs** (Si jun zi tang), or **Eight Precious Herbs** (Ba zhen wan).

Food Therapy: Refer to this category under Deficient Spleen Qi and Deficient Liver Blood.

Other Therapies: Refer to this category under Deficient Spleen Qi and Deficient Liver Blood.

Exercise: Walking, Four Purifications Pranayam; Eight Brocades with a special emphasis on exercises number 2 and 3; Qi Gong.

> **Liver Invading the Spleen Symptoms:**
> (Incoordination Between the Liver and the Spleen)
> stuffiness and fullness of epigastrium
> hypochondriac pain
> nausea
> no appetite
> loose stools
> feeling of heaviness
> thirst but desire to only drink in small sips
> sallow complexion
> **Pulse:** slippery and wiry
> **Tongue:** thick, sticky, yellow coat

Herbal Therapy: **Bupleurum and Peony Combination** (Xiao yao san) and **Four Major Herbs** (Si jun zi tang)

Food Therapy: Refer to this category under Deficient Spleen Qi and Liver Qi Stagnation.

Other Therapies: Refer to this category under Deficient Spleen Qi and Liver Qi Stagnation.

Exercise: Four Purifications and Shitali pranayam; Eight Brocades with emphasis on exercise number 5; Qi Gong.

Spleen and Kidneys

The Spleen is the material foundation for the acquired constitution, while the Kidney provides the inherited constitution. Kidney Yang can be likened to the pilot light of the stove while Spleen Yang and the Stomach are the burners under the pot. A Deficiency of the Yang of the Kidney will also contribute to a depletion of Spleen Yang and vice versa. If Kidney Yang is insufficient to warm the Yang of the Spleen, or when a long-term Deficiency of Spleen Yang produces Dampness which can eventually injure the Kidney Yang, this pattern results. It can also occur from prolonged intake of cold, raw and damp foods, excessive sexual activity and old age.

Spleen and Kidney Yang Deficiency Symptoms:
chronic diarrhea
chilliness
feeling of cold in the back
watery stools with undigested food
diarrhea at dawn
borborygmus
cold and painful sensation in the abdomen
edema
coldness of body and limbs
abundant-clear or scanty-clear urination
poor appetite
mental listlessness
abdominal distention
gas and bloating
physical weakness
difficulty breathing or breathlessness
lack of desire to talk
desire to lie down
Pulse: weak, deep, slow
Tongue: pale, swollen, wet

Herbal Therapy: Vitality Combination (Zhen wu tang).

Food Therapy: Refer to this category under Deficient Spleen Yang and Deficient Kidney Yang.

Other Therapies: Refer to this category under Deficient Spleen Yang and Deficient Kidney Yang.

Exercise: Four Purifications and Ujjayi pranayam; Eight Brocades with a special emphasis on exercise number 7; Qi Gong.

Spleen and Heart
This is described under the Heart combined patterns.

LIVER

The main functions of the Liver are to ensure the smooth and regular flow of Qi and Blood and to store Blood. Any dysfunctions of either of these functions has ramifications which can affect the entire body or any of its Organs. Disharmonies include Stagnation of Liver Qi or Blood, Excessive Heat, called Fire, in the Liver, Liver Wind, Damp Heat in the Liver, Cold in the Liver Meridian, and Deficiency of Liver Blood or Yin.

Causes for Liver Disharmonies:

Pathogenic Influences: The two External Pernicious Influences which affect the Liver are Wind and Dampness. Although Wind does not invade the Liver directly, it can aggravate an existing condition of Interior Wind in the Liver. When it does, it causes Liver Qi to stagnate, which can further result in Blood Stagnation. It can also cause skin rashes and hives which appear and move quickly.

Emotions: Anger, frustration, resentment, irritability, mood swings and depression indicate, and can cause, Liver imbalances such as Liver Fire Rising or Qi Stagnation. Therefore, it is important to discover the underlying cause for these feelings and find outlets which are constructive and beneficial.

Diet: Many foods lead to a build-up of Heat and congestion in the Liver, causing the Liver patterns which have far-reaching effects in the body. These include excessive consumption of fried and fatty foods, nuts and nut butters, avocados, cheese and dairy, chips of all kinds, turkey and red meats, alcohol, hot and spicy foods, caffeinated foods and drinks including coffee, black tea, cocoa, colas and chocolate, drugs and stimulants. The foods which decongest and aid the liver include vegetables, bitter foods and dark leafy greens such as kale, collards, dandelion, mustard, beet and mustard greens. Lemons also clear Heat and congestion from the Liver. A good morning liver cleanse is a fresh squeezed lemon in water with 1 or 2 teaspoons of olive oil and a couple of "00" sized capsules of cayenne pepper. This is followed with fennel seed tea.

Lifestyle Habits: Excessive activity, sex, exercise, regularly going to bed late at night (after 11 PM), working at jobs one doesn't like, repressing and stuffing emotions and not getting enough physical activity all imbalance the Liver. To rebalance the liver, go to bed by 11 PM at the latest, express and release emotions in a constructive way and do some movement through walking, dancing or another physical activity. Creativity is an important release for pent up Liver energy, as is self-expression in constructive and creative ways.

Stagnation of Liver Qi

This is not only the most common Liver pattern, but also one of the most common disharmonies in the body. When Liver Qi does not flow smoothly or regularly, it becomes Stagnant, and Excess and Heat result. This affects not only the Liver, but the other Organs and the Seven Emotions as well. Liver Qi Stagnation can result from suppressed or overly expressed anger, resentment and frustration, from a diet rich in stimulants, drugs, fatty and oily foods, recreational drugs, alcohol, coffee, black tea and from overwork without sufficient rest. Since there are so many ways this pattern can appear, it is divided into categories of related symptoms. As with all patterns, it is not necessary for all these symptoms to appear to indicate this disharmony. Three or more of the signs indicate its involvement.

It is very important when administering herbal therapy that tonics are not given for this condition, as it only creates Stagnation and Excess and so worsens the condition (like adding more cars to a bad traffic jam). In fact, it is for this reason that an important therapeutic herbal strategy is to first give moving herbs from the category of Regulating Qi and Blood along with clearing Heat herbs before or while giving tonics.

Symptoms:
1) overall
distension of hypochondrium and chest
hypochondriac pain
sighing
hiccuping

2) emotions
depression
moodiness and mood swings
frustration
inappropriate anger
a lump or plum-pit feeling in the throat
unhappiness
feeling of difficulty in swallowing

3) gynecological
PMS tension and irritability
swollen breasts before periods
irregular periods; painful periods

4) digestion
nausea
vomiting
sour belching
abdominal pain
poor appetite
epigastric pain
diarrhea or alternating diarrhea and constipation
churning feeling in the stomach
feeling of pulsation in epigastrium
abdominal distension
borborygmi

5) in the meridians
Iumps in the neck, breast, groin or flank
Pulse: wiry

Tongue: body color may be normal

Herbal Therapy: Bupleurum and Dang Gui Formula (Xiao yao san or Rambling Powder): **Bupleurum and Peony Formula** (Jia wei xiao yao san)

Food Therapy: Avoid fried and fatty foods, nuts and nut butters, avocados, cheese and dairy, chips of all kinds, turkey and red meats, alcohol, hot and spicy foods, caffeinated foods and drinks including coffee, black tea, cocoa, colas and chocolate, drugs and stimulants. Eat plenty of grains, legumes, vegetables and dark leafy greens, such as kale, collards, dandelion, mustard, beet and mustard greens. Lemon juice also helps decongest the liver.

Other Therapies: Work with the emotions of anger, frustration, resentment, irritability, mood swings and depression by finding constructive outlets to express and release them. Above all, do not repress or stuff your emotions, as this is what helped create these physical symptoms in the first place. Avoid excessive activity, sex and exercise. Regularity of habits helps to regulate Liver Qi. Go to bed by 11 PM at the latest, and if there is accompanying Kidney Yin Deficiency, go to bed by 9 - 9:30 PM.

Find work and jobs which you enjoy and are fulfilling. Alternate work with rest and play, as over-working can cause this pattern. Developing and expressing creativity is very important, as this opens the Liver Qi and helps it flow. Self-expression does this as well. Do cupping over the back, breathing exercises, singing and wear a harimaki. Gall Bladder and Liver flushes, GLA oils, flax seed, evening primrose, borage, black currant seed oils are also appropriate.

Exercise: In our modern lives, we have little need for natural exercise. This greatly contributes to energy being unused and unexpressed, which leads to its Stagnation. As a substitute, we go to gyms or have exercise equipment and video tapes at home, yet it does not compare to the amount of walking, lifting and carrying which was a normal part of life before motor vehicles. Thus, daily active movement is essential to a healthy Liver and the body overall.

Further, one of the best expressions of frustration, anger and resentment rather than "stuffing" them, which only turns them inward to harm the body, is to apply them in constructive movement. Anger is energy, so cleaning up the kitchen or unloading old drawers or closets, giving expression to creative endeavors or running around the block all help to express and release this energy in healthy ways. Movement through walking (especially in the woods), dancing, Tai Chi, Qi Gong, Yoga or regular exercise helps keep Liver Qi healthy.

Stagnation of Liver Blood
    When Liver Qi stagnates, it can also cause Stagnant Blood. Symptoms of Blood Stagnation are fixed, usually sharp, stabbing pains (especially in the chest). These can be aggravated by, as well as caused from, long-standing emotional problems and are a consequence of prolonged Liver Qi Stagnation.

Symptoms:
dark and clotted menstrual blood
irregular menses
painful menses
vomiting of blood
epistaxis
abdominal pain
"masses" in the abdomen, such as fibroids
Pulse: Wiry
Tongue: purple with purplish spots, especially on the sides

Herbal Therapy: Disperse Vital Energy in the Liver Powder (Chai hu su gan san); **Bupleurum and Dang Gui Formula** (Xiao yao san or Rambling Powder)

Food Therapy: Refer to this category under Liver Qi Stagnation.

Other Therapies: Refer to this category under Liver Qi Stagnation; moxibustion or castor oil packs over the abdomen

Exercise: Four Purifications and Ujjayi pranayam; Eight Brocades, especially exercises numbers 2, 3, 4 and 5.

Liver Fire Blazing Upwards
    This is an Excess Heat condition of the Liver precipitated by prolonged repressed or overly expressed anger, resentment or frustration or by Stagnant Liver Qi generating Fire. It can also arise from excessive intake of alcohol, drugs, caffeinated foods and drinks, hot foods such as lamb and beef and fried and greasy foods.
    When Heat accumulates in the Liver, it has a tendency to rise, causing symptoms in the head, face and eyes. Further, Heat consumes Fluids, resulting in Dryness signs. It can also drive the Blood out of its pathways, producing bleeding through various bodily orifices (much like earth "fluids", lava, are pushed out of a volcano when heated).

Symptoms:
red face and eyes
irritability
propensity to outbursts of anger
deafness, tinnitus or sudden ringing in the ears
dizziness
dry mouth
splitting headaches and migraines
insomnia
dark scanty urine
thirst
bitter taste
tight neck and shoulders
dream-disturbed sleep
constipation with dry stools
nose bleeds
vomiting of blood
coughing up of blood
Pulse: full, wiry and rapid
Tongue: red body with redder sides, dry, yellow coat

Herbal Therapy: Major Bupleurum Combination (Da chai hu tang)

Food Therapy: Avoid excessive intake of alcohol, drugs, caffeinated foods and drinks including coffee, black tea, cocoa, colas and chocolate, hot foods such as lamb and beef and fried and greasy foods, chips of all kinds, nuts and nut butters, avocados, cheese and dairy, turkey and red meats, hot and spicy foods, drugs and stimulants. The foods which decongest and aid the Liver include vegetables, bitter foods, dark leafy greens, such as kale, collards, dandelion, mustard, beet and mustard greens, lemon, watermelon, cucumber and mung beans. Drink dandelion and chicory tea.

Other Therapies: It is extremely important in this pattern to find constructive and beneficial ways to express and release the pent up anger, frustration, irritability and resentment so it is not taken out on oneself or others in any forms of abuse. Find work which is satisfying and enjoyable. Discover creative outlets and actively pursue them. Regularly do cupping over the back, breathing exercises and meditation or contemplation.

Exercise: Movement and exercise of all types can be a valuable release of energy for this pattern and a constructive outlet for repressed anger, frustration and resentment. Further, meditation, contemplation and prayer help to subdue Fire.

Liver Wind Agitating Internally
Internal Wind is characterized by either movement or lack of movement, such as spasms, tics, tremors, numbness, dizziness, convulsions or paralysis. It can arise from three different causes: extreme Heat, Deficiency of Liver Blood and Deficiency of Liver Yin with Liver Yang rising.

Extreme Heat Generating Wind
During acute febrile diseases it is possible for Exterior Heat to invade and penetrate deeply into the Blood level. This can then stir up the Wind, causing an Excess type of Internal Wind. It is more common in children during measles, encephalitis and meningitis.

> **Symptoms:**
> high temperature
> convulsions
> rigidity of the neck
> tremor of limbs
> tetany
> coma in severe cases
> **Pulse:** full, rapid and wiry
> **Tongue:** stiff, deep red, thick yellow coat

Herbal Therapy: Gastrodia and Uncaria Combination (Tian ma gou teng yin)

Food Therapy: Only very simple and bland foods should be eaten during this period, such as rice cereal and soups. In some cases fasting on fruit or vegetable juices might be appropriate. Avoid all else, including iced and refrigerated drinks, as these can create more heat.

Other Therapies: Seek appropriate medical attention.

Exercise: Bed rest.

Deficient Liver Blood Generating Wind
When Liver Blood is Deficient, the Blood vessels become "empty" and are then "filled" with Wind. Blood then fails to nourish the sinews, tendons and muscles. It occurs from chronic Blood Deficiency.

> **Symptoms:**
> shaking of head
> **tremors of limbs**
> tics

numbness of limbs
Pulse: choppy
Tongue: pale and deviated

Herbal Therapy: Dang Gui Four (Si wu tang) with gastrodia

Food Therapy: Refer to this category under Deficient Liver Blood.

Other Therapies: Refer to this category under Deficient Liver Blood; meditation, contemplation and prayer help calm Wind; moxibustion over the lower abdomen and kidneys; regular oil massage.

Exercise: Aerobic and strenuous exercise stir up more Wind and so should be avoided. Gentle movement and stretches are beneficial, such as Yoga, Tai Chi and Qi Gong.

Deficiency of Liver Yin with Liver Yang Rising and Generating Wind
Prolonged Yin Deficiency causes Liver Yang to rise upwards. It is sometimes termed Arrogant Liver Yang, and combines both Excess and Empty (Deficient Yin) Fire. Thus, signs of both are present. Because Liver Yang can generate Wind, Wind stroke may occur. It can occur from excessive exercise, physical exertion or sexual activity over a long period of time, from Blood Deficiency, particularly in women with chronic menorrhagia, and from prolonged anger, resentment and frustration.

Symptoms:
sudden unconsciousness
convulsions
deviation of eye and mouth
hemiplegia aphasia or difficult speech
dizziness
Pulse: rapid, floating and empty or wiry and fine
Tongue: red and peeled, deviated

Herbal Therapy: Rehmannia Six Combination (Liu wei di huang wan) with lycii berries and chrysanthemum (or Qi ju di huang wan)

Food Therapy: Eat a simple diet of grains, legumes, cooked vegetables and greens. Avoid foods which are cold and raw, fried and greasy, caffeinated drinks including coffee, black tea, cocoa, colas and chocolate, nuts and nut butters, avocados, cheese and dairy, chips of all kinds, turkey and red meats, alcohol, hot and spicy foods, drugs and stimulants. The foods which decongest and aid the Liver include vegetables, bitter foods, dark leafy greens, such as kale, collards, dandelion, mustard, beet and mustard greens. Lemons also clear Heat and congestion from the Liver.

Other Therapies: Rest is extremely important, as is avoiding excessive exercise, physical exertion and sex. Over-doing anything will only perpetuate this pattern. Meditation, contemplation and prayer help replenish Yin. Be sure to appropriately express and release any repressed anger, frustration and resentment, and allow creative expression. Limit mental activity until the Yin is restored. Being asleep by 9 - 9:30 PM is very beneficial. Avoid saunas and hot tubs.

Exercise: Gentle stretches are beneficial, such as Yoga, Tai Chi and Qi Gong, but avoid strenuous exercise and exertion.

Damp Heat in the Liver

This pattern arises from excessive Heat in the Liver and Dampness due to Spleen Deficiency. When Damp Heat accumulates it disrupts the flow of Qi, causing Qi Stagnation symptoms. Since Dampness has a tendency to flow downwards, it frequently settles in the Lower Burner, causing urinary bladder infections and vaginal discharge, itching and infection. This is commonly caused by poor diet impairing the Spleen function, such as prolonged and excessive intake of cold and raw foods, plus excessive consumption of hot and greasy foods, refined sugar, coffee and alcohol. Irregular diet and lifestyle habits can also contribute. Any causes of Liver Qi Stagnation, such as anger, plus overexposure to hot and damp climates and environments also cause this pattern.

> **Symptoms:**
> fever
> fullness of chest and hypochondrium
> nausea
> jaundice
> vomiting
> loss of appetite
> abdominal distention
> bitter taste scanty
> dark urine, possibly with burning upon urination
> vaginal discharge and itching pain,
> redness and swelling of the scrotum
> **Pulse: slippery**, rapid and wiry
> **Tongue:** red body with sticky **yellow coat**

Herbal Therapy: Gentiana Combination (Long dan xie gan tang) and **Capillaris Formula (**Yin chen hao tang)

Food Therapy: Follow a balanced diet of grains, legumes, cooked vegetables, greens, winter squash and warm or room temperature drinks. Eat all cooked foods. Avoid cold and raw foods and drinks, consumption of hot and greasy foods, dairy, nuts and nut butters, chips of all kinds, caffeinated foods and drinks, red meat, fruits, juices, iced drinks, ice cream and popsicles, salads, uncooked foods and the excessive use of sugar and other sweeteners. Avoid eating an irregular diet and at irregular times.

Other Therapies: Same as Liver Qi Stagnation.

Exercise: Same as Liver Qi Stagnation, so long as the exercise does not overexert the body.

Stagnation of Cold in the Liver Meridian
This pattern occurs when External Cold invades the Liver Meridian. Because this meridian encircles the groin, pain and contraction of the scrotum occur.

> Symptoms:
> hypogastric pain referring to the scrotum and testes,
>   relieved by warmth
> straining of testes or contraction of the scrotum
> in women there may be shrinking of the vagina
> **Pulse**: deep, slow, wiry
> **Tongue**: pale, wet, white coat

Herbal Therapy: **Evodia Combination** (Wu zhu yu tang)

Food Therapy: All cooked foods and absolutely nothing raw or cold in energy or temperature, rice, millet and other grains, legumes, winter squash, cooked vegetables, greens.

Other Therapies: Moxibustion over the navel, lower abdomen and kidneys; cupping over the back; breathing exercises; singing; harimaki; find constructive ways to meet one's emotional and creative needs.

Exercise: Light walking, swimming, bicycling and dancing; Yoga, Tai Chi, Qi Gong.

Deficiency of Liver Blood
Since the Liver stores Blood, any Deficiency of Blood often appears in the Liver also. This will affect areas the Liver relates to, such as the tendons, eyes, nails and menstruation. It arises from the causes of Deficient Blood, such as poor diet, Deficient Spleen Qi so Blood cannot be produced, hemorrhaging, and a Deficiency of Kidney Qi or Essence,

Symptoms:
blurred vision
dull-pale complexion
scanty periods
numbness of limbs
pale lips
muscular weakness
muscle spasms
cramps
withered and brittle nails
"floaters" or black spots in the eyes
insomnia
Pulse: choppy or fine
Tongue: pale body, especially on the sides, dry

Herbal Therapy: Dang Gui Four (Si wu tang)

Food Therapy: Lamb, dang gui and ginger soup, bone soups, milk, black and aduki beans, congee, all cooked foods; do not skip meals.

Other Therapies: Contemplation, meditation and prayer; moxibustion over the lower abdomen and Kidneys; harimaki; breathing exercises; rest; oil massage; working on emotional issues such as discovering what one is lacking emotionally, creatively and physically and finding beneficial ways to meet those needs. Avoid saunas and hot tubs, over-working and over-doing, physical exertion and too much movement. Excessive sexual activity and late nights.

Exercise: Light aerobic and stretching exercises including Yoga, Tai Chi and Qi Gong.

Deficient Liver Yin
This is an empty Fire pattern arising out of Deficient Liver Blood or Deficient Kidney Yin. It has similar symptoms to Deficient Liver Blood with the additional signs of Dryness and Yin Deficient Heat. Excessive activity, overwork, "burning the candle at both ends" without sufficient rest, and poor and irregular diet lead to this imbalance. Many menopausal symptoms fit this category.

Symptoms:
dry eyes
dry throat
night sweats
scanty menstruation
muddled vision
sallow complexion
dream-disturbed sleep
insomnia

numbness
blurred vision
amenorrhea
dizziness
malar flush
afternoon fever
hot palms, soles and chest
nervousness
depression nervous tension
Pulse: wiry, rapid and thin or floating and empty
Tongue: red, especially on the sides, and peeled

Herbal Therapy: Rehmannia Six Combination with Lycii berries and Chrysanthemum (Qi ju di huang wan) or **Ming mu di huang wan** patent medicine.

Food Therapy: Eat plenty of grains, legumes, a little meat, cooked vegetables, greens, milk and black and aduki beans. Avoid spicy, greasy and fried foods, caffeinated foods and drinks including coffee, black tea, cocoa, colas and chocolate, nuts and nut butters, chips of all kinds, avocados, dairy (except warm milk with cardamom and honey), alcohol, drugs, chips of all kinds, turkey and red meats and stimulants. The foods which decongest and aid the Liver include vegetables, bitter foods, dark leafy greens, such as kale, collards, dandelion, beet and mustard greens. Lemons also clear Heat and congestion from the Liver.

Other Therapies: Rest is extremely important in nourishing Yin, as is meditation, contemplation and prayer. Avoid excessive mental and sexual activity, overwork and "burning the candle at both ends". Get regular oil massage. Go to bed by 9 - 9:30 PM. Do cupping over the back. Avoid saunas and hot tubs.

Exercise: Stretching and light movement are beneficial, such as Yoga, Tai Chi, Qi Gong, swimming and walking. Avoid strenuous exercise or over-exertion.

Arrogant Liver Yang

Also termed Liver Yang Rising, this is a combined Excess Heat and Deficient Yin pattern. in terms of Five Elements, Water is insufficient to nourish Wood and so Liver Yang rises. This pattern appears without true Heat because of the presence of Deficiency. Usually Liver Yin Deficiency appears with Kidney Yin Deficiency, although it may also appear with a Kidney Yang Deficiency. Because Kidney Yang shares the same root as Kidney Yin, a Deficiency of one suggests to some degree a Deficiency of the other. Thus, a Kidney Yang Deficiency eventually creates a Yin Deficiency and possible Liver Yang rising.

Symptoms:
headache in vertex, temples, eyes or lateral side of head
irritability
dizziness
tinnitus
deafness
tight neck and shoulders
dry mouth and throat
irritability
insomnia
shouting in anger
Pulse: wiry
Tongue: red, especially on the sides

Herbal Therapy: Rehmannia Six Combination with Lycii berries and Chrysanthemum (Qi ju di huang wan), or **Ming mu di huang wan** (patent medicine) and **Major Bupleurum Combination** (Da chai hu tang).

Food Therapy: Refer to this category under Deficient Liver Yin.

Other Therapies: Refer to this category under Deficient Liver Yin.

Exercise: Refer to this category under Deficient Liver Yin.

Combined Patterns
Liver and Spleen: Explained previously under Spleen.
Liver and Lungs: Explained previously under Lungs.

Liver and Kidneys
The Liver stores Blood while the Kidneys store Essence. Liver Blood depends on Essence for nourishment, while Essence depends on Blood for replenishment. Both have a common source: Grain Qi derived from the Spleen. A long term Liver Blood Deficiency can cause depletion of Kidney Yin. In terms of Five Elements, the Kidneys nourish the Liver. Thus, any depletion of the Kidneys affects the Liver. Usually this appears as a Liver and Kidney Yin Deficiency, or Yin Deficiency with Liver Yang Rising. However, if Kidney Yang is depleted, Kidney Yin will tend to be Deficient and then affect Liver Yin. Furthermore, prolonged emotional problems due to anger, frustration and depression cause this pattern.

Liver and Kidney Yin Deficiency Symptoms:
dry eyes
dry throat
night sweating
scanty menstruation

sallow complexion
dull occipital or vertex headache
insomnia
dream-disturbed sleep
dizziness
malar flush
numbness of limbs
blurred vision
propensity to outbursts of anger
soreness of lower back
tinnitus
feeling of heat in palms, soles and chest
difficult-dry stools
nocturnal emissions
amenorrhea
delayed menstrual cycle
infertility in women
Pulse: wiry, rapid and thin or floating and empty
Tongue: red, peeled and cracked

Herbal Therapy: Rehmannia Six Combination (Liu wei di huang wan) and **Rehmannia Six Combination with Lycii berries and Chrysanthemum** (Qi ju di huang wan) or **Ming mu di huang wan** patent medicine.

Food Therapy: Refer to this category under Deficient Liver Yin and Deficient Kidney Yin.

Other Therapies: Refer to this category under Deficient Liver Yin and Deficient Kidney Yin.

Exercise: Refer to this category under Deficient Liver Yin and Deficient Kidney Yin.

KIDNEYS

The main functions of the Kidneys are to store Essence, govern birth, growth and reproduction and to rule water. Because the Kidneys store Jing, which the body can never have in excess, Kidney disharmonies are most always from Deficiency rather than Excess. Furthermore, since the Kidneys are the root of Yin and Yang and Source Qi for the entire body, disharmonies of the Kidneys are rarely isolated but usually involve other Organs. Likewise, chronic illnesses of other Organs usually include some impairment of the Kidneys, either of Kidney Yin or Kidney Yang.

Central to the treatment of the Kidneys is the recognition of the interdependence of Kidney Yin and Kidney Yang, since they arise from the same source, Essence. A depletion of one signals, to a lesser degree, a depletion of the other and vice versa. Thus, both must be treated together for best results.

Causes for Kidney Disharmonies

Hereditary Weakness: Because the fetus is determined by the Essence of both parents, if Essence is weak in any way, especially at the moment of conception, the person can inherit a weakened constitution prone to many ailments or congenital diseases. This can appear as poor bone development, mental retardation and childhood asthma or diabetes, for instance.

Emotions: The emotions of the Kidneys are fear, anxiety, shock, apprehension, paranoia, panic, suspicion and distrust. These can ultimately lead to a feeling of inadequacy, inferiority, lack of self-trust, a victim complex, procrastination and avoidance, injuring the Will which resides in the Kidneys. Fear, anxiety, insecurity and shock all weaken Kidney Qi, causing frequent urination and bed wetting, especially in children. Ultimately the Qi rises and can lead to Empty Fire of the Kidneys.

Diet: Diet is very important to Kidney health. Adequate whole grains, protein, especially beans, cooked vegetables and greens support the Kidneys. Considering that Kidney Yang is the "pilot light" of the body, the excessive intake of cold and raw foods, juices, fruits, iced drinks and foods such as ice cream or frozen yogurt create Cold in the Kidneys and injure the Yang. When the pilot light cannot stay lit, it cannot warm the Yang of the other Organs such as the Spleen and Heart, causing poor digestion, diarrhea and slowed circulation. Further, alcohol, coffee and other caffeinated drinks or foods and tobacco smoking all seriously deplete the Kidneys and thus, the Yin, Yang and Essence of the body.

Lifestyle Habits: The Kidneys are among the Organs most affected by stress and excessive activity of any sort. Stress depletes the Yin and Essence, thus lowering immunity and causing insomnia, poor memory and sexual difficulties. Excessive mental, physical and sexual activity (orgasm), inadequate sleep, overworking, staying up late at night, eating on the run or late at night, hurried meals, lack of rest, relaxation and exercise and excessive mental work all compromise Kidney Yin and Essence. Further, the stress, anxiety and worry usually accompanying overwork additionally deplete Kidney Yin and Essence. Additionally, excessive standing weakens Kidney Qi, resulting in weakness, tiredness and pain in the lower back. Perhaps more than any other Organ syndrome, supportive lifestyle habits are vitally important to preserving Kidney Qi and promoting health and longevity.

Long term illness eventually affects the Kidneys, either Kidney Yin or Kidney Yang. Further, with age there is a natural decline of Kidney Essence. Most of the signs of old age are due to a waning of Kidney Essence, such as hearing difficulties, poor eyesight, brittle and fragile bones and declining sexual function.

Kidney Yang Deficiency

A depletion of Kidney Yang results in signs of Internal Cold and weakness. This has far reaching effects, since a Kidney Yang Deficiency indicates that the Life Gate Fire is also Deficient, and thus the fundamental warmth for the body is impaired. Therefore, the Organs lack warmth and cannot fully perform their functions. Additionally, Essence cannot warm the sexual function and uterus, possibly causing infertility and lowered libido. It further results in insufficient Qi to give strength to the bones. In severe cases, the Yang fails to transform Fluids, which accumulate to form edema and to cause water retention in other Organs, particularly the Heart and Lungs. When this occurs there will be accompanying signs of breathlessness on exertion, cough, asthma and thin, watery, frothy sputum (Lungs), or breathlessness, palpitations and cold hands (Heart). This pattern is frequently seen with Deficient Heart or Spleen Yang or Lung Qi.

Kidney Yang Deficiency is caused by overexposure to cold climates and environments, excessive intake of cold and raw foods and drinks and Kidney depleting substances such as alcohol, coffee, sugar; excessive sexual activity, especially if one is exposed to cold immediately after sexual intercourse, chronic Dampness and old age.

Symptoms:
cold and sore lower back
copious, clear pale urine
cold limbs
fear of cold
weak legs
soreness and weakness of lower back
cold knees
lack of Shen
bright, white or darkish face
lassitude
apathy
edema of the legs
loose stools
subdued, quiet manner
impotence or frigidity
sterility or infertility
premature ejaculation
spermatorrhea
nocturnal emissions without dreams
chronic vaginal discharge or leukorrhea
loose teeth
loss of hearing or deafness
night time urination
frequent and copious urination
clear urination

weak stream urination
dripping urine
urinary incontinence
Pulse: deep, slow
Tongue: pale

Herbal Therapy: Rehmannia Eight Combination (Ba wei di huang wan) and/or **Eucommia and Rehmannia Combination** (Restore the Right - You gui wan); **Circuligo and Epimedium Combination** (Er xian tang).

Food Therapy: Eat a balanced diet of all cooked foods and those with a warm energy such as whole grains, legumes (especially aduki beans), meat (especially lamb, beef and pork), cooked vegetables and greens. Drink walnut tea or use walnuts in cooking. Asparagus, black cherry juice, raspberries and millet all aid Kidney Qi. Avoid any intake of cold and raw foods and drinks, frozen yogurt, ice cream, popsicles, iced and refrigerated drinks, juices, sodas, coffee and other caffeinated foods and drinks, sugar, alcohol, soy milk and tofu.

Other Therapies: Avoid excessive sexual activity, exposure to cold (especially over the lower abdomen and back), and excessive use of hot tubs and saunas, being sure to dunk or thoroughly rinse in cool water after they are used. Wear a harimaki, apply moxibustion or ginger fomentations over the lower abdomen and Kidney regions and do breathing exercises.

Exercise: Get plenty of physical exercise as appropriate for your body's capability. Do the Four Purifications and Ujjayi (in the Winter) and the Eight Brocades, especially exercise numbers 7 and 8.

Kidneys Failing to Receive Qi
    This pattern results from a dysfunction of the Kidneys' capacity to receive and hold Qi. When the Kidneys cannot receive and hold down Qi, it accumulates above, resulting in symptoms such as difficulty in breathing, especially on exertion, and sweating. It is considered a type of Kidney Yang Deficiency and so includes signs of that pattern. It develops from prolonged chronic conditions, excessive physical exercise, particularly during puberty, excessive lifting and standing and hereditary weakness of the Lungs and Kidneys.

Symptoms:
shortness of breath on exertion
sweating
clear urination
difficulty in inhaling

rapid and weak breathing
cough
asthma
cold limbs, especially after sweating
swelling of the face
thin body
mental listlessness
clear urination during asthma attack
soreness of the back
Pulse: weak, tight, deep
Tongue: pale

Herbal Therapy: Rehmannia Eight Combination (Ba wei di huang wan) with Gecko

Food Therapy: The same as Deficient Kidney Yang.

Other Therapies: The same as Deficient Kidney Yang.

Exercise: The same as Deficient Kidney Yang.

Kidney Yin Deficiency
    This pattern is characterized by a Deficiency of Yin and Essence of the Kidneys. Yin Deficiency gives rise to false Heat symptoms, such as night sweats, thirst and five palm heat. These signs are from a depletion of Fluids and Essence. There may also be an insufficiency of Marrow to fill the brain, causing memory weakness and forgetfulness. Deficient Kidney Yin is most often seen with Deficient Heat, Deficient Liver Yin or Deficient Lung Yin. It occurs from prolonged overwork, "burning the candle at both ends", excessive activity or sexual involvement, chronic long term illnesses, consumption of Body Fluids by Heat in fevers, prolonged blood loss, overdosage of Kidney Yang tonics, smoking and Kidney-depleting foods such as coffee, alcohol, sugar, and fruit juices.

> **Symptoms:**
> dry mouth at night
> night sweats
> thin, shriveled constitution
> dry throat thirst
> dizziness
> vertigo
> heat in palms, soles and chest
> malar flush
> afternoon heat flushes
> tinnitus
> ache in bones
> poor hearing or deafness
> weak and sore back
> little sperm

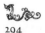

premature ejaculation
nocturnal emission
constipation
dark, scanty urination
forgetfulness or poor memory
Pulse: floating, empty and rapid
Tongue: red with no coat, cracks

Herbal Therapy: Rehmannia Six combination (Liu wei di huang wan); **Anemarrhena and Phellodendron Combination** (Zhi bai di huang wan).

Food Therapy: Eat plenty of whole grains with protein complement such as legumes or meat, cooked vegetables and greens to support the Kidneys. Pork, duck, milk and congee are especially beneficial. Avoid coffee and other caffeinated foods and drinks, alcohol, sugar and tobacco smoking.

Other Therapies: As mentioned above, lifestyle habits are very important in preserving Kidney health. Prolonged stress, staying up late, sexual activity, mental work, eating late at night, overwork and lack of rest, relaxation and exercise all compromise Kidney Yin, and thus these activities should be moderated. Wear a harimaki, do breathing exercises and do cupping over the back. Avoid saunas and hot tubs.

Exercise: Rest is one of the best and most important ways to replenish Yin. Since over-exertion depletes Yin, exercise should be mild and gentle, such as swimming, walking, Yoga, Tai Chi and Qi Gong. Aerobics and any exercise which causes sweating should be avoided.

Deficient Kidney Jing
  Deficient Kidney Jing usually incorporates Deficiency of Kidney Yin and, to some extent, Kidney Yang. Its signs manifest in relation to growth, development, reproduction, sexuality, bones, marrow, the brain, teeth, memory and head hair. Its depletion is caused by poor hereditary constitution in children, old age, excessive sexual activity or any of the causes of Kidney Yin or Yang Deficiency over a prolonged time.

Symptoms
In Children:
poor bone development
softness or late closure of the fontanel
mental dullness or retardation

In Adults:
weak knees and legs

falling hair
weakness of sexual activity
premature aging or senility
bad or loose teeth
poor memory
brittle bones
softening of the bones
premature graying of the hair
soreness of the back
Pulse: floating, empty
Tongue: red and peeled

Herbal Therapy: Five Seeds of Creation (Wu zi wan)

Food Therapy: Refer to this category under Deficient Kidney Yin and Kidney Yang.

Other Therapies: Refer to this category under Deficient Kidney Yin and Kidney Yang.

Exercise: Refer to this category under Deficient Kidney Yin and Kidney Yang.

Kidney Yin Deficient, Empty Fire Blazing
    When Kidney Yin is severely depleted, it leads to the signs of empty Fire rising. The rising Deficiency Heat can disturb the Mind and cause mental restlessness or insomnia. There is also a depletion of Body Fluids, causing Dryness, and a possibility of Heat causing the Blood to move out of the vessels. This pattern results from the same causes of Yin Deficiency with the addition of chronic emotional problems.

Symptoms:
malar flush
dry throat, especially at night
mental restlessness
feeling of heat in the afternoon
low grade or afternoon fever
insomnia
mental restlessness
night sweats
scanty dark urine
blood in the urine
dry stools
soreness of the lower back
nocturnal emissions with dreams
excessive sexual desire
Pulse: floating, empty, rapid
Tongue: red, peeled, cracked

Herbal Therapy: Anemarrhena, Phellodendron with Rehmannia Combination (Zhi bai di huang wan)

Food Therapy: Refer to this category under Kidney Yin Deficiency.

Other Therapies: Refer to this category under Kidney Yin Deficiency.

Exercise: Refer to this category under Kidney Yin Deficiency.

Combined Patterns
Kidney and Heart: Described under Heart.
Kidney and Liver: Described under Liver.
Kidney and Lung: Described under Lung.
Kidney and Spleen: Described under Spleen.

YANG ORGANS
SMALL INTESTINE
The Small Intestine functions to control receiving and transforming food and fluids and to separate fluids. It then sends the waste to the Large Intestine and the impure Fluids to the Urinary Bladder. Thus, disorders of the Small Intestine result in digestive, intestinal and urinary symptoms. Most patterns of disharmony are included in Yin Organ imbalances. One pattern in particular, however, is especially distinguished for itself, Heat in the Small Intestine.

Heat in the Small Intestine
When the Heat from the Heart interferes with the Fluid separating function of the Small Intestine, it then gets sent to the Urinary Bladder, where it is improperly processed and causes Heat in the Bladder. It is caused and aggravated by hot, spicy, fatty and greasy foods and drinks, long term anxiety, especially over life direction and pressures, and spreading oneself too thin from overworking.

> **Symptoms:**
> abdominal pain
> tongue ulcers
> scanty, dark and painful urination
> mental restlessness
> pain in throat
> deafness
> heat sensation in the chest
> thirst
> **Pulse**: rapid, full
> **Tongue**: red with redder swollen tip, yellow coat

Herbal Therapy: Gentiana Combination (Long dan xie gan tang)

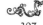

TRIPLE WARMER

There are no Triple Warmer patterns of disharmony because it is not a distinct Organ from the other Organs in the body. Instead, Triple Warmer syndromes are involved in disharmonies of the Yin and Yang Organs within the Upper, Middle and Lower Warmers. Upper Warmer dysfunctions generally include invasion of an Exterior Pernicious Influence, such as Wind Cold or Wind Heat, which blocks the circulation of the Lung's Defensive Qi and causes sneezing, runny nose, sore throat, body aches, fever, headaches, earaches and so on. Middle Warmer disharmonies occur from digestive disturbances and food retention. Lower Warmer imbalances include improper transforming, separating and excreting of fluids and waste.

STOMACH

The Stomach is in charge of receiving and digesting food and fluids. It then sends the pure portion to the Spleen and the impure to the Small Intestine for further digestion. The patterns of disharmony include Deficiency and Coldness, a Deficiency of Yin, Heat, rebellious Qi and Food Stagnation. Because Stomach Qi Deficiency and Stomach Coldness are so similar to Spleen Qi Deficiency and Spleen Yang Deficiency, they are not included here.

Stomach Yin Deficiency

The Stomach is the origin of Fluids and hates to be Hot or Dry. When there are insufficient Fluids for the stomach, Dryness and Heat result. However, as in all Yin Deficiency, it is not a true Heat, but occurs as a result of lack of moisture and coolness. Thus, there will be Yin Deficient signs such as thirst, feeling of heat and no appetite, but there will be no desire to drink, the feeling of Heat will occur mainly in the afternoon and the appetite is low instead of high as with true Stomach Heat. Long term irregular eating habits, such as skipping meals, eating on the run, having late night meals, eating while reading or conducting business, working immediately after eating and a poor diet all cause this pattern.

Symptoms:
epigastric pain
dry mouth
no appetite
fever or feeling of heat in the afternoon
dry mouth and throat
thirst but with no desire to drink or only in small sips

feeling of fullness after eating
constipation with dry stools
Pulse: floating and empty
Tongue: red and peeled in the center

Herbal Therapy: Ophiopogon Combination (Mai men dong tang)

Stomach Fire

Stomach Fire signals a true Excess of Heat in the Stomach, creating symptoms such as mouth ulcers, bad breath, intense thirst and bleeding of the gums. In this case the excessive Heat burns off the Fluids, creating extreme thirst and constipation. Over time the Heat can cause obstruction to Stomach Qi, resulting in vomiting, sour regurgitation and nausea. Excessive intake of hot, spicy, greasy and fried foods along with alcohol, tobacco and sugar cause Stomach Fire.

Symptoms:
burning sensation in the epigastrium
extreme thirst, especially for cold drinks
frontal headaches
craving for cold drinks and foods
gum swelling, pain and bleeding
constant and ravenous hunger
constipation
nausea
vomiting
sour regurgitation
feeling of dryness in mouth
Pulse: full, slippery, rapid
Tongue: red with dry thick yellow coating

Herbal Therapy: Clear the Stomach Powder (Qinq wei san)

Rebellious Stomach Qi

When the Qi of the Stomach is obstructed or interfered with from strong emotions such as anxiety and worry, it "rebels", or ascends rather than descends. This frequently appears with other patterns, such as Stomach Fire or Cold invading the Stomach. It results in vomiting, nausea, belching and stomachache.

Symptoms:
hiccuping
nausea
vomiting
belching
stomach ache

distention
Pulse: tight in Stomach position
Tongue: no changes

Herbal Therapy: Clove and Persimmon Calyx Combination (Shi di tang)

Food Stagnation
This pattern occurs from food being improperly digested and thus, retained in the Stomach. It causes a blockage and feeling of fullness and Stagnation. Stomach Qi then becomes obstructed and ascends rather than descends. Insomnia can occur from this because the ascending Qi disturbs the Mind. Most people can probably remember overeating a holiday meal with the accompanying bloating, belching, pain and poor sleep that resulted. Overeating, eating too quickly or worrying while eating all cause this condition.

> **Symptoms:**
> epigastric fullness
> sour regurgitation
> no appetite
> fullness and distention of the epigastrium relieved by vomiting
> vomiting
> nausea
> foul breath
> belching
> insomnia

Herbal Therapy: Citrus and Crataegus Formula (Bao he wan)

Cold Invading the Stomach
The Stomach is one of three Organs which can be directly invaded by Exterior Cold (along with the Large Intestine and Uterus). It is an acute condition caused by exposure to cold from improper dressing and excessive consumption of cold foods and iced drinks.

> **Symptoms:**
> sudden pain in the epigastrium
> vomiting of clear fluid
> feeling cold
> desire for warmth and warm foods and liquids
> feeling worse after swallowing cold fluids which are quickly vomited
> **Pulse:** deep, slow and tight
> **Tongue:** thick white coat

Herbal Therapy: **Agastache Formula** (Huo xiang zheng qi san); **Tea of Ginger** or a combination of ginger, cinnamon and anise seed.

LARGE INTESTINE

The main function of the Large Intestine is to receive the contents of the Small Intestine, absorb excessive water from it and discharge the waste from the body through the anus. Dysfunctions have to do with disturbances in bowel movements, including the substance and amount of feces and the times of defecation.

Damp Heat in the Large Intestine

Excessive intake of spicy and greasy foods along with prolonged emotional issues, such as anxiety and worry, cause Dampness and Heat in the Large Intestine. This interferes with its function of absorbing Fluids and excreting stools, causing diarrhea with mucus and a foul odor.

> **Symptoms:**
> abdominal pain, worse with pressure or heat
> diarrhea with mucus and blood in the stools
> foul odor of stools
> burning of anus
> scanty dark urine
> fever
> sweating which doesn't decrease with the fever
> thirst without desire to drink
> feeling of heaviness of body and limbs
> stuffiness of chest and epigastrium
> **Pulse**: slippery and rapid
> **Tongue**: red with greasy yellow coat

Herbal Therapy: Coptis, Scute and Pueraria Combination (Ge gen huang qin huang lian tang)

Heat in the Large Intestine

Different from the previous pattern, this dysfunction signals true Heat in the Large Intestine which burns off Fluids and causes Dryness. It arises from excessive intake of spicy and hot-natured foods (such as lamb) and fluids (such as alcohol and coffee).

> **Symptoms:**
> dry stools
> burning sensation in anus and mouth
> constipation
> dry tongue
> scanty dark urine
> **Pulse**: full and rapid
> **Tongue**: thick yellow and dry coat

Herbal Therapy: Major Bupleurum Combination (Da chai hu tang) for a stronger patient; **Cannabis Seed Pills** (Ma zi ren wan - also known as **Apricot Seed and Linum**) used as a nutritive, demulcent laxative for weaker, more Deficient patients.

Cold Invading the Large Intestine

Exterior Cold can directly invade into three Organs: The Large Intestine, Uterus and Stomach. This is an acute condition caused by the invasion of Exterior Cold directly into the Large Intestine, either from exposure to a cold climate or environment, or from improper clothing that doesn't protect the body adequately. The Cold interferes with the movement of Qi and causes it to stagnate, resulting in pain.

> **Symptoms:**
> sudden abdominal pain
> diarrhea with pain
> feeling of cold
> cold sensation in abdomen
> **Pulse**: deep, wiry
> **Tongue**: thick white coat

Herbal Therapy: White Atractylodes and White Peony Powder (Tong xie yao fang); Decoction of Ginger and Garlic. For more severe conditions add 3 to 9 gms of prepared aconite.

Large Intestine Cold

This differs from the previous pattern in that it is an Interior Deficient Cold pattern, similar to Spleen Yang Deficiency. The excessive intake of cold and raw foods and fluids and prolonged exposure to cold weather without adequate clothing causes this pattern.

> **Symptoms:**
> loose stools
> cold limbs
> dull abdominal pain
> borborygmi
> pale urine
> cold limbs
> **Pulse:** fine and deep
> **Tongue:** pale

Herbal Therapy: Refer to this category under Cold Invading the Large Intestine.

Collapse of Large Intestine
A Deficiency of Spleen, Stomach and Large Intestine Qi causes this pattern. The Large Intestine Qi sinks, causing chronic diarrhea, hemorrhoids and prolapsed anus.

Symptoms:
chronic diarrhea
prolapse of anus
hemorrhoids
tiredness after bowel movements
cold limbs
mental exhaustion
desire to drink warm liquids and have the abdomen massaged
no appetite
Pulse: deep and weak
Tongue: pale

Herbal Therapy: Ginseng and Astragalus Combination (Bu zhong yi qi tang)

THE GALL BLADDER

The Gall Bladder receives bile manufactured by the Liver, stores it, and then secretes it into the Small Intestine to aid digestion. It is also connected to the ability to make decisions and the courage to carry them out. The Gall Bladder is dependent upon smooth Liver Qi to carry out its functions, and like the Liver, is affected by similar disharmonies. Anger, frustration, resentment, the excessive consumption of fried and fatty foods and over-exposure to hot damp climates imbalances Gall Bladder functions.

Damp Heat in the Gall Bladder
Damp Heat arises from the excessive intake of hot, greasy and fried foods and from prolonged suppressed anger, resentment and frustration. The Dampness occurs from an underlying Spleen Qi Deficiency unable to transform Fluids. Both can occur from over-exposure to damp and humid environments.

Symptoms:
hypochondriac pain and distension
bitter taste
vomiting of bitter fluid
nausea
jaundice or yellow complexion
poor digestion and absorption
loss of appetite
diarrhea
nausea

belching
inability to digest fats
scanty and dark yellow urine
fever
thirst without desire to drink
Pulse: slippery, wiry
Tongue: thick sticky yellow coat, either on both sides or on the
    right side

Herbal Therapy: Capillaris Formula (Yin chen hao tang) or
Gentiana Combination (Long dan xie gan tang)

Deficiency of Gall Bladder

Since the Yang of the Liver and Gall Bladder can never really be
Deficient, this describes more a type of personality rather than a
Deficiency of Gall Bladder Yang. This also relates to the Hun and its
capacity to give direction and self-expression. If the Liver is weak, or if
Blood is Deficient so it cannot root the Hun, the Gall Bladder will be
timid and fearful. Of course, life situations and family relationships can
also contribute to forming this type of character.

> **Symptoms:**
> timidity
> sighing
> lack of courage and initiative
> nervousness
> propensity to being easily startled
> dizziness
> blurred vision
> **Pulse:** weak
> **Tongue:** pale or normal

Herbal Therapy: Bamboo and Poria Combination (Wen dan tang
- Gall Bladder Warming Decoction)

URINARY BLADDER

The function of the Bladder is to receive, store and excrete urine.
This capacity relates to Kidney Yang providing the Qi and Heat for
Fluid transformation, the function of the Small Intestine in separating
the pure Fluids from the impure, and the Lower Warmer and its
involvement in Water metabolism. Because the Kidneys can only be
Deficient, any Excess patterns pertaining to the urinary system are
attributed to the Bladder.

Causes of Bladder imbalances include prolonged exposure to damp and hot or cold environments and climates, sitting on cold or damp surfaces such as concrete, excessive fear, anxiety, insecurity, suspicion or jealousy or excessive sexual activity.

Damp Heat in the Bladder
This is an Excess Heat and Dampness pattern which obstructs the smooth flow of Fluids in the Lower Burner and causes burning and other heat sensations. It is due to excessive exposure to external damp heat or damp cold, or from prolonged suspicion or jealousy.

> **Symptoms:**
> burning on urination
> dark yellow and/or turbid urine
> difficult urination (stopping mid-stream)
> frequent and urgent urination
> blood in the urine
> sand in the urine
> fever
> thirst
> **Pulse:** rapid, slippery
> **Tongue:** red, thick sticky yellow coat on root with red spots

Herbal Therapy: **Polyporus Combination** (Zhu ling tang) or **Gentiana Combination** (Long dan xie gan tang).

Damp Cold in the Bladder
This pattern is distinguished by the presence of Cold and Damp in the Bladder. The Coldness and Dampness obstruct the Water passages of the Lower Burner and interfere with the Bladder functions. It is caused by excessive exposure to cold and damp environments and climates, sitting on cold and damp surfaces and injury of Kidney Yang.

> **Symptoms:**
> pale and turbid urine
> feeling of heaviness in hypogastrium and urethra
> difficult urination (stopping mid-stream)
> frequent and urgent urination
> **Pulse:** slow, slippery
> **Tongue:** white sticky coating on root

Herbal Therapy: Poria Five Herbs formula (Wu ling san)

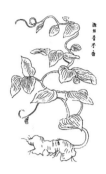

TWELVE

EIGHT METHODS
OF HERBAL TREATMENT

Chinese medicine refers to Eight Therapeutic Methods of Treatment: sweating, vomiting, purging, harmonizing, warming, removing, supplementing and reducing.

SWEATING

Sweating, or diaphoretic therapy, is used for External diseases. These are further differentiated into External Cold or External Heat with Wind, as a proliferating disease condition often combines with External conditions. Thus, sweating is used to treat either Wind-Cold or Wind-Heat. The major symptoms for External Wind Cold are chills, fever, headache, aching stiffness, especially of the neck and shoulders, a white-coated tongue and a floating and tense pulse. Diaphoretic formulas include **Ephedra Combination** (Ma huang tang), **Pueraria Combination** (Ge gen tang) and **Cinnamon Combination** (Gui zhi tang).

The symptoms for External Wind Heat are high fever, chills, thirst, red tongue with a thin yellow coat and a rapid pulse. The formulas indicated for this are **Lonicera and Forsythia Combination** (Yin qiao san) or **Morus and Chrysanthemum Combination** (Sang ju yin). **Contraindications:** Do not use sweating therapy where there is anemia, a severe loss of bodily fluids from vomiting and diarrhea, or a Deficiency of Blood and/or Yin.

VOMITING

Vomiting (emetic) therapy is used for food and narcotic poisoning, mucus accumulation causing lung congestion, and abdominal pain. Currently in TCM, vomiting is less used for mucus conditions than it is in Ayurvedic East Indian medicine. Because of the possibility of undesirable reactions to vomiting therapy, other less drastic methods are used to eliminate mucus in TCM.

Vomiting is, however, the most important method in TCM for treating food and narcotic poisoning. Chinese herbal medicine uses **Melon Pedicel Formula** to induce vomiting, but more simply one can use **Syrup of Ipecac**, made from the South American herb commonly available from most pharmacies.

Another Western emetic herb is lobelia inflata. The seeds are the most effective, but currently are rarely available in trade. Either the seeds or the aerial portions of the whole herb can be rendered into an acetic or vinegar extract. Lobelia has both antispasmodic and stimulant properties and is sometimes called the "thinking herb" because it is often effective when we are unable to envision a satisfactory final outcome for a particular problem. It is also given for the most acute stage of asthma. First have the patient drink one or two quarts of strong peppermint tea. Follow this with a teaspoon of lobelia tincture. Repeat the lobelia every 10 minutes for two more times. At this point the patient should vomit, alleviating the asthma and, in some cases, completely curing it from a single lobelia emetic treatment. To achieve such results, one should wait until the asthma reaches its most acute stage before giving the lobelia emetic.

Contraindications: Vomiting should never be done to counteract caustic poisons such as swallowing lye or various other petroleum or chemical poisons. Rather, the approach should be to dilute the poisonous substance with a protecting demulcent substance such as licorice tea, marshmallow root or slippery elm gruel. For such serious poisoning, proper medical assistance should be obtained as soon as possible.

PURGATION

Purgation is indicated for elimination of toxins through the colon. Purgatives are used for Excess conformation with gastric and intestinal pains, constipation, dry stools and Stagnant blood in the lower abdomen with possible lower abdominal pain.

The most commonly used purgatives are rhubarb root, buckthorne, cascara sagrada, aloe and senna. These are all characteristically bitter, cold and detoxifying. Chinese purgative formulas include **Major and Minor Rhubarb Combination** (Da cheng qi tang and Xiao cheng qi tang) and **Rhubarb and Moutan Combination** (Da huang mu dan pi tang).

In East Indian Ayurvedic medicine the safest and most mild purgative is **Triphala,** made from Terminalia emblica, T. belerica and T. chebula. This formula is safe because it will not cause laxative dependency, and it can be used for both Excess and mildly Deficient individuals to

aid internal cleansing and detoxification, since it does not aggravate any existing weaknesses or deficiencies. Other purgatives are warm or hot in energy and have a more drastic action. These are used for Excess conformation diseases associated with Fluid accumulation under the heart, sweating and asthma. Purgatives are also used to expel worms, often in combination with anthelmintics.
Contraindications: These include all surface conformation diseases since purgatives can drive the External disease inward; also for half-External and half-Internal conditions (requiring harmonizing therapy instead); and in individuals with loss of Fluids and associated constipation, delicate health and/or lack of vitality. They should not be used during menstruation, pregnancy or the postpartum period.

HARMONIZING

Harmonizing therapy is used for lesser Yang (Shao Yang) diseases involving the Liver or Gall Bladder. It is the most commonly used herbal therapy for restoring general balance. It is given for diseases of a polarized, half and half conformation.

Harmonizing therapy is indicated for Liver and Gall Bladder diseases such as hepatitis, symptoms of Liver Qi Stagnation with chest and abdominal discomfort, nausea, intermittent fever such as malaria, individuals who are prone to extreme mood swings and depression and premenstrual syndrome in women. It is also indicated for lingering colds and fevers where the symptoms are mixed External, Internal, Hot, Cold, Excess and Deficient.

Some of the most commonly used Harmonizing formulas are **Minor Bupleurum Combination** (Xiao chai hu tang), **Bupleurum and Cinnamon Combination** (Chai hu gui zhi tang) and the purgative, **Major Bupleurum Combination** (Da chai hu tang).
Contraindications: Harmonizing therapy is contraindicated for individuals with a clear External, Internal or Excess conformation.

WARMING

Warming therapy uses warm stimulants to treat Cold conditions. It supplements and strengthens Yang Qi, making it useful for helping to restore lost vitality. It is useful for Coldness, vomiting, abdominal pain, weak pulse, and a general Cold, weak conformation.

Coldness occurs in individuals with a loss of Yang, causing digestive weakness, loose stools, clear urine, weakness of body and spirit, cold extremities, poor appetite, abdominal distention and stomach pains.

Biomedically, it is often associated with conditions such as hypoglycemia, hypothyroid and hypoadrenalism.

For this, Internal Warming stimulants such as red and black pepper, dried ginger, cinnamon, cloves, galangal and prepared aconite are used. For general coldness and hypofunction, one can use **Aconite, Ginger, and Licorice Combination** (Si ni tang). For Cold, Yang-Deficient digestion (Deficient Spleen Yang), use **Vitality Combination** (Zhen wu tang) or **Ginseng and Ginger Combination** (Li zhong tang). For Deficient Kidney-adrenals use **Rehmannia Eight** (Ba wei di huang wan).

Contraindication: Do not use where there is Internal Excess Heat or Internal Heat with External chills; in individuals with Yin Deficiency and symptoms of False Yang; where there are signs of spitting up of blood or blood in the stools; and during diarrhea with fever.

COOLING

Cooling is a method of detoxification used to remove fever and inflammation, helping the body to overcome negative Pathogenic Influences such as viruses and bacteria.

In TCM, four stages of heat are outlined:

The first stage is called the Wei Level, which corresponds to the External Wind Heat conformation of high fever, mild chills, sore throat, headache, thirst, pink tongue with a yellow coat, and a floating, rapid pulse. **Lonicera and Forsythia Combination** (Yin qiao san) is indicated for this stage.

The second stage is at the Qi Level. Here there is high fever, no chills, irritability, excess perspiration, great thirst, constipation, abdominal pain, flushed face, abhorrence of heat, cough with yellow phlegm and dark, concentrated urine. The tongue is red with a yellow coat and the pulse is strong and full. This corresponds to the Sunlight Yang (Yang Ming) stage of disease. Formulas used are **White Tiger Combination** (Bai hu tang), **Coptis and Scutellaria Combination** (Huang lian huang qin tang), **Coptis and Rhubarb Combination** (San huang xie xin tang - a combination of equal parts coptis, scutellaria and rhubarb) and **Gentiana Combination** (Long dan xie gan tang).

The third stage of Heat is at the Ying or Essence Level. This stage corresponds to Yin Deficient or auto-consumptive Heat. There may be symptoms of late afternoon and evening fever, insomnia, irritability, delirium and dry, scarlet tongue with a rapid and thin pulse. It requires herbs and formulas that are demulcent, nutritive and cooling such as marshmallow root, Irish moss and comfrey root in Western herbal medicine and raw rehmannia, lycii bark, pseudostellaria root in Chinese herbal medicine. **Anemarrhena, Phellodendron and Rehmannia Combination** (Zhi bai di huang wan) can be used for this stage of Heat.

The fourth stage is Heat at the <u>Blood or Xue Level</u>. Symptoms are high fever, delirium or unconsciousness, coma, insomnia, signs of bleeding such as vomiting of blood, nose bleeding, blood in the stool, easy bruising underneath the skin, spasms from heat and exhaustion. The tongue is dark red with prickles and the pulse is thready and rapid. This is the deepest level of Heat penetration and requires herbs that clear Heat and cool the Blood, such as rhinoceros horn (for which three or four times water buffalo horn can be substituted), raw rehmannia and scrophularia. The formula that is used is **Rhinoceros Horn and Rehmannia Combination** (Xi Jiao di huang tang).

Contraindications: Cooling therapy is contraindicated for individuals with delicate health who have cold extremities, loose stools, diarrhea, low energy, Blood Deficiency and anemia.

TONIFICATION

Tonification therapy is indicated for individuals who are weak and are in need of some level of nutritional supplementation. In Chinese herbalism there are four kinds of Deficiencies: Qi, Blood, Yin and Yang.

Qi Deficiency is accompanied with such symptoms as low energy, weakness, prolapse, shallow breath, timidity and soft spoken voice. Herbs such as ginseng, astragalus and atractylodes are indicated. The basic formula for Qi Deficiency is **Four Major Herb Combination** (Si jun zi tang).

Blood Deficiency is diagnosed in individuals with pale complexion, weakness, dizziness, thirst, palpitations and scanty or stopped menstruation. **Dang Gui Four** (Si wu tang) is the base formula indicated.

Yin Deficiency presents with a thin, emaciated appearance, possible night sweats, insomnia, dizziness, exhaustion, excessive palpitations, five burning spaces (a sensation of heat on the soles of the feet, hands and chest), nocturnal emissions and spitting of blood. **Rehmannia Six Combination** (Liu wei di huang wan) is commonly used for Kidney and Liver Yin Deficiency.

Yang Deficiency is indicated by feelings of cold and chills, especially of the lower body, knee pains, aching lower back pain, irregular bowel movements, lower abdominal pains, frequent urination, impotence, frigidity and diarrhea. **Rehmannia Eight Combination** (Ba wei di huang wan) is commonly used.

Since food is considered the supreme tonic, appropriate tonic foods (rice or proteinaceous foods) are most effective if they are prepared with corresponding tonic herbs. An example of this is to precook the herbs, such as ginseng, astragalus, dang gui, lycii berries and jujube dates, according to the needs of the individual, and then cooking rice in the resultant tea or using it as a stock for soup. Cooking herbs with sweet glutinous rice is called Congee, and is superior to taking only the food or the herbs by themselves.

Contraindications: Tonification is contraindicated for individuals with an Excess conformation or Stagnation of Qi.

REDUCING

Reducing therapy is used to remove Stagnation of Qi, Blood or Phlegm. Unlike purgation therapy, reducing therapy dissolves, or breaks up, accumulations such as cysts, tumors, abnormal swellings, obesity, ulcers, blood clots and extravasated blood. Unlike purging, reducing therapy tends to be slower and more gradual (over a period of weeks or months) before results are noticed. Formulas such as **Cinnamon and Poria Combination** (Gui zhi fu ling tang) and the patented **Yunnan Baiyao** are used for Blood Stagnation; **Stephania and Astragalus Combination** (Fang ji huang qi tang) together with **Siler and Platycodon** (Fang feng tung shen san) are given to reduce obesity; and **Crataegus and Citrus Combination** (Bao he wan) is used for food Stagnation; and **Bupleurum and Chih Shih** (Szu ni tang) is given for Qi Stagnation.

Contraindications: Do not use the reducing method when there is weakness of Qi with abdominal distention, low grade fever, thirst, loss of appetite, diarrhea, weak digestion, and gynecological problems with loss of blood and amenorrhea.

COMBINING METHODS

Because contemporary diseases are often quite complex, different combinations of the Eight Methods are often used:

Sweating and purging are used when chills, fever, headaches and stiffness are associated with constipation. The rule is first sweat, then purge.

Warming and removing are used when there are upper or lower body chills or fever following infectious diseases. Warming herbs are combined with removing herbs to offset side effects and prevent loss of vitality.

Attacking and supplementing are used when the disease exhibits signs of both weakness and Excess congestion. If one gives only supplements the disease might not be uprooted; if one gives only purging, further prostration could occur. In these cases a combination of ginseng and similar tonics can be given along with purgatives.

Treatment Principles

1. Supplement weakness before purging and eliminating. This is done to protect the righteous energy from degenerating.

2. Treat External diseases first before treating extravasated Blood.

3. Treat the outer stem before treating the root. Treat External diseases before working on Internal weaknesses. Even for those who experience weakness and Deficiency, cool natured, antibiotic herbs should be given to resolve inflammatory conditions either before or simultaneous with the use of appropriate tonics. About three days to one week can be followed in this approach. If this doesn't work, then the treatment principle should be reversed. Some formulas, such as Minor Bupleurum Combination, can treat both inside and outside conformations at the same time.

4. Always treat cautiously at first to be sure that the condition is one of either Excess or Deficiency, Hot or Cold. If there is any question, begin treating as if it were a Deficient disease so as not to aggravate the illness.

5. If during the course of treating an Internal chronic disease the patient develops an acute condition, treatment for the chronic condition should be suspended and treatment of the acute given instead. When the acute condition is alleviated, then resume treatment of the chronic one.

6. Most often an appropriate herbal treatment exhibits its positive effects within three days, in which case it should be continued. If no improvement is noted, it may, however, still be the right treatment and so should be continued anyway. A healing crisis syndrome can occur at this point. If so, treatment can be temporarily suspended or the dosage lowered for a time. A healing crisis is always accompanied by concomitant signs of improvement. It is also characterized by a shortened retracing of earlier disease syndromes.

7. Because conditions change, especially in acute diseases, it is important to have regular follow up evaluations. This may be necessary during the two or three days of acute diseases or once or twice monthly during certain chronic conditions. A patient taking a Reducing formula should be reevaluated weekly or every other week.

8. It is often a part of good herbal strategy to first prescribe a purgative formula such as one of the rhubarb formulas for anywhere from three days to a week before or while giving the primary formula that seems indicated. In most cases such an eliminative formula can be

tolerated without any significant imbalance even by relatively Deficient individuals. If this is followed, the primary tonic formula will be more effective than if it were taken immediately. Alternatively, a balanced eliminative formula, such as the Ayurvedic Triphala, is very balanced, safe and can be safely prescribed as a single dose each evening throughout the primary course of treatment.

9. Often patients respond more effectively when more than one formula is taken simultaneously. This can be prescribed by telling them to take the more tonic formula a half hour to twenty minutes before eating and the more eliminative formula after meals. This is especially effective if one uses pills or extracts, but can be done with teas as well.

10. Foods and drinks of contrary energies and properties should be avoided during herbal therapy. For instance, foods with strong Cooling properties should be avoided if one is taking Warming tonic herbs and formulas. Conversely, strong heating foods such as sugar, coffee and alcohol should be avoided if one is taking cooling herbs and formulas. Stimulating foods and drinks should be avoided while taking sedative herbs, and greasy or oily foods should be avoided while taking digestives.

11. Herbs with strong moving properties such as Blood or Qi regulating herbs (strong carminatives or emmenagogues) are contraindicated during pregnancy. Similarly, highly toxic herbs should be avoided by pregnant or nursing women. There is only one molecule of difference between mother's milk and blood. Anything taken by the mother should be safe for the nursing child. Generally this is true if there is an indication that either individual could be benefited by a particular herb or formula. Strong or toxic herbs are contraindicated for children, the very weak or aged.

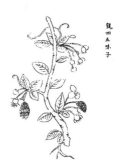

THIRTEEN

WHOLE NUTRITION

Like herbs and disease, every type of food has an inherent Cool or Warm energy. The Cooling or Warming energy of food affects the body by creating more Coldness or Heat in it. While Western cultures are accustomed to thinking of nutrition as food groups, Eastern cultures recognize the energy of food regardless of the group it is in.

Learning the energy of food is important in order to regain and maintain the body's health. If a person has a lot of Heat in the body and continues to eat warming and heating foods, then the body will only create more Heat and its associated problems. The same is true for a person with Coldness. If he eats a lot of cooling foods, then the Coldness leads to Deficient Yang and Cold Damp conditions.

As a result, even when a person is taking herbs for healing, if she is eating in a way that energetically opposes what the body needs and what the herbs are intended to do, then the herbal treatment will either be less effective, will take longer to heal or will have no effect at all. Often we know we have the right diagnosis and herbal treatment, yet the patient is either not getting better or is progressing too slowly. The cause for this can be an inappropriate diet which is sabotaging our treatments.

As an example, one patient had low energy and frequent colds. He was given warming and building herbs and a balanced diet to eat. Yet, in two weeks time little progress was made. When questioned about the diet, he admitted to consuming fruit and juices, believing they were healthy and important foods to eat. Yet, these same foods were continually causing his poor digestion, mucus, lowered immunity and tiredness. When he eliminated these foods, within a week he felt stronger and had better digestion and more energy.

Another patient had skin problems, frequently breaking out on her face and shoulders. Again an appropriate energetic diet was given along with heat clearing and detoxifying herbs. Within a few weeks she was feeling better and her face had cleared, but she continued to break out on her back and shoulders. When questioned further, it was discovered that she still ate her weekly dose of chocolate chip cookies, white sugar included. When these were stopped, her skin fully cleared up.

Thus, every food eaten affects the body in some way. Food can tonify Yang, Qi, Yin and Blood. Likewise it can cause Coldness, Dampness, Dryness, Heat and Stagnation. Because most people eat two to three times a day, then two to three times a day the energy of the body is being affected by the energy of the food ingested. "You are what you eat" is not such a strange adage from this perspective.

A BALANCED DIET

A balanced diet is one which uses foods energetically. It incorporates more foods with a neutral to Cool and neutral to Warm energy, a little less food with Warm or Cool energies and sparing use of foods with Hot and Cold energies. If these energies are placed on a continuum, it is easier to visualize how they affect us.

| Hot | Warm | Neutral-Warm | Neutral-Cool | Cool | Cold |

When eating according to the energy of foods, an energetically balanced diet includes grains, beans, mostly cooked vegetables, white meat, and small amounts of fruit and red meat, if desired. Most people eat in an energetically imbalanced way, eating large amounts of red and white meats, few vegetables and fruits and little or no grains or beans.

We can determine ourselves how food makes us feel by noticing the effects it has after eating it. These effects can be evident immediately, such as the spiciness of hot peppers, or it may take three days or more, such as the effects of Cold-energied ice cream. Most foods affect us within three days to a month. An excess amount of one type of food builds over time until we feel the effects of that food more readily. Ultimately, we become so sensitive to certain foods that we become "allergic" to them.

Another way of looking at the Warm-Cool energy of food is in terms of acid-alkaline. In general, foods that are Cool or Cold tend to make the body more alkaline. Foods that are Warm or Hot tend to make the body acidic.[1]

The taste of each food also indicates its Warming, Cooling or neutral energy. Foods which are bitter, like endive or spinach, tend to be cooling and eliminate toxins. Sour foods are refreshing and cool, like sauerkraut, and small amounts aid digestion. Spicy foods are stimulating and Heating. They move Blood and Qi. Salty foods, like seaweed and miso, are Cool and softening because they hold Fluids in the body. Full sweet foods, or complex carbohydrates which break down slowly, are

Warm to neutral in energy. These complex carbohydrates help nourish bones, muscles and Blood.

The energy of a food is its natural inherent energy regardless of how it is eaten or prepared. It can be modified somewhat by eating it raw (more Cooling) or cooking it (more Warming). Overall, adding heat, pressure, cooking time and spices makes a food less Cooling and more Warming. Adding water, refrigeration or freezing, eating it raw and unspiced makes food less Warming and more Cooling.

Yet, despite preparations, a Cool food can never be warm and vice versa. For example, a pear which has a Cool energy, can be baked with walnuts and cinnamon to make it less Cool in energy. Likewise, eating Warm-energied shrimp in a raw state gives it a less Warm energy since the shrimp isn't cooked.

Empty-Full

Along with Warming and Cooling energies, foods have a quality of being either empty or full. Empty and full refer to the effects that a food has on the body and not its nutritional contents. Like energy, empty-full is on a continuum so that a food is not absolutely empty or full, but is slightly empty or strongly full. This is an important concept to grasp in terms of food because it gives us a broader and deeper understanding of how food affects the body.

Relative to each other, fruit and juices are empty, vegetables are neutral to somewhat empty, meat and dairy are full and grains and legumes are neutral. From this it appears that protein-rich foods are full and more water-containing foods are empty.

meat & eggs	dairy	grains & legumes	vegetables	fruit
full		neutral	neutral-empty	empty

←————————————————————▲————————————————————→

Prolonged eating of mostly empty foods creates elimination in the body. This can affect the Qi, Blood, strength and working capacity of the Organs, and it ultimately results in some sort of Deficiency. People who predominantly eat empty foods often feel tired, unfocused and depleted.

For instance, fruit and juices are empty foods, although they range from Warm to Cold in energy. They generally lower the body temperature and metabolism by creating elimination. Small amounts of fruit eliminates toxins and moistens Dryness. Yet, if eaten too frequently or predominantly, they can create poor digestion, gas, bloating, loose stools, runny nose, possible low back pains, Dampness, lowered immunity and resistance and feelings of being ungrounded and unfocused.

On the other hand, prolonged eating of mostly full foods creates Excess in the body. This usually leads to congestion and Stagnation of Qi, Blood and Organ functions. It ultimately results in some type of Excess condition, either Heat, Dampness or both. People who predominantly eat full foods often feel congested, stuck, explosive and hypertensive.

For example, red meat and dairy are full foods, although they are neutral to Warming in energy. Appropriate amounts strengthen Blood and Qi and build strength and endurance. However, excessive eating of red meat or dairy, particularly if the diet is lacking in vegetable and fruit, ultimately creates too much congestion, resulting in a red neck and face, irritability, a loud voice, aggressive behavior, constipation and toxicity in the Blood and Organs.

Putting the concept of empty-full together with Warming and Cooling energies helps us look at food in a different way. For instance, some foods may be Warm in energy but also empty. The spice, cayenne, is Hot, but it doesn't build or strengthen. Instead, it is stimulating and dispersing and in excess can cause elimination. On the other hand, some foods may be Cool in energy but also full, such as barley. It expands the intestines and so helps stop diarrhea. It also strengthens the Spleen Qi. Likewise, American ginseng is a Cool herb, but it tonifies Yin and Qi.

Thus, along with the energy of a food, it is important to look at its empty-full effects. Overall, it is a question of balance. It is best to eat a diet comprised predominantly of foods with a neutral-Warm and neutral-Cool energy and neutral, neutral-empty, and some of the full quality. Eating large amounts of the more extreme foods, those that are Hot, Cold, full and/or empty, creates imbalance and disease.

Grains, Legumes, Nuts & Seeds

	ENERGY	
WARM	**NEUTRAL**	**COOL**
sweet rice	adzuki bean	barley
black bean	kidney bean	wheat
pine nuts	string bean	mungbean
sesame seed	rice	tofu
walnut	yellow soybean	buckwheat
chestnut	black soybean	millet
	sunflower seed	soybean
	almond	
	peanut	
	corn	
	peas	
	rye	

Grains, legumes, nuts and seeds are predominantly neutral-Warm and neutral-Cool in energy. They are neutral in quality. Grains give complex carbohydrates to the body, which break down slowly and provide long lasting energy and strength. Beans, nuts and seeds provide a protein balance to grains, and should be eaten regularly by those who don't eat meat. For those who do, they can be used as a periodic protein substitute to alleviate the potential of creating too much congestion and toxins from eating meat all the time. Eating too many nuts, nut butters and seeds, however, creates Damp Heat in the Liver and Gall Bladder and leads to Stagnant Liver Qi.

Some people need more protein than others. Protein gives strength, endurance, immunity, resistance and Heat to the body. But in excess, it creates toxins, congestion, irritability and Heat conditions. Each person needs to determine his/her own level and needs. Quite often vegetarians don't eat sufficient protein for their bodies needs. Eating grains and beans together creates a complete protein, yet it is still based on all carbohydrates. For many, this is insufficient and their bodies actually need animal protein to regain health and balance. Don't go by an intellectual idea or theory, but experiment with how you feel when you don't eat enough or eat too much protein. Find what amount helps you feel good, strong, energetic and flexible. Bear in mind that your protein needs change from day to day and week to week according to what is going on in your life.

Bread is not a substitute for grains, as floured foods, even if whole grain, cause Dampness and Stagnation. One meal with bread in a sandwich is fine, but beyond that, whole grain cereals and pilafs should be used instead of refined or floured grains.

Vegetables

ENERGY

WARM	NEUTRAL	COOL	COLD
onion	carrot	cucumber	tomato
garlic	celery	eggplant	bemboo shoots
winter squash	beet	lettuce	seaweed
mustard leaf	potato	radish	snow pea
kale	pumpkin	spinach	
	sweet potato	button mushroom	
	yam	alfalfa sprouts	
	shiitaki	summer squash	
	cabbage	celery	
		asparagus	
		broccoli	

Vegetables range from slightly neutral-Warming to neutral-Cooling. They are neutral to empty in quality. In general, compact vegetables which take a long time to grow and mature and grow into the Fall and Winter are slightly Cooling in energy. Vegetables which grow quickly, expand easily, have a high water content and occur mostly in Summer are more Cooling in energy. Cooking vegetables makes them a little less Cool, but their inherent energy is still Cooling to the body. Eating them raw partakes of their full Cooling energy.

Vegetables are an important addition to any type of diet; in fact, most people don't eat enough of them. They should comprise about 40-50% of each meal, as they neutralize the acid-forming potential of grains and meat. Greens and sea vegetables should be included in abundance. They aid in the digestion of grains, give important vitamins and minerals and clear Heat from the Liver, Heart and Blood. Raw vegetables are Colder in energy and take strong Spleen Qi to metabolize, whereas slightly cooked ones are much easier to digest, so more nutrients are assimilated from them.

A large controversy exists around raw versus cooked foods. Raw food proponents believe that cooking vegetables kills their live vital energy and renders them useless to health in the body. Frankly, there are as many sick raw vegetarians as there are meat eaters, and generally it is more difficult to bring them back to health.

Raw and Cold food in excess does several things: it thins the Blood, it creates Coldness and Dampness and it depletes Spleen Qi and Yang. Aches and pains, stiffness, anemia, arthritis, gas, bloatedness, lethargy and other problems can result. Raw foods in an already cold diet of fruits, juices, salads and no meat, quell the metabolic ability of the body to break the food down and assimilate it. If this breakdown and assimilation cannot occur, or happens poorly, then the vitality of raw foods is totally lost.

In addition, the body needs little hydrochloric acid to digest vegetables. When only eating vegetables, the body tends to produce small amounts of hydrochloric acid. Over time this situation decreases the digestive ability of the body, since other foods need more hydrochloric acid to break down. Overall, therefore, the body may be able to assimilate and get more out of cooked rather than raw vegetables.

On the other hand, vegetables should never be over-cooked or mushy. Overcooking destroys important nutrients. Cooked and still slightly crunchy vegetables are less Cold and digest and assimilate well. A little raw food is beneficial, and meat eaters can healthily include salads, fruits and juices to help counteract their Warmer diet.

Fruits & Juices

ENERGY

WARM	NEUTRAL	COOL	COLD
cherry	fig	apple	banana
coconut	grape	mango	grapefruit
guava	olive	tangerine	persimmon
peach	papaya	mandarin orange	watermelon
raspberry	pineapple	pear	cantaloupe
date	plum	strawberry	
kumquat	apricot	loquat	
	coconut meat	lemon	
		orange	

Fruit and juice have a neutral-Warm, neutral-Cool or Cold energy. Their predominant emptiness creates elimination and Dampness in the body. In excess and over time, however, they also cause Deficient Qi, resistance and immunity, resulting in loose stools, diarrhea, frequent and recurring colds and flu, poor digestion, mucus, chronic asthma and other lung problems, low back pain, sciatica, impotence, infertility, nasal drip and other such problems. Used correctly, meat eaters can benefit from these foods, especially for fasting purposes. In the Summer and when fruit is in season, a little is important for all of us, yet even then if eaten to excess, it can cause abnormal Dampness in the body, injuring Spleen Qi and causing water retention. Vegetarians should eat these foods more sparingly, especially fruit juices, and bake or stew their fruit, adding cinnamon and walnuts to make it less Cool. Vegetable juices are less empty than fruit juices.

Dairy

ENERGY

WARM	NEUTRAL
butter	cow's milk
	cheese
	yogurt

Dairy products can add valuable protein to the diet, especially for vegetarians. Yet most dairy products are full in quality and so in excess, are very congesting to the energy; they create mucus, thus causing Stagnation and poor digestion. Therefore, these highly concentrated foods should be eaten in moderation. For a body that is Dry and underweight, a little milk can actually moisten and build. For this, use raw milk, warm it up and add a little cinnamon or ginger. It can then be followed by a half teaspoon of honey to counteract the mucus producing aspects of milk. An alternative is goat's milk which is less fatty and more similar to human milk.

For those who have a lot of mucus in general, are overweight, have Dampness, are prone to cysts, tumors or fibroids, have chronic coughs or runny noses, or experience such obvious problems as asthma or allergies, dairy will only aggravate these conditions. Often children's asthma, coughs, runny noses, diarrhea or constipation will disappear by simply eliminating dairy and juices from the diet.

Meat

	ENERGY	
WARM	NEUTRAL	COOL
lamb	beef	clam
chicken	duck	crab
fresh ham	eggs	
mussel	pork	
shrimp	carp	
anchovy	oyster	
	goose	
	tuna	
	sardine	
	herring	
	whitefish	

Meat ranges from neutral-Warm to neutral-Cool in energy, yet it is full in quality. Meat is a powerful food-medicine and should be treated as such. It tonifies Qi and Yang. Excessive prolonged eating of red meat eventually results in toxins and Stagnation with their accompanying problems.

For people who have eaten a lot of meat, it may be best to eliminate meat from the diet for a while until the body becomes balanced. If you are going to eat meat, it should be organic, always cooked and eaten with a little raw ginger root. Ginger aids in the assimilation and detoxification of meat in the body.

The issue of whether to eat meat or not is a personal one. In general, vegetarians need to eat a more limited diet, since without meat most other foods are cooling. If a balanced diet is followed consisting mainly of grains, beans, cooked vegetables, some dairy items, a little fruit in season and an adequate protein level, then balance can be maintained. This does not allow for many empty foods to be included in the diet such as fruits, salads, juices and other raw uncooked foods.

Warming and building herbs can be included to help provide warmth, resistance and immunity. Likewise, for those who desire to eat meat, some empty foods can be incorporated more abundantly to help balance the fullness of meat and create elimination of possible toxins. However, as meat is a strong food, for the body to stay in balance it should always be accompanied by a large quantity of cooked and some raw vegetables and small quantities of fruit. This is a vast reduction from the Western tradition of eating meat almost three times a day with little or no fruit or vetables included. If eaten this frequently and in this quantity, toxins, Stagnation and Heat result in hypertension, heart attacks, cancer, arthritis, strokes, constipation, aggressiveness, irritability, red face and neck and rheumatism, for example.

Extreme Foods

ENERGY			
WARM	NEUTRAL	COOL	COLD
coffee	honey	beer	sugar cane
tobacco	white sugar		green tea
vinegar			salt
wine			
brown sugar			
malt & maltose			
molasses			

There are several other foods worth discussing here, including sugar, salt, alcohol, caffeine and tobacco. All of these are extreme foods. Eating one usually sets up a craving for the other and creates an endless cycle. For example, after eating sugar for a while, the body craves salt and vice versa. Yet this type of "balance" is extreme, like the seesaw described earlier.

Refined sugar cane is an empty food. It leeches important vitamins and minerals from the body, such as calcium. It is also well known as a leading cause for disease. It creates Stomach Heat and over time, Deficient Spleen Qi and Dampness. Heavy meat eaters often crave sugar because its emptiness offsets the fullness of meat. Sugar also causes salt cravings, and the heavy eating of salty foods conversely causes sugar cravings, the Warming and Cooling energies of each counterbalancing the other. Whole sugars such as maple sugar, honey, barley and rice malts and raw sugar cane are much better for the body, though they should be used sparingly as they are empty.

Salt is necessary along with potassium to maintain the proper balance of "Intra" and "Extra-cellular fluid" and body softness. Too much is harmful. Again use whole, un-refined salt from natural rock salt or sea salt that has a balance of other minerals. such as iodine, for the thyroid function. If using sea salt first pan roast it to evaporate the chlorine.

Alcohol, caffeine and tobacco all cause Heat and irritation in the body. In meat eaters this creates excessive amounts of Heat. In vegetarians, alcohol, caffeine and tobacco can provide Heat which the body craves if provided with a very Cooling diet. This quite often makes it much more difficult, if not impossible, for vegetarians to quit smoking cigarettes and drinking coffee without a diet change, even more so than meat eaters. In addition, alcohol, because of its sugar content, creates the same problems as sugar in the body.

Caffeine depletes Kidney Qi, Yang, Yin and Essence. It also creates Damp Heat in the Liver and leads to Liver Qi Stagnation with its associated problems of digestion, depression and gynecological issues. In time this leads to Adrenal exhaustion. Drinking coffee to push through tiredness ultimately leads to an exhaustion which is very difficult to replenish. It may take years for this to show up, and then it occurs suddenly. Those who drink several cups of coffee per day and are frequently tired or have low immunity, or those who drink coffee or black tea at night and have no problem falling asleep (i.e., the caffeine no longer keeps them awake), are near to adrenal exhaustion.

Tobacco restricts the circulation and promotes excessive coldness in the extremities. It also robs the cells of their much needed oxygen supply, which causes a weakening of their functions throughout the whole body. It then injures the Blood. It further causes Deficient Lung Yin which can lead to cancer.

Water is worth mentioning here because it, too, can cause disease in the body when taken improperly. Most meat eaters tend to drink lots of iced water to eliminate some of the fullness and acidity they feel inside. Yet iced water is one of the largest contributors to a Cold Damp Spleen and Stomach Heat, causing gas, bloatedness, frontal headaches, bleeding gums, bad breath or lethargy after eating. Imagine throwing iced water on a fire and the resulting steam and eventual dead fire if enough is used. The same occurs in the Stomach where the digestive fires are very much needed. Likewise, excessive drinking of carbonated water causes symptoms of gas, bloatedness, hiccup, poor digestion, dizziness, spaciness and lethargy.

Quantity is another issue. Eight glasses of water a day are fine for meat eaters. This much is needed to flush the Heat, toxicity, acids and irritations of the meat from the body. However, for those who eat little or no meat at all, too much water causes Dampness in the digestive system, quelling the fire and causing the Kidneys to constantly work unnecessarily. If eating little or no meat, four glasses a day of room temperature or hot water or herb tea is adequate. Cold water is aggravating to all bodies, and even more so to vegetarians. This goes for cold juices, too!

Whole Foods

It is important here to distinguish between whole healthy foods and disease causing foods. Whole foods are those which come to us in their purest form from nature with the least possible interference. This means they are preferably organic and without chemicals, additives or preservatives. They are also unrefined and in their whole natural state. Brown rice, maple syrup, and earth salt are examples of whole foods. Refined white rice, white sugar and table salt are examples of processed, disease-causing foods. The following chart suggests many healthy foods to eat and unhealthy foods to avoid.

Whole Foods Chart

HEALTHY FOODS	UNHEALTHY FOODS
whole grains	white sugar
beans	white flour
vegetables (esp organic)	white bread
sea vegetables	"junk food'
seeds, nuts	additives
greens	preservatives
small amounts of sea salt	refined salt
a little honey, maple syrup	artificial colorings/
or grain syrup as needed	flavorings
fruit in season, baked if needed	chemicals in foods
salads in season	soda
a little meat as needed (optional)	deserts containing white
small amounts of dairy	sugar
	tobacco
	caffeine

Food should never be cooked in aluminum pots and pans. Aluminum is toxic and contaminates the food. Gas or wood heat is best for cooking. Electric heat is fine for strong bodies, but for those with lowered immunity and severe or degenerative disease, it can alter the food enough to interfere with the healing process. Microwaves ideally should never be used, as they rearrange the molecular structure of the food, altering the electromagnetic field and making the food something different than nature created. Food doesn't cook evenly and tastes strange to some.

SOUP

Herbal soups are traditionally made in China on a weekly basis to keep the body and immunity strong and to prevent colds, flu and other seasonal 'bugs.' Soups are similar to congee in that the herbs are cooked with food. However, they are made into a soup form and not cooked down for hours. Soups generally contain some form of meat, vegetables, grains and water along with the herbs. Typical herbs include codonopsis, jujube dates, peony, Fu Ling, lycii berries, atractylodes, ginseng, astragalus, cornus, dioscorea and Dong Quai.

To make an herbal soup, place herbs, or tea made from the herbs, meat (if desired) and water in large pot. Bring to boil, then lower heat and cook slowly for 1 hour. Add raw vegetables during last 10 minutes, or sauteed ones (they maintain their own flavor and so taste better this way) at the end. Add cooked grain. Cook all together another 5-10 minutes. Serve and eat.

CONGEE

Congee is a well-cooked soupy grain or type of fortified porridge. Because it is considered very easy to digest, it is a very therapeutic food which is perfect during convalescence from sickness, for treating acute diseases, strengthening the digestion and assimilation, general debility and low vitality. It also helps those who cannot digest carbohydrates or keep any food down. By combining herbs with foods such as rice, we are supporting the nutritional needs of the body to help overcome imbalances. There are further benefits in combining tonic herbs with foods. By cooking them together, both seem to be better absorbed, with less chance of adverse reactions to either. Traditional Chinese families serve it to the whole family on a weekly basis, with herbs added to enhance the immune system and strengthen digestion.

The tradition of using herbs with food was first recorded more than 2500 years ago in China. During the first Tang and Sung dynasties, Chinese physicians made extensive use of food and herb combinations and began to record specific therapeutic recipes. One text, compiled during the Sung dynasty, was called *The Peaceful Holy Benevolent Prescriptions* and consisted of a collection of 129 prescriptions. Most of these are still commonly prescribed and used, including Apricot Porridge for the treatment of cough, Sour Jujube Seed Porridge for insomnia and Ginseng Porridge for Qi deficiency.

Grains are seeds that embody the entire Yin-Yang life cycle of a plant and tend to be more balanced than most foods. They are therefore especially suitable as a staple for regular daily consumption as well as for the treatment of disease. A congee is made with a grain, usually white rice, water and your personally chosen herbs. It has a long cooking time over low heat, which slowly and thoroughly breaks down the grain so that it is extremely easy to digest and assimilate. Thus, the body gets the most nutrients out of it as possible, which is perfect for weak digestive power that can't break down or assimilate food well.

Ideally enamel, clay, glass or good quality stainless steel is used. Do not use aluminum, iron or metal pots other than stainless steel. The herbs chosen can vary from week to week to satisfy your current needs. Sometimes herbal tablets are broken down and used instead of fresh herbs, although the fresh ones are best.

Basic Sweet Rice Congee

To make congee, fill a large pot with 9 cups water, 1 cup grain (white rice is best), 1 ounce (28 grams) of whole herbs and 1 - 2 oz. meat, if desired. Cover pot and bring to a boil, then turn down heat to lowest possible setting. Cook slowly and gently, about 6-8 hours. Congee is done when soupy with a thick porridge consistency. This basic sweet rice congee strengthens the stomach, tonifies Qi, improves digestion and acts as a tonic for diarrhea and symptoms of nausea and vomiting. White rice is used because it is easier to digest.

Nowadays, special stainless steel electric rice cookers are available from Oriental hardware stores which are wonderful for making congees. Alternatively, a crock pot could be used.

Variations:
1. **Jujube Date Congee**
The most common addition to congee is about 15 to 30 jujube dates. This is good for Qi and Blood Deficiency.

2. **Ginseng Congee for Deficient Qi**
Add 3 to 6 grams Chinese ginseng or 15 to 30 grams Codonopsis pilosula. Sweeten with pure brown sugar or barley malt syrup to taste. This is ideal for individuals with Qi Deficiency who have symptoms of chronic fatigue, weakness and general debility. It is highly tonifying, in that it supports righteous energy and helps prevent senility and premature aging.

3. Garlic Congee
Boil 30 grams of peeled and sliced garlic for one minute and then remove the garlic. Add one or two cups of brown rice and continue to boil. After fifteen to twenty minutes, add the sliced cooked garlic to the rice. This can be taken once or twice daily for breakfast or supper. Because garlic is heating, it is not recommended for patients with chronic gastritis or peptic ulcers. Garlic congee can be used for consumption, dysentery, chronic bronchitis, tuberculosis, hypertension and arteriosclerosis.

4. Codonopsis, Dang Gui, Astragalus, Lycii and Jujube Congee
Another Qi and Blood tonic can be made by cooking 9 grams each of astragalus root, codonopsis root and lycii berries with 15 jujube dates and 3 grams Dang Gui.

5. Amaranth Seed Congee
The Andean amaranth seed makes a good substitute for sweet rice in congee. A combination of dried apricots and amaranth seeds is particularly tasty with a higher than normal protein content and therapeutically beneficial for the lungs and gastrointestinal tract.

Other Possible Formulas:
Poor digestion, gas, bloatedness, lowered energy and immunity: ginseng, Dang Gui, codonopsis, red date and astragalus.
Cough, asthma, mucus, bronchitis: apricot kernel, comfrey root.
Fever, detoxification, diarrhea and dysentery: mung beans mixed with rice and cumin, turmeric and coriander browned in ghee; it becomes an Indian Dahl called Kicharee, or the "Food of the Gods".
Edema, gout, retention of urine or frequent urination and other kidney-bladder problems: aduki bean, cooked Rehmannia (Di Huang), Polygonum multiflorum (He Shou Wou) and Cornus (Shan Zhu Yu).
Coldness, poor circulation and as a blood rejuvenative after menstruation: lamb, Dang Gui and ginger.
Malnutrition, hypoglycemia, tiredness, diarrhea and weakness: beef, ginseng, licorice and ginger.

FOOD AND THE ORGANS
Each Organ has an associated taste which, in small amounts, tonifies it and, in large amounts, depletes or stagnates its energy. This taste can be used both diagnostically and therapeutically. For instance, if someone craves sour foods a lot, such as lemons, mustard or vinegar, it can point to Deficient or Stagnant Liver Qi. On the other hand, for someone who

has Damp Heat in the Liver, we could suggest a lemon water drink along with the herbal formula to help clear the Damp Heat created by their diets.

The bitter taste is cooling, drying, detoxifying and anti-inflammatory. It stimulates the secretion of bile, which in turn sparks the digestive fires and stimulates normal bowel elimination. It also helps protect the body against parasites, clears Heat from the Blood and eliminates cholesterol. As such, this taste strengthens the Heart and Small Intestine. Sweet cravings can be alleviated through ingestion of something bitter. It also dries Dampness and secretions in the body, such as diarrhea, leukorrhea and skin abscesses.

The bitter taste is generally lacking from Western diets, although it is frequently ingested in Europe in the form of "bitters" which are drunk before meals to stimulate and aid digestion. Several good bitters products are now available and, along with the regular daily intake of dark leafy greens, provide an excellent source of the bitter taste in the diet.

The sweet taste, associated with the Spleen, refers to complex carbohydrates and protein. It is warming, nourishing, strengthening and builds Qi and Blood. It also alleviates sweet cravings which are too often perpetuated by being fed the simple carbohydrates: sugar, fruit and juices. While unrefined sugar cane and fruits can provide important nutrients, and malt is frequently added to formulas to build a weakened and underdeveloped body, in excess these simple carbohydrates cause Stomach Heat, a Cold Damp Spleen and Deficient Spleen and Kidney Qi. Instead, getting plenty of whole grains with an adequate protein complement three times a day strengthens the Spleen and eliminates sweet cravings.

The acrid, pungent or spicy taste is warm to hot in energy. It stimulates the circulation of Qi, Blood and Fluids, counteracting poor digestion and circulation, Coldness and Dampness. It disperses energy to the exterior of the body, opening pores and facilitating sweating. Thus, it is especially useful for External Wind Cold conditions of colds, flu and mucus congestion. It also stimulates the circulation of Fluids, secretions and saliva. The acrid taste has a direct effect on the Lungs and Colon. Since acrid foods, such as chili peppers and cayenne seasoning, are dispersing, in excess they can exhaust Deficient Qi and tighten the tendons, decreasing flexibility. Therefore, they should be used in moderation.

The salty taste, cold in energy, stabilizes and regulates the Fluids and softens hardened lymph nodes, tight muscles, constipation, hard lumps and cysts. Because the salty taste is associated with the Kidney-

Adrenals and Urinary Bladder, a salt craving often indicates impending adrenal exhaustion. In small amounts it tonifies the Kidneys, and so a pinch of salt is often added to herbal formulas to help direct their actions to the Kidneys. In excess, however, salt can cause water retention, high blood pressure and injure the Blood. Herbs high in mineral salts do not create these complications and so can be regularly included in the diet with great benefit. These include all seaweeds and pot herbs such as nettles.

The sour taste is Cooling, Drying and astringent. It dries Dampness and tightens the tissues and muscles, thus toning them. It helps stop excessive perspiration, loss of Fluids and excess secretions of mucus and bleeding. It also stimulates digestion and metabolism and aids in breaking down fats through its stimulation of bile, thus aiding their absorption. The sour taste, associated with the Liver and Gallbladder, in small amounts eliminates Excess Heat and Dampness in the Liver, Gallbladder, Stomach and Small Intestine, while large amounts can toughen the flesh and coat the mucus linings of the stomach and intestines, thus causing poor digestion and absorption.

Food Therapy

When treating health imbalances, it is wise to adjust the diet accordingly to assist your treatment plan. As mentioned earlier, an inappropriate diet can sabotage herbal treatments, causing them to appear ineffective when, in fact, the diet is at fault. A body that has too much Heat can be balanced by eating more Cooling foods and less heating ones, whereas the continued eating of Cooling foods and drinks only perpetuates the person's condition, and vice versa. Because all people's bodies are different, everyone requires different types of foods to stay in balance, and even this may vary from season to season and year to year. Therefore, there is no such thing as one type of diet that is healthy for all people. Instead, each person should learn what his/her current bodily needs are and eat the right foods for those personal conditions.

For instance, if experiencing Heat signs of constipation, irritability, frequent sweating and always feeling warm, then eliminate those foods with a Hot energy, eat a few with a Warm energy and focus more on neutral, cool and a small amount of Cold-energied foods. Likewise, for someone experiencing Deficient Qi and Coldness with symptoms of frequent cold and flu, lowered immunity, runny nose, tiredness, weakness and feelings of chill and cold, eliminate all Cold foods, eat some Cool foods, but only in cooked form, and focus more on balanced, Warm and some Hot energy foods.

If the plan is to maintain existing good health or if one is recovering from an illness, then follow the balanced diet outlined at the beginning of this Chapter. This diet incorporates 40-60% whole complex carbohydrates with adequate protein complement three meals a day, 40-50% vegetables including dark leafy greens and seaweeds, and a small portion of meat, dairy and fruits as appropriate per person.

Often people with Deficient Qi and Blood do not get enough food per meal, skip meals or have inadequate protein in their diets. It is not unusual to discover a person with Deficient Blood and Qi to skip breakfast or only eat a muffin or bagel, have a salad for lunch and then eat dinner late at night because they are working or studying all day. Often just getting these people to eat an adequate diet clears up the symptoms without even giving herbal formulas. If the problem has occurred for too long, however, it is often necessary to tonify Spleen Qi and Yang, to stimulate the appetite and digestion to strengthen their metabolism.

Following is a chart outlining energetic diet plans for the general conditions of Coldness, Heat, Dampness, Dryness, Deficiency and Excess. These can be tailored according to the specific symptomology and differential diagnosis of each person, creating a personal therapeutic diet appropriate to accompany the herbal treatment program. Then, specific foods are listed, giving their energy, tastes, Organs and meridians entered and their therapeutic effects. Thus, specific foods can be emphasized in the diet to enhance the overall healing program.

Name	Energy/Taste	Elements	Therapeutic Conditions
Aduki bean	neutral	Heart sweet, sour Sm. Intestine	Edema, beriberi, mumps jaundice, diarrhea, discharge of blood from anus, reduces weight. Avoid: dryness or emaciation.
Almond	neutral; sweet	Lungs, Spleen-Pancreas	Relieves cough, resolves Phlegm, lubricates Lungs; tonifies Qi and Blood.
Apple	cool; sweet	Spleen-Pancreas	Lubricates, clears Heat, counteracts depression, moistens; low blood sugar, indigestion, morning sickness, chronic enteritis.
Asparagus	cool; sweet, bitter	Lungs, Kidneys	Clears Heat, dries Dampness, lubricates Dryness; tonifies

			Yin; cough, mucus discharge, swelling, various kinds of skin eruptions, shortage of mother's milk, diabetes, TB, wasting Heat disease Avoid: Deficiency Cold diarrhea; Wind Cold Cough.
Banana	cold; sweet	Spleen, Stomach	Lubricates, clears Heat, counteracts toxins; constipation, lubricates Intestines, bleeding piles, hemorrhoids, alcoholism, tonifies Yin. Avoid: Cold Damp conditions.
Barley	cool; sweet, salty	Spleen, Stomach	Regulates Stomach, promotes urination, clears Heat, lubricates Dryness, expands Intestines; edema, dysuria, indigestion, burns, diarrhea.
Beef	neutral; sweet	Spleen, Stomach, Large Intestine	Tonifies Qi, Blood, and Yin; strengthens tendons and bones, tonifies Stomach and Spleen; emaciation, edema, diabetes, weak knees and low back pain with emaciation; various parts are good for corresponding Organs.
Beet	neutral; sweet	Spleen	Tonifies Qi and nourishes Blood, Fluids; opens Meridians; rheumatic pains, poor circulation, expels Cold.
Black Pepper	neutral; sweet	Lungs, Spleen, Stomach, Large Intestine	Regulates Qi, warms the body, carminative, removes Blood Stagnation and Coldness, dries mucus; vomiting of clear liquid, diarrhea from Coldness, food poisoning, locally on toothache, weak nerves. Avoid: Yin Deficiency and Internal Heat
Black Sesame Seeds	neutral; sweet	Kidneys, Liver	Liver and Kidney tonic, lubricates the Organs; treats vertigo, constipation, gray

hair, weak knees, rheumatism, dry skin, shortage of mother's milk; black sesame seeds are better for the Kidney-Adrenals, and the yellow for the Spleen-Pancreas. Avoid: Spleen Dampness and watery stools

Black Soya Bean	neutral; sweet	Spleen, Kidneys	Promotes Blood circulation and urination, de-toxifies, nourishes Kidney and Liver Blood, expels Wind; lower back and knee pains, infertility, seminal emission, blurred vision, difficult urine, edema, jaundice, rheumatism, muscular cramps, lockjaw, drug poisoning, Wind Bi.
Buckwheat	cool; sweet	Large Intestine, Stomach, Spleen	Clears Heat, lowers Rebellious Qi, improves appetite; eliminates swelling and accumulations; boils, chronic diarrhea, dysentery, skin lesions and eruptions. Avoid: vertigo, indigestion or Wind or Hot diseases.
Butter	warm; sweet	Spleen, Stomach	Removes Stagnant Blood, expels Coldness; scabies, skin eruptions, body odor.
Cabbage	neutral; sweet	Spleen, Stomach, Large Intestine	Promotes urination, beneficial to Kidneys and brain after long consumption; constipation, thirst due to intoxication, ulcers, depression, coughs and colds, hot flashes. Avoid; Qi Deficiency, Spleen/Stomach Yang Deficiency, nausea.
Carrot	neutral; sweet	Lung, Spleen	Diuretic and digestive; improves eyes, removes swellings and tumors, indigestion, cough, dysentery, difficult urination, skin eruptions, chronic diarrhea and dysentery.
Cayenne	hot; pungent	Spleen, Heart	Warms, removes Blood Stagnation, disperses congestion, expels Cold; poor appetite, cold abdominal pains, diarrhea,

			vomiting. Avoid: Yin Deficiency, Excess Fire, Cough, eye disease.
Celery	cool; bitter, sweet	Stomach, Liver, Kidney	Clears Heat, dries Damp, calms Liver, expels Wind, promotes urine; hypertension, headache, dizziness, discharge of blood in urine, conjunctivitis, carbuncle. Avoid: scabies.
Cheese	neutral; sour, sweet	Liver, Lungs, Spleen	Tonifies Qi, Blood, and Yin, quenches thirst; Deficiency fever, Dryness, constipation, skin eruptions, itchy skin. Avoid: weak digestion or mucus conditions.
Cherry	warm; sweet	Heart, Spleen	Moves Blood in lower half of body, expels Cold and Wind Damp; rheumatism, arthritis, lumbago, paralysis, numbness, frostbite.
Chicken	warm; sweet	Spleen, Stomach	Tonifies Qi, moves Blood, expels Cold, tonifies Jing; underweight, diarrhea, edema, poor appetite, vaginal bleeding and discharge, lack of mother's milk, general weakness, frequent urination, weakness after childbirth, diarrhea, dysentery, diabetes, edema, anorexia. Avoid: Excess conditions, External diseases.
Clam	cold; salty	Stomach	Clears Heat, lubricates Dryness, tonifies Yin, softens hardness; diabetes, edema, scrofula, leukorrhea, hemorrhoids, vaginal bleeding.
Coconut Meat	neutral; sweet	Spleen, Stomach	Tonifies Qi & Blood, expels Wind; malnutrition in children.
Coconut Milk	warm; sweet	Spleen, Stomach	Tonifies Qi & Blood, expels Cold, moves Blood; diabetes, quenches thirst.
Corn	neutral; sweet	Stomach, Spleen, Large Intestine	Regulates digestive Organs; weak Heart, difficult urination, sexual

weakness.

Crab	cold; salty	Stomach	Clears Heat, moistens Dryness, tonifies Yin, moves Blood; fractures, poison ivy, burns. Avoid: Wind disease, Spleen/ Stomach Yang Deficiency; do not over-consume as it is considered toxic.
Cucumber	cool; sweet	Stomach, Spleen, Large Intestine	Detoxifies, clears Heat, promotes urination, quenches thirst; sore throat, pink eyes, inflammation, burns.
Date (red)	warm; sweet	Spleen, Stomach	Tonifies Qi and Blood; weak stomach, palpitations, nervousness, hysteria from weakness.
Duck	neutral; sweet, salty	Lungs, Kidneys	Tonifies Qi, Blood, and Yin, lubricates Dryness; treats swelling and edema, hot sensations, cough. Avoid: Spleen Deficiency, Stagnant Qi, symptoms of hemorrhage.
Eggplant	cool; sweet	Large Intestine, Spleen, Stomach	Clears Heat, removes Stagnant Blood, relieves pain, swelling; dysentery, bleeding discharges from anus, urine and dysentery, boils, skin ulcers and mastitis, prevents strokes. Avoid: women without Stagnant Blood in uterus should avoid over-consumption.
Fig	neutral; sweet	Large Intestine	Detoxifies, Stomach tonic; heals swelling, constipation, hemorrhoids, sore throat, diarrhea, dysentery.
Garlic	warm; pungent	Lungs, Stomach, Spleen	Warms, expels Cold, promotes Qi and Blood circulation, destroys worms and kills parasites, anti-viral, anti-bacterial; arthritis, Cold abdominal pain, edema, diarrhea, dysentery, whooping cough, TB, pneumonia, hepatitis.

			Avoid: Yin Deficiency with False Fire Rising; canker sores.
Ginger (dried)	hot; pungent	Lungs, Stomach, Spleen	Warms, carminative, expels Cold, moves Blood, benefits digestion, relieves cramps; colds, coughs, cold limbs, diarrhea, vomiting, nausea, mucus, rheumatism, cold abdominal pain. Avoid: Yin Deficiency, Internal Heat, Hot Blood hemorrhage.
Gluten, Wheat (seitan)	cool; sweet	Stomach, Spleen,	Tonifies Qi, clears Liver Heat; reduces fever, sedates hypertension, quenches thirst.
Goose	neutral; sweet	Lungs, Spleen	Tonifies Qi, harmonies Stomach; diarrhea, diabetes. Avoid: Damp Heat conditions.
Grapes	neutral; sweet, sour	Lungs, Spleen, Kidneys	Red variety is very tonifying to Qi and Blood, strengthens bones and tendons, promotes urine, harmonizes stomach, relieves anger and irritability; Blood and Qi Deficiency, cough, palpitations, night sweats, rheumatism, difficult urination, edema.
Herring	neutral; sweet	Lungs, Spleen	Tonifies Deficiency, moistens Dryness; Deficiency fatigue. Avoid: skin eruptions or when recovering from chronic diseases.
Honey	neutral; sweet	Lungs, Spleen, Large Intestine	Tonifies Qi and Blood, lubricates Dryness, relieves pain; Dry cough, constipation, stomach ache, sinusitis, mouth cankers, burns, neurasthenia, hypertension, TB, heart disease, liver disease; aconite poisoning.
Kelp	cold; salty	Stomach, Spleen	Clears Heat, moistens Dryness, tonifies Yin, softens hardness; scrofula, goiter, edema, leukorrhea, orchitis. Avoid: Stomach & Spleen Yang Deficiency and/or Dampness.

Kidney Bean	neutral; sweet	Spleen, Kidney	Tonifies Yin, promotes urination, clears Heat, diuretic, reduces swelling; edema.
Kudzu root powder	cool; sweet	Stomach, Large Intestine	Clears Heat, tonifies Yin; quenches thirst, Stomach & Intestinal flu, hangover, toothache, Hot skin eruptions.
Lamb (mutton)	hot; sweet	Spleen, Kidneys	Tonifies Qi, warms and expels Coldness, removes Blood Stagnation; indigestion, fatigue, emaciation, coldness, lumbago, general weakness, underweight, abdominal pain, cold sensations post partum, sore loins; strengthens sexual power and penis erection. Avoid: Cold External diseases, Internal Heat.
Lemon	cool; sour	Liver	Produces Fluid, considered good for pregnancy; cough with mucus discharge, diabetes, indigestion, laryngitis, reduces fat.
Lettuce	cool; sweet, bitter	Large Intestine	Clears Heat, dries Damp, promotes urination and milk secretion, calming, inhibits bleeding. Avoid: eye disease; over-consumption can cause dizziness and blurred vision.
Lotus root	cool; sweet	Stomach, Spleen, Heart	Cools Blood, tonifies Yin, clears Heat, strengthens appetite, tones Spleen, produces muscles; thirst, dryness, weakness, bleeding; cooked root is used for anorexia, diarrhea and Lung ailments.
Loquat	neutral; sour, sweet	Spleen, Liver, Lungs	Lubricates Dryness and Lungs, quenches thirst; cough, constipation, laryngitis.
Mango	cold; sweet, sour	Stomach	Quenches thirst, strengthens Stomach, relieves vomiting, promotes urination; cough, indigestion, bleeding from gums. Avoid: common cold,

indigestion,			during convalescence; over-consumption can cause itching or skin eruptions.
Milk	neutral; sweet	Lungs, Stomach,	Tonifies Blood and Qi, produces Fluids, lubricates Dryness and Intestines, tonifies Deficiencies; indigestion (take scalded and warm), upset stomach, difficulty swallowing, diabetes, constipation. Avoid: for weak Spleen-Stomach with Dampness.
Millet	cool; sweet, salty	Stomach, Spleen, Kidneys	Tonifies Qi, clears Heat, benefits Kidneys and Middle Warmer, lubricates; indigestion, counteracts toxins, diabetes, vomiting, diarrhea, indigestion. Avoid: undigested food in stools, Spleen & Stomach Yang Deficiency.
Mung Bean	cool; sweet	Stomach, Heart	Promotes urination, clears Heat, detoxifies, relieves hypertension, Summer Heat; diarrhea, dysentery, diabetes, boils, edema, burns, lead and drug poisoning; sprouts are good for alcoholism.
Mushroom (common button)	cool; sweet	Lungs, Large Intestine, Stomach, Spleen	Clears Heat, calms Spirit, reduces tumors; edema, mucus discharge, vomiting, diarrhea. Avoid: Cold Stomach, skin problems or allergies.
Mustard greens	warm; pungent	Lungs	Carminative, regulates Qi, removes Blood Stagnation, expels Cold, dries mucus; cough, mucus discharge, chest congestion. Avoid: skin eruptions, eye disease, hemorrhoids, anal hemorrhage, Heat conditions, bleeding, pink eye.
Nori	cold; sweet, salty	Lungs	Clears Heat, tonifies Yin, softens hardness, diuretic; goiter, beriberi, edema, dysuria, hypertension.

Olive	neutral; sweet, sour	Lungs, Stomach	Moistens, clears lungs; sore throat, coughing blood, alcoholism.
Onion	warm; pungent	Lungs, Stomach	Tonifies and regulates Qi, removes Blood Stagnation, expels Cold, diaphoretic, counteracts toxins, diuretic, expectorant; external applications for trichomonas vaginitis and ulcers; pneumonia, common cold, headache, constipation, cold abdominal pain, dysuria, dysentery, mastitis, nasal congestion, facial edema.
Oyster	neutral; sweet, salty	Kidney, Liver	Tonifies Blood and Yin, hormone tonic; stress, insomnia, nervousness. Avoid: skin diseases.
Papaya	neutral; sweet	Spleen, Heart	Promotes digestion, destroys intestinal worms; stomach ache, dysentery, difficult bowel movements, rheumatism, Wind Bi.
Peach	warm; sour, sweet	Spleen	Promotes Blood circulation, removes Blood Stagnation, expels Cold, lubricates; dry cough, hernial pain, excessive perspiration, indigestion Avoid: excess can produce Internal Heat.
Peanut	neutral; sweet	Lung, Spleen	Lubricates Lungs, good for stomachache; Dry cough, upset stomach, promotes mothers' milk. Avoid: Cold Damp conditions, Qi Stagnation.
Pea	neutral; sweet	Stomach, Spleen	Lowers rebellious Qi, diuretic, induces bowel movements; spasms, carbuncle, counteracts skin eruptions.
Pear	cool; sweet	Lungs, Stomach	Clears Heat, produces Fluids, lubricates Dryness, transforms Sputum; Hot cough with mucus, constipation, alcoholism,

			indigestion, difficulty when swallowing, difficult urination, diabetes.
Persimmon	cold; sweet	Lung, Heart, Large Intestine	Clears Heat, tonifies Yin, lubricates Lungs, quenches thirst; cough, canker sore, chronic bronchitis. Avoid: Spleen/ Stomach Yang Deficiency, diarrhea, malaria.
Pineapple	neutral; sweet	Spleen	Quenches thirst, promotes digestion, relieves diarrhea; anorexia, edema, thirst, sunstroke, oliguria. Avoid: Damp and/or Cold conditions.
Pinenut	warm; sweet	Lung, Liver, Large Intestine	Tonifies Qi, removes Blood Stagnation, expels Cold, moistens, expels Wind; Wind Bi (rheumatism), vertigo, dry cough, constipation.
Plantain (banana)	cold; sweet	Large & Small Intestine	Clears Heat, tonifies Yin, expels sputum, sharpens vision, anuria, dysuria, leukorrhea, hematuria, pertussis, jaundice, edema, dysentery, epistaxis, conjunctivitis, eye pain, skin ulcers. Avoid: spermatorrhea.
Plum	neutral; sweet, sour	Kidneys, Liver	Clears Liver, clears Heat, moistens, promotes urination and digestion; Liver disease, diabetes, fatigue. Avoid: excess can cause bloating and gas.
Pork	neutral; salty, sweet	Kidney, Stomach Spleen	Lubricates Dryness, tonifies Yin; diabetes, weakness, emaciation, dry cough, constipation Avoid: Hot sputum or Qi Stagnation.
Potato	neutral; sweet	Spleen, Stomach	Heals inflammation, tonifies Qi and the Spleen; lack of energy, mumps, burns.
Pumpkin	neutral; sweet	Spleen, Stomach	Dries Dampness, tonifies Qi, induces sweating; bronchial asthma.

Radish (seed)	warm; sweet, pungent	Lungs, Stomach	Detoxifies, promotes digestion, eliminates Hot mucus discharge, expels Cold; abdominal swelling due to indigestion, laryngitis due to continual cough with mucus discharge, vomiting of blood, nosebleed, dysentery, headache, bloating, hoarseness, diabetes, occipital headache, epistaxis, dysentery, trichomas vaginitis. Avoid: Coldness from Deficiency.
Raspberry	neutral; sweet, sour	Liver, Kidneys	Tonifies Liver & Kidneys, checks frequent urination, sharpens vision; impotence, dizziness, spermatorrhea, polyuria, enuresis, Deficiency fatigue, blurred vision. Avoid: painful or difficult urine.
Rice, brown	neutral; sweet	Spleen, Stomach	Tonifies Qi and Spleen, harmonizes Stomach, relieves depression, quenches thirst; diarrhea, morning sickness, thirst.
Rice, white	slightly cool; sweet	Spleen, Stomach	Similar to brown rice but clears Heat from acidity.
Rice, sweet	warm, sweet	Lungs	Tonifies Qi and assists Yang, expels Cold, moves Stagnant Blood; diabetes, polyuria, diarrhea, excessive sweating. Avoid: Stomach/ Spleen Qi Deficiency, Damp Heat or Wind disease.
Rye	neutral; bitter	Heart	Dries Dampness, diuretic; post partum hemorrhage, migraine; can be toxic.
Salt	cold; salty	Large Intestine, Small Intestine, Stomach, Kidneys	Detoxifies, lubricates Dryness, causes vomiting, cools Blood; abdominal swelling and pain, difficult bowel movement, dysuria, pyorrhea, sore throat, toothache, corneal opacity, skin eruptions, constipation, bleeding from gums, cataract.

Sardine	neutral; sweet, salty	Spleen, Stomach	Moistens, tonifies Yin, warms Middle Burner, strengthens tendons and bones, activates Blood, diuretic; digestant, urinary strain. Avoid: over-consumption can cause Fire and Sputum.
Seaweed	cold; salty	Kidney, Stomach	Lubricates Dryness, softens hardness (lumps and tumors), tonifies Yin, eliminates mucus, promotes water passage; goiter, abdominal swelling and obstruction, edema and beriberi.
Sesame Oil	cool; sweet	Stomach	Detoxifies, lubricates Dryness, promotes bowel movements, clears Heat, produces muscles; dry constipation, abdominal pain caused by indigestion, roundworms, skin eruptions, ulcers, tinea, scabies, dry and cracked skin. Avoid: diarrhea with deficiency of Spleen Qi.
Shiitake mushroom	neutral; sweet	Stomach, Liver	Tonifies Blood, benefits the Stomach, anti-inflammatory; cholesterol, hypertension, common cold, chickenpox, cancer, Kidney problems, gallstones, hemorrhoids, lack of vitamin D, softening of the bones, cataract, pyorrhea, ulcers, neuralgia, anemia, measles.
Shrimp	warm, sweet	Spleen, Stomach	Tonifies Qi and Yang, removes Blood Stagnation, expels Cold, eliminates Wind, expels Sputum, promotes lactation, destroys worms. Avoid: Hot skin diseases & while recuperating from chronic illness.
Soybean	cool; sweet	Large Intestine, Spleen	Clears Heat, sedates Yang, strengthens Spleen, moistens Dryness; diarrhea, emaciation, skin eruptions, hemorrhage from trauma, Qi Stagnation, cough &/or heavy sensations in the body.

Spinach	cool, sweet	Large Intestine, Small Intestine	Lubricates Dryness, arrests bleeding, clears Heat, homeostatic; nosebleed, discharge of blood from anus, thirst in diabetes, constipation, alcoholism, scurvy, hemorrhoids. Avoid: spermatorrhea.
Squash (winter)	warm; sweet	Stomach, Spleen	Tonifies Qi and Blood, assists Yang, heals inflammation, relieves pain, moves Blood, expels Cold; pulmonary abscess, roundworms. Avoid: Dampness &/or Qi Stagnation.
Strawberry	warm; sweet, sour	Liver, Kidneys	Removes Blood Stagnation, expels Cold; polyuria, vertigo and motion sickness.
String Bean	neutral; sweet	Spleen, Kidneys	Tonifies Yin, Kidneys, strengthens Spleen; polyuria, diarrhea, diabetes, spermatorrhea, leukorrhea. Avoid: Qi Stagnation and constipation.
Sweet Potato	neutral; sweet	Spleen, Kidneys	Tonifies Qi and Spleen, removes Blood Stagnation, expels Coldness, produces Fluid, induces bowel movements; jaundice, emaciation, skin eruptions, Stomach and Kidney weakness, premature ejaculation. Avoid: Qi and Food Stagnation.
Swiss Chard	cool; sweet	Large Intestine, Lungs, Stomach	Clears Heat, detoxifies, hemostatic; delayed eruptions of measles, dysentery, amenorrhea and carbuncle.
Tangerine	cool; sour, sweet	Lungs, Kidneys, Lungs, Stomach	Regulates Qi, clears Heat, quenches thirst, lubricates Lungs, relieves coughing; chest congestion, vomiting, hiccuping, stimulates appetite, diabetes. Avoid: cough and sputum from External Wind & Cold.
Tomato	cold; sweet, sour	Stomach, Liver	Clears Heat, tonifies Yin, quenches thirst, promotes

digestion; thirst and anorexia.

Trout	hot; sour	Liver, Gall Bladder	Assists Yang, expels Cold, regulates Qi, harmonizes Middle Warmer, warms Stomach. Avoid: over-consumption can cause scabies and skin eruptions.
Tuna	neutral; sweet	Stomach	Tonifies Qi and Blood, transforms Damp; beriberi, Damp Bi.
Vinegar	warm; sour, bitter	Stomach, Liver	Disperses coagulations, removes Blood Stagnation, detoxifies, arrests bleeding, dries Dampness, induces perspiration, expels Cold, hemostatic, vermifuge; post partum syncope, genital itching, abdominal swelling and obstruction, jaundice, food poisoning. Avoid: Spleen/ Stomach Yang Deficiency, muscular atrophy, rheumatism, tendon trauma, and beginning of a common cold.
Walnut	warm; sweet	Lungs, Kidneys	Tonifies Kidneys, lubricates Intestines, checks seminal emission, expels Cold, solidifies sperm, warms Lungs, calms; asthma, cough, lumbago, impotence, spermatorrhea, frequent urination, dry stools, kidney and bladder stones, constipation. Avoid: Yin Deficiency with False Fire Rising.
Water Chestnut	cold; sweet	Lungs, Stomach	Clears Heat, relieves fever and indigestion, promotes urination, disperses accumulations; hypertension, diabetes, jaundice, conjunctivitis, measles, dysentery with bloody stools, smoker's sore throat. Avoid: anemia, Coldness or Blood Deficiency.
Watercress	cool; pungent	Lungs, Stomach	Removes Blood Stagnation, clears Heat, benefits water; jaundice, edema, urinary strain, leukorrhea, mumps, oliguria.

Avoid: Spleen/Stomach
Deficiency or frequent urination.

Watermelon	cold; sweet	Stomach, Heart, Bladder	Clears Heat, lubricates Intestines, relieves Summer Heat, relieves mental depression, quenches thirst, diuretic; oliguria, sore throat, canker sores, diminished urination. Avoid: Excess Dampness, anemia, frequent urination or Coldness in the Middle Warmer.
Wheat	cool; sweet	Spleen, Heart, Kidney	Nourishes Heart, Calms Spirit, clears Heat, quenches thirst.
Whitefish	neutral, sweat	Lungs, Stomach, Liver	Tonifies Spleen, relieves indigestion, promotes water flow.
Yam	neutral; sweet	Lungs, Spleen, Kidney	Tonifies Spleen, Lungs, Kidneys, benefits semen; diarrhea, dysentery, diabetes, leukorrhea, spermatorrhea, polyuria, cough. Avoid: Excess diseases.

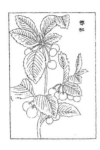

FOURTEEN

HERBAL PREPARATIONS & TREATMENTS

METHODS OF PREPARING AND TAKING CHINESE HERBS

Chinese herbs are taken in many forms. Some of these are based on what is most effective for optimum absorption while others are simply based on convenience. Chinese herbs are taken as decoctions, pills, alcoholic liquors, maceration, pastes, dried and liquid extracts and with food.

Herb Teas

Decoctions and Infusions

Teas are generally regarded as the most assimilable form for taking herbs. There is a difference between Western and Chinese approaches to making medicinal herb teas. In Western herbalism, the concern is the overall amount of either a single or compound herbal formula, which is usually about one ounce to a pint of water. In Chinese herbalism, however, there is a prescribed effective dose for each ingredient which is combined with little concern for the total amount or weight. The average dose for most Chinese herbs ranges from 3 to 9 grams; 9-15 grams is indicated for heavier roots and barks and 9 to 30 grams for dense minerals and shells. For more toxic substances the dose is usually less than 3 grams, depending on the degree of toxicity. This means that a compound Chinese herb formula may have a considerably higher volume of total herb material than the equivalent Western herbal preparation. If herbs are used fresh rather than dried, one must increase by half or double the amount to compensate for the water content of the fresh herbs.

Vessels Used For The Preparation Of Chinese Herbs

Teas should be made in such non-metallic containers as glass, earthenware or enamel pots. Stainless steel is all right to use if the others are not available. Whenever possible, spring or purified water, rather than tap water, should be used. Metal cooking vessels are inappropriate because they can react with the biochemical constituents of the herbs and alter their properties.

Decoctions: The Most Common Method for Preparing Chinese Herb Teas

There are many methods of preparing herbal teas, called "tangs" (literally translated as "soups" or decoctions) based upon the predilection of the herbalist. One standard method is to combine the ingredients of each formula in 3 to 4 cups of water. This is then brought to boiling and allowed to slowly simmer for approximately 45 minutes to an hour or until the original volume of fluid has been reduced to approximately 2 cups. One cup is taken morning and evening for chronic or three times daily for acute conditions. Again for chronic conditions, the remaining strained herbs of the original tea can be reused and cooked again the next day using two cups of water cooked down to one. The reserved two cups of the first preparation is then combined with the second to make a total of three cups.

Since length of cooking may extract even deeper constituents, there may be a saturation level where the fluid has become too saturated in one decoction. To effectively extract any further, the double decoction method is often used. In this, one follows the preceding double decoction method to arrive at a total of 3 cups of tea which are combined together.

There are many other methods, including presoaking heavier roots, barks and substances for an hour or two before bringing to a boil, further decocting or reducing the herbs even a third time, and so forth. However, the methods described are the ones that will yield good results.

Certain ingredients require different cooking times and processes. For instance, some herbs, especially the surface relieving diaphoretics whose potency is dependent upon volatile oils, are volatilized and destroyed in a lengthy decoction process. They are added last to be steeped after the heavier ingredients have been extracted. These include herbs such as mint, chrysanthemum flowers, fresh ginger and cinnamon twigs. On the other hand, heavier herbs, especially minerals such as dragon bone, oyster shell and iron, require longer extraction, up to one or two hours of preparation. In the case of toxic herbs, such as unprepared aconite, it is important to slowly simmer them at least an hour in boiling water to neutralize or lessen their toxicity. This is even recommended for the preparation of prepared or previously detoxified herbs such as prepared aconite (Fu Zi).

In cooking a formula that combines minerals or toxic herbs with those that have volatile oils, one needs to first decoct the longer cooking herbs first and then add those ingredients that require less cooking time.

Infusions

An infusion is used for herbs whose volatile oil content is important to their primary therapeutic application. This might include diaphoretic and carminative herbs. To prepare an infusion, boiling water is poured over the herbs in a pot which is then covered with a lid to prevent the escape of volatile oils. The amount of time an herbal formula is allowed to steep is anywhere from 15 to 20 minutes or until cool enough to drink.

Dose and methods for taking herb teas: Most commonly teas are taken warm. Sometimes to enhance diuretic action, diuretic formulas can be taken cool. Normally the dose for adults is 2 to 3 cups daily while for children the dose may be half or even less according to size and age. In acute conditions more frequent small doses throughout the day is more effective. For long term chronic conditions, 2 to 3 cups of the tea is taken as a daily dose. It is good to schedule periodic days off from taking the herbs. A good general principle is to abstain from taking herbs one regular day each week. For convenience and long term usage, herbs can be taken in various other forms such as dried or alcoholic fluid extract, pills, capsules or powdered herbs mixed with honey.

Storage: Herbs should be stored in airtight jars or containers and protected from direct light to slow oxidation. Sometimes it is unavoidable that certain herbs are prone to insect infestation and should be discarded. However, at the first sign, the jarred herbs can be placed in the freezer overnight which will kill off any larvae. Adding a few strongly aromatic leaves of bay, for instance, will also help prevent infestation by insects.

General Dosage Guidelines

Historically, weights varied at different periods. Since the Tang dynasty, one liang equaled 31.25 grams. This being an awkward number, the People's Republic of China standardized modern equivalents as follows:

1 liang = 30 grams
1 chien = 3 grams
1 fen = 0.3 grams
1 li = .03 grams

Most average strength Chinese herbs are 6-9 grams dosage. Herbs that are light in weight or strong are 3-6 grams. Heavier minerals and herbs are precooked and range from 9 to 30 grams. If one is studying Japanese-Chinese herbalism (Kanpo), the average dose is approximately one third that of the Chinese.

Dosage was originally determined according to the patient's condition and tolerance. The following can be considered a guideline to proper dosing:

1. Strong and toxic substances, such as cinnabar, should be prescribed in the smallest possible dose.
2. Heavy roots are taken in higher dosage than light flowers or leaves.
3. Most heavy minerals and shells are used in still higher dosage.
4. Tonics, sedative, tranquilizing herbs are prescribed in higher doses, while sweating, Qi moving (carminative), Blood moving, Drying and fragrant herbs are prescribed in smaller doses.
5. A single herb or substance is generally prescribed in higher dosage than when it is in a formula. However, the primary herb(s) in a formula is always prescribed in a higher dose relative to the assistant and counter-assistant herbs.
6. Fresh herbs containing more water need to be taken in double the indicated dose.
7. The dose for a more serious disease should be as high as the patient can tolerate.
8. For children under one year the dose is 1/10 that of an adult dose; From 2-3 years the dose is 1/4 the adult dose; from 3-6 years it is 1/3 the adult dose; from 10 years to adult the dose is approximately 1/2 the adult dose.

HOW AND WHEN TO TAKE HERBS

Tonics are generally taken before meals. Herbs that are Cooling and detoxifying can be more irritating and may be taken after meals. Purgatives and anthelmintics should be taken on an empty stomach for maximum effect. Sedative and tranquilizing herbs should always be taken before rest and at least three times throughout the day to support and strengthen the nervous system for proper rest to occur in the evening. Pain-relieving herbs can be taken as often as needed.

Herbs should be taken Warm for Cold conditions and Cool for Hot conditions such as fevers. Individuals who experience nausea should take the herbs in small repeated dosages according to tolerance.

Other methods for taking Chinese herbs

Besides water based teas, herbs can be taken as powders, pills, capsules, syrups, plasters, liniments, alcohol based herbal wines and extracts and combined with food. Commercially manufactured Chinese herbal formulas made both here, in China, Taiwan and Hong Kong can be very effective. However, one must realize that quality control standards in China are not as stringent as in the West. Further, the Chinese do not share our bias for or against the inclusion of Western pharmaceutical drugs with their herbal products. The majority of patented Chinese herb products are relatively safe and effective, but there has been in recent times a good deal of publicity about certain imported so-called herbal products that contain Western drugs.

Western herb companies are now producing highly effective Chinese herbal products often combined with herbs from the West and other parts of the world. Conforming more to prevailing marketing standards, these are worthy of their increasing popularity.

Another problem that many have with imported Chinese herbs is that they are not necessarily grown organically, are fumigated or sprayed to prevent insect damage and retain an appearance of freshness. Commonly the spray to retain color and freshness is sulfur-based, which can cause an adverse reaction for those with asthma. Increasingly the practitioner and consumer of Chinese herbs is being provided with the opportunity of at least purchasing unsprayed and unfumigated herbs. In general, begin with the minimum indicated manufacturer's dose and increase as individual tolerance will allow.

Following the principle of Five Elements and based on empirical experience, certain formulas are more effective when combined with certain ingredients. For instance, a formula intended for the Kidneys is more effective if it is taken with a pinch of salt or soya sauce. Circulatory, arthritic or rheumatic formulas are better if taken with a teaspoon of rice wine or alcohol, which helps to carry it into the circulation more efficiently. A Spleen Qi tonic is enhanced when taken with a teaspoon or so of honey, barley malt or a small amount of rice.

Herbs taken to cleanse the liver should not be taken as an alcoholic extract. If one desires to take a tincture without the alcohol, most of it can be evaporated by putting the appropriate amount of extract in a cup of boiling water for a few minutes.

Powders, called **"san"**, are taken by simply mixing them with a little warm water. Another method is to mix the herbal powders with honey to form either several small **pills**, called **"wan"**, or one large pill mass. The average dose for most herbal powders is approximately 6 grams at a time at least twice a day, more or less according to constitution, body size, age and sensitivity.

Alcoholic extracts, called **"chih"**, are usually made with a high potency alcohol such as a particular type of Chinese rice wine. To make these, the whole or powdered herbs are allowed to macerate in the rice wine or alcohol for anywhere from two weeks to a year.

Chinese herbs are also taken as nutritive tonics in **soup,** or in a **rice soup,** called **"congee"**, using herbs such as jujube dates, astragalus root, dioscorea, lycii berries, ginseng or codonopsis root. These are commonly cooked with glutinous sweet rice using one part (by volume) rice to 7 to 10 parts water. This is cooked slowly for 8 to 10 hours and is taken in the morning or at various times throughout the day as an easily digested porridge. Other foods, such as meat and various appropriate root vegetables, can be added. This method is least likely to generate an adverse reaction and is particularly good for those who have poor digestion or are wasting, thin, emaciated and/or weak. Today it is most convenient to use a timed "slow cooker" or high quality stainless steel rice cooker for these kinds of preparations.

A popular innovation is the use of **concentrated dried extracts**. These are made through a special closed extraction process where the herbs are decocted in an enclosed vessel so as to fully capture their volatile components, which are then reintroduced back into the final dried powdered concentrate. Depending upon the quality of the original herbs, these extracts can produce equivalent results to whole bulk herbs. A concentration of approximately 5 parts herb makes one part of the powdered extract. Many of the classic formulas are available in this form as well as single herbs to prepare individual formula combinations. The ready availability of these products in many Western countries makes them convenient for practitioners and students with limited funds and space for storing a pharmacy of 250 to 300 herbs. They can be ingested as a powder or granule, mixed with water or placed into gelatin capsules. Dosage for most conditions is 500 mg. per 20 pounds of body weight. For acute conditions more should be taken for one to three days and then tapered off as the symptoms subside.

Finally, when visiting a traditional Chinese pharmacy, one will at first be amazed at the wide variety of herbal products that are available. Besides those mentioned, one can find a variety of external liniments, rubbing oils, salves and various plasters that can be used externally for injuries and to promote healing.

Fomentations and Baths

An herbal fomentation, also known as an herbal compress, is made by moistening a flannel or some other absorbent cloth in an herbal tea and laying on the body, usually as warm as the individual can bear. Herbal baths are made by boiling a pot of herb tea and pouring it into the bathwater and then soaking all or part of the body in it. It is amazing how absorbent the skin surface can be when something the body needs is applied onto it. Further, there is some protection from any adverse reactions since the skin also acts as a natural barrier to prevent the undue absorption of an herb. This makes fomentations particularly useful for the highly sensitive or babies and small children.

In helping restore vitality to a part of the body that has been immobilized or weakened by a disease, the hot fomentation can be alternated with a shorter application of cold water. Heat serves to relax the body and open the pores, while cold stimulates the body and causes contraction. The alternation of hot and cold will revitalize the area.

Ginger Fomentation: A ginger fomentation is an excellent remedy for sore throats, lower back pain, lung congestion and phlegm, sprains, cramps, pains, menstrual cramps, coldness, swellings, colds, flu, coughs, excessive mucus and strained muscles. It is also very effective for drawing out blood toxins and stimulating the circulation. Placed over the lower abdomen and perineum during childbirth, it helps prevent tearing and stops pain.

It can also be placed over the chest for congested lungs, cough, asthma and bronchitis (all from Coldness); over the abdomen for pains, spasms, poor digestion, coldness, bladder infections (from Heat locked in by Cold, usually from deficient Kidney Yang) and menstrual cramps; over the lower back for pain and ache, lowered immunity, Deficient Qi and poor digestion; and over any other part of the body where there is congestion, Stagnation, sprains, swellings, cramps, pain or coldness.

To make a ginger fomentation, first make an infusion out of fresh grated ginger, using about 2" of the root to 1 Quart of water. Next, dip a small cloth (such as washcloth) into the tea and let soak for 5 minutes to absorb tea. Using a pair of tongs, lift the cloth out of the tea. Quickly wring it out and put it over the part of the body where a fomentation is desired. Immediately cover the cloth with a towel. Place a hot water bottle or heating pad over the towel and cover everything with another towel so all is kept warm. Leave on at least 20 minutes.

You may want to put a fomentation on more than once. Have the second cloth soaking in the tea while resting with the first one on. After

20 minutes change cloths and then leave the second compress on for another 20 minutes. A ginger fomentation can be applied two times in one day, or left on overnight. Be sure to keep it warm.

Castor Oil Compress

Castor oil compress is a fabulous way to rejuvenate scarred and failing tissues and organs. The oil is very close to natural oils in the body and so penetrates the cells easily, healing and rejuvenating them. It detoxifies, heals cysts, growths, warts, treats epilepsy, paralysis and other nervous system disorders, stimulates the body's deep circulation and heals body tissues such as detoxifying and healing liver disorders or chronic bladder infections (place over the liver and bladder respectively for these). Apply the compress over the affected area, be it the liver, bladder, kidneys, cyst or other growth.

Repeated applications are necessary over time to heal these conditions. Often a pattern is followed of applying the castor oil compress for 4 days in a row and then leaving it off for 3 days. This is repeated for several weeks to months or until the condition is healed.

Castor oil compress is made a little differently than other fomentations. In a pan, soak with castor oil a piece of felt, cloth or cheesecloth cut to fit the desired area. Heat in the oven till very warm but still touchable. Place over the desired area, cover with plastic wrap, then follow the above directions for a ginger fomentation. Generally, this compress is left on for several hours or overnight.

Plasters and Poultices

A plaster is the application of powdered herbs mixed with a binding agent, such as a little water and flour, and spread onto a cloth and applied directly over an affected area. An herbal poultice is more bulky, consisting of an herbal mash that is wrapped up in a protective cloth or combined in a thick base material such as slippery elm or an oil and then placed on the skin. It is first placed in the cloth or oil because the herbs used in a poultice are stronger and might burn or extremely irritate the skin if they were put directly on it. Mustard and garlic are two common examples.

Poultices and plasters are both good for muscle spasms, swelling, arthritis, rheumatism, tumors, fevers, mucus congestion in the chest, bronchitis and pneumonia. They can be used in treating enlarged glands and organs (neck, breast, groin, kidney, liver, prostate) and various eruptions (boils, abscesses). The major difference is that a poultice can use more healing or vulnerary herbs and often uses cool natured herbs as well, while a plaster more typically uses herbal essential oils and/or stimulant herbs such as cinnamon bark, cayenne pepper or mustard seed to create a warming counter-irritant effect.

To make the poultice, first choose herbs and powder them in a blender or seed/coffee grinder. Add a little bit of hot water, herbal tea, liniment or a tincture to powdered herbs and mix to form a thick paste. If all herbs are not powdered, make them into tea first and add some to the rest of the powdered herbs. Spread the paste on a thin piece of cheesecloth and wrap up until the paste is well enclosed in cloth. Place on the skin where wanted and keep warm with a hot water bottle or heating pad. Change frequently if needed. Poultices may be applied continuously and over-night as needed. Some need to be reapplied and kept on for several days. Usually, however, they are applied from 20 minutes to several hours or longer.

Onion Poultice

Onions are a natural antibiotic and so aid infections and inflammations. Made into a poultice and placed over the lungs, they are a tremendous aid to pneumonia, lung infection, bronchial inflammation, asthma and will clear the lungs of mucus congestion and coldness. Slice 3 large onions (preferably organic) and steam or sauté in a little water until slightly soft. Wrap in a cheesecloth and place over the desired area, covering it with a towel and a hot water bottle or heating pad.

Mustard Plaster

A mustard pack, or plaster, is a well known folk remedy. It is excellent for aches, sprains, spasms, cold areas needing circulation and to cause mucus expectoration. It is made with 1 tablespoon mustard powder, 4 tablespoons whole wheat flour and enough water to form a paste. If the skin is sensitive or if it seems too strong, use an equal amount of egg white instead of the water to prevent blistering. After removing the plaster, the skin may be powdered with flour and the area wrapped with dry cotton.

Mustard plasters are usually placed on the chest to draw out mucus congestion, dispel coldness, aid asthma, eliminate coughs, and heal colds and flus. It can also be placed where needed to treat body and joint pains and treat watery, oozing and chronic sores or boils.

Other plasters are made by mixing powdered herbs such as ginger, cinnamon or cayenne, with honey spread on a cloth with another cloth between the plaster material and the skin to protect it from over-stimulating the tissues. Herbal plasters are also purchased in traditional Chinese pharmacies throughout the world.

APPENDIX

ACCESSORY HEALING THERAPIES FOR THE HERBALIST

Quite often, it is not enough to just take herbs internally. Rather, additional therapies are needed as important supplementary healing approaches. These help correct any internal imbalances which cause the illness, as well as speed up the healing process. Many of the following therapies have been used around the world and by various cultures for thousands of years. Some are shared by different cultures although located quite far apart, such as cupping therapy. Others are unique to the culture itself, such as dermal hammer. Some therapies treat the subtle aspects of our beings, affecting our healing process through the emotions and mind. While some therapies have direct effects on the body, others are less physically tangible.

Moxibustion

Moxibustion is a method of burning herbs on or above the skin, usually at specific acupuncture points. The heat warms and circulates Qi, Blood and Fluids in the body, and is useful in the treatment of disease and maintenance of health. Quite often pain and disease result from Stagnation of Qi, Blood and Fluids, and moxibustion stimulates with heat to alleviate the original blockage and correct the flow. Moxibustion is wonderful for sprains, traumas and injuries. In addition, it stimulates and supports the immunity of the body, and eliminates Cold and Damp, thus promoting normal functioning of the Organs.

Although it can be made from a variety of herbs, moxa (short for moxibustion) is generally made from the mugwort plant (*Artemesia vulgaris*). This herb, while its heat is mild, burns easily and penetrates deeply beneath the skin into the body. It comes in a variety of forms, either as the loose wool, in cones or as sticks, often called moxa cigars. It can be burned either directly on the body or over the surface. Loose green moxa is not aged as long as yellow moxa, which is generally 7-14 years old. (The yellow moxa burns hotter and is normally used for direct moxibustion. The better quality yellow moxa wool burns cleaner, faster and at a lower temperature.)

Here we will only learn how to use moxa sticks over the surface of the body. This is a safe and universally useful method. The sticks may be purchased at Oriental medical suppliers and are not expensive. Moxa sticks may be made at home by picking and drying mugwort, then grinding it into a fine powder, sifting and filtering it to remove coarse materials and then repeating this entire process until a fine, soft, wooly powder results. It is then tightly rolled up in tissue paper to form a 6" long thick "cigar".

To use, remove the commercial paper wrapper (not the white inner paper) from the stick and light one end. Hold it about 1 inch from the surface of the skin over the chosen area, the distance varying with the tolerance of the person and the amount of heat stimulation desired. With this method the stick is held still and only moved when the heat level becomes intolerable. It is not necessary to withstand the heat beyond tolerance levels or to become burned. Heating to the threshold level and then moving the stick away for a moment is sufficient.

If several points or areas are to be warmed, then the stick may be moved to the next place, coming back to the original point later. Normally, the moxa stick is burned a total of from 5 to 15 minutes over each area, or until the skin becomes red in the vicinity of the point.

Another method is to use a circular motion, with the stick moving around and over the desired area. This spreads the focus of the heat over large surface areas, and is especially good for soft tissue injuries, skin disorders and larger areas of pain. A third method is called "sparrow pecking" - the moxa stick is rapidly "pecked" at the point without touching the skin. This enables the heat to penetrate deeply when strong stimulation is desired. A point is done when it develops a red or pink "flush."

Whatever the method being used, be sure to periodically tap the ashes off the stick into a container, or they will fall on the person's skin and burn them. (The ashes may be kept in a jar and used to stop bleeding, externally or internally). Putting out the moxa stick is just as important as learning to use it. If not safely extinguished, it can easily continue to smolder and potentially cause a fire. Make sure the stick is no longer smoking before you leave it and turn your attention elsewhere.

To extinguish moxa sticks, either twist them down into a container of rice or sand, place them in a jar and screw the lid on tight or wrap a piece of tin foil tightly around the lit end. With any of these methods you will not lose any of the stick. It is possible to cut off the burning end, dousing the cut end in water; however, much of the stick is then lost. Often one can find a small-holed candle holder which just fits the stick, and placing the lit end of the moxa down inside will effectively put it out. A major caution here is not to put the moxa stick out in dirt.

Though this seems as if it will work, it doesn't. The moxa stick continues to quietly burn, potentially causing a fire.

The usefulness of moxa is endless. When used over the following areas, it can help the conditions indicated:

Chest: lung congestion, cough, cold, flu, allergies, asthma, bronchitis, mucus, difficulty in breathing and other Lung complaints.

Upper abdomen: poor digestion, gas, poor appetite, nausea, vomiting, local spasms and cramps and food congestion. Caution: do not use over the right upper abdomen near the rib cage as this is the residence of the Liver, an organ already too prone to Heat.

Middle abdomen: poor digestion, gas, diarrhea, local cramps and spasms, weakness, low energy, fatigue.

Lower abdomen: gas, diarrhea, local cramps and spasms, bladder infections (without the appearance of Blood), low energy, body coldness, lowered immunity, menstrual cramps and difficulty, frequent urination, night time urination, weakness, leukorrhea and other discharges, poor circulation and prostate difficulty.

Upper back: this will treat the same conditions as listed under chest, only this area is perhaps not as sensitive or vulnerable to treat on most people. To strengthen immunity, especially treating the spine between the 7th cervical and first thoracic vertebrae.

Middle back (waist level): Kidney and Bladder disorders, frequent and night time urination, low back pain, bone and disc problems, hair loss, knee and other joint pains, lowered immunity and resistance, poor circulation, coldness, infertility, weakness, low energy. Heating this area will raise the resistance and energy level of the entire body, thus aiding all other bodily organs and systems. It is especially good for vegetarians who tend to have more Internal Coldness than others.

Lower back: low back pain, menstrual difficulties, leukorrhea, bladder infections and diarrhea.

Joints: local pain and swelling, arthritis, aches, soreness, local injuries, Coldness and congestion.

Other body parts: moxa is useful over other body parts where there is tension, soreness, ache, arthritis, cramps or spasms or any type of blockage, and where healing is not occurring.

Cautions: A few cautions do exist in using moxa, including not over the Liver as indicated above: Do not burn the person; Do not use when a fever exists; Do not use over areas of inflammation or infection; Do not use over the lower back or abdomen of pregnant women; Avoid use in the vicinity of sensory organs or mucus membranes; If an area is numb or there is little feeling or poor circulation, take special care not to over-use on those areas because the person cannot feel as well in those places and burning could easily occur.

If for some reason the person does get burned, then a blister will form. Take care not to let small blisters break. The fluid will be absorbed without infection. Large blisters may break and so should be dressed to prevent infection.

Note: An interesting note here is the use of moxibustion for injuries. Western medicine usually defines any injury as inflammation and thus promotes the use of ice over the affected area. Seemingly heat would be contraindicated in these situations. Yet, from the viewpoint of Chinese medicine the opposite is true. While ice numbs and stops the heavy influx of inflammation and infection-fighting cells, thus decreasing the pain, the long term results are blocked energy and Blood (caused by Cold), a slower healing process and a longer duration of pain. Ice and coldness slow down circulation and congeal the Blood, just as ice on a river stops the flow of water on the top. The flow of energy is then blocked, also.

With the application of heat (the sooner the better), fresh energy and Blood are immediately brought to the location for healing with continued circulation. The heat also alleviates the pain and actually quickens the healing process, especially over the long run. This is true of wounds, too. The only time moxa should not be used in these cases is where a true inflammation occurs (with redness and swelling), and this will be indicated by extreme redness of the skin and possible pus formation. For injuries such as broken bones, ice can be used first, alternating with moxibustion.

Other: If moxibustion is not available and heat is needed, a hot water bottle, stones, bags of sand or salt heated in an oven or on a woodstove are good alternatives.

Cupping

Cupping is a folk technique which has been, and still is, widely used by people in Greece, Turkey, Poland, Czech Republic, Iraq, Germany, France, South America, Japan, Indonesia, India and China. It is the treatment of disease by suction of the skin surface. A vacuum is created in small jars which are then attached to the body surface. The vacuum pulls the skin into a mound formation in the cups, pulling inner congestion and Heat (both Excess and Deficient) in the body upwards and out. After the cups are removed, the skin will appear slightly discolored or even bruised. This may take several days to clear, but the painful condition will usually be significantly relieved.

To do cupping, you will need several jars or cups with even and smooth rims. Good cups to use are the small brandy snifters, votive candle holders or baby food jars. However, wine glasses or other light weight and thin glasses may also be used. Specially made bamboo cups or glass or plastic cups made for this purpose may also be purchased at Chinese medical supply stores. You will also need some cotton balls, forceps or other metal holder, such as tweezers or stick for the cotton, or alternately a candle and some rubbing alcohol as well as matches or a cigarette lighter.

Have the person and all your tools in place before starting. Then attach the cotton ball to a stick or forceps and lightly dip it in alcohol. Ignite the cotton and while burning, insert it into the cup. Hold the cup so its mouth opening is down or the flame can burn your hand. Be sure to hold the cotton in the body of the cup and not near the opening so the lip of the cup doesn't get hot. If you are using a candle, hold the cup over the flame for a short time, then quickly place on the skin as above. This will evacuate some of the air, causing a partial vacuum within the cup. Often the vacuum can be "seen" by a slight clouding in the cup. Withdraw cotton stick and quickly place mouth of cup firmly against the skin at the desired location. Suction should hold it in place. Check by lightly tugging at the cup.

Another method is to hold the cup downward, close to the area where it is to be applied, and simply pass a lighted match or cigarette lighter in the cup and quickly lower it down onto the skin. The Ayurvedic method is to wrap a small coin, such as a penny, in a thin piece of cotton or gauze, tying it securely with a thread or rubber band. Cut the remaining fabric about 1/2" from the point of tying, creating a small wick. Dip this end into some oil or alcohol, light with a match and put on the body where the cup is to be placed. Then immediately place the cup over the ignited covered coin. This will automatically put the flame out and create a perfect suction. The wrapped coins may be reused several times, dipping their wicks in oil again before each use.

Be careful not to leave the cotton stick in the cup too long, as this will cause a hot cup and could burn the person. Conversely, if the cotton stick is not left in long enough, suction will not occur and the cup will fall off when tugged gently. Practice will yield desired results, and it is easier to do than it may sound.

As an alternative, a plastic or glass cupping set can be purchased. It contains a plunger which slides on top of the cup and sucks out the air with pumping strokes. This method is very quick, easy and portable. For purchasing, see the Appendix, Sources and Resources.

To remove cups, let air into the cup by holding it in one hand while the other hand presses the skin at the rim of the jar. You may need to gently slide your pressing finger down and under the rim in order to break the seal. The cup should then pop off.

Cups should be retained in place from 5 to 15 minutes, depending on the strength of suction. Especially in hot weather, or when cupping over shallow flesh, the duration of treatment should not be too long. Often I have seen the cups pop off for no apparent reason. Body hair can break the suction, so it may be necessary to shave the area where they are to be applied. A characteristic dark discoloration usually occurs under the cups to indicate where the congestion and pain was centered. This may take 1 - 10 days to disappear. I have also seen small blisters appear which should be dressed and treated to prevent infection. **Because of this it is a good idea to advise the patient accordingly before administering this therapy.**

Cupping is done over areas where there is swelling, pain, congestion or Stagnation, either of Qi, Blood or Fluids. Thus, it is good for edema, swellings, asthma, bronchitis, dull aches and pains, arthritis, abdominal pain, stomachache, indigestion, headache, low back pain, painful menstruation, coughs from excessive mucus, and places where bodily movement is limited and painful. They are also placed over the upper and middle back for colds and flu.

Cautions: Cupping should not be done during high fever, convulsions or cramps, or over allergic skin conditions, ulcerated sores, or on the abdomen or lower backs of pregnant women. It will also be difficult or impossible to apply over areas with irregular body angles, where the muscles are thin, the skin is not level or where there is a lot of body hair.

Scraping

Scraping, called "Gua Sha," has a similar purpose to cupping: that is to create a counter-irritation on the surface of the skin to relieve subcutaneous Stagnation and inflammation. Various tools can be used ranging from a special round piece of Jade, a coin or the edge of a Chinese ceramic soup spoon. The method is to simply apply oil on the skin and scrape vigorously over affected areas of pain or spasm such as cervical whiplash, shoulder, arm, or leg spasm or even over areas of the abdomen. The process can be sensitive, but for most it is bearable because relief is immediate. There may be some minor bruising or reddening of the skin surface which usually vanishes in a few days. However, the patient should be advised in advance of this likely outcome.

The main difference between cupping and scraping is that cupping has a more localized benefit, whereas scraping can cover a broader area and can even be used along meridians to open the flow of Qi and Blood.

Dermal Hammer

A dermal hammer is an acupuncture tool which has a long handle supporting a head which holds a cluster of small individual needles. The needles are not sharp, but dull, and they can puncture the skin or not, depending on the use. Several needles striking the skin simultaneously cause less pain and stimulate a wider surface area than does a single needle. They are more suitable for use on small children, those sensitive to pain and those who desire to treat themselves.

Other names for dermal hammers are seven star needle and plum-blossom needle, both having a different number and arrangement of needles. They may be purchased at Chinese medical supply stores. As an alternative, you can make a similar, though less effective, device (because it is missing the springing action of the handle), by bundling together about 10-30 toothpicks and binding them with a rubber band.

The dermal hammer is rarely used over a single point, but rather is applied over a broad area, tapping across the skin more in the manner of pecking than puncturing. Where an area has been stimulated, the skin becomes reddened and moist. In general, it should not be painful or cause bleeding.

Dermal hammers are tapped over local areas of pain and congestion, over numbness, areas of hair loss, around sites of wounds and localized diseases, blocked areas of Stagnant Qi and Blood, aches, spasms and local skin diseases. Tapping may be administered on the meridian and relevant points to open the flow of Qi and therapeutically benefit the corresponding internal Organ. With this approach many internal and chronic diseases can be treated, such as headache, dizziness, vertigo, insomnia, menstrual disorders, hypertension and gastrointestinal disorders. Any acupuncture, acupressure or Shiatsu text will give diagrams of the acupuncture meridians and points.

To use, hold the dermal hammer by its handle 1-2 inches from the skin, then lightly and repeatedly tap over the desired area with a flexible movement of the wrist. If you know acupuncture points or meridians it may be done over them, but just the general area to be treated will do. The tapping should be done continuously for 5-10 minutes, until the skin becomes red and moist. **Do not break the skin and cause bleeding.** (If you do, the dermal hammer must be sterilized before using on someone else.) Treatment may be repeated several times a day for many days or until the problem is alleviated.

If many areas of the body are to be treated or acupuncture meridians used, then generally the tapping follows a traditional sequence: first do the center of the body, then sides; first do the top of the body then move down to the feet; first do the back, then front. This sequence is traditional, whether using needles, moxa or dermal hammer.

Sterilization: Dermal hammers should be sterilized by cooking in a pressure cooker at 15 lbs. pressure for 20 minutes before and after each use.

Cautions: Do not use on anyone who has a blood-carried disease, such as hepatitis or AIDS. Do not break the skin and cause bleeding. If you are experimenting with the dermal hammer and cause the skin to bleed, be sure to sterilize it before using it on someone else. Do not use in areas where there are ulcerations or traumatic injuries, or during acute infectious disease or acute abdominal disorders.

Magnet Therapy

Magnet therapy, a method of treating disease with magnets, dates far back into antiquity: the Chinese, ancient Egyptians and Greeks utilized naturally occurring lodestone taken internally as a mineral and applied externally to treat a wide variety of complaints. Today, permanent magnets of very high gauss strength are electronically manufactured using a variety of alloys.

Being one of the most powerful methods of alternative treatment, magnet therapy is often effective in relieving inflammation and pain more quickly and efficiently than either herbal medicine or acupuncture. Properly speaking, magnet therapy warrants a full discussion of its own beyond the scope of this work, to which we direct the reader to Michael's book, *Biomagnetic Therapy and Herbal Medicine* (see bibliography). However, since at least in principle, it is the simplest and one of the safest methods of treatment, making a powerful adjunctive treatment modality for herbalists, the basic theory and method of using magnets is presented as follows:

Essentially magnet therapy consists of placing permanent magnets (as opposed to magnets generated by an active electrical field) of selected strengths and sizes over affected areas of the body to treat disease. The main considerations for magnet therapy are: 1. Determining what areas of the body require treatment, 2. Selecting the size and strength magnets, 3. Determining, if relevant, the appropriate North or South polarity of the magnet to apply directly to the body.

1) Determining Areas of the Body to be Treated with Magnets:

The first method is to apply magnets directly to the most highly reactive or sensitive areas called "trigger points". Another approach uses acupuncture points both near and distal to the site of the affected area. This can be combined with the use of magnets over the site of vital Organs that may be involved with the presenting condition.

For instance, if the problem involves a headache, magnets can be applied to the temples, forehead or the base of the occiput. Usually, this alone is enough to relieve most headaches. However, if it is unresponsive or tends to be chronic, we might select areas over the Liver, Stomach or relevant acupoints along the spine or meridians involved.

2) Choosing the Appropriate Type, Size and Strength Magnet

Magnets come in various types, sizes and strengths. Magnetic strength is classified as follows:

Low gauss	300 - 700 g	High gauss	3000 - 6000 g
Medium gauss	1000 - 2500 g	Super gauss	7000 - 12000 g

Generally speaking, it is best to begin by applying low gauss magnets. Use low strength magnets on the sensitive, weak, small children or very aged. The inexperienced should only use lower strength magnets on the head or chest.

There are large bulky circular or bar magnets that are intended to be applied to the affected area for a prescribed period of time two or three times a day for usually around 30 minutes. This method is most suitable for high strength magnets.

Smaller acupoint magnets come with a self sticking adhesive. These are intended to be applied to specific trigger points, acupoints, or affected areas.

Flexible bipolar magnets are flat and generally much wider and cover a larger area. They are generally of lower gauss strength, but their bipolar configuration increases their therapeutic effect of helping to increase Blood circulation by dilating Blood vessels. Because they are bipolar and do not necessitate determining the use of the magnet's North or South polarity, they are simpler to use by the inexperienced or novice.

3) Determining the correct application of the North and South

Correctly applying the North or South facing magnet, especially in higher strength magnets, is essential to successful treatment. The

North facing side of a magnet is Cooling and anti-inflammatory. It is used for acute pain, inflammation and to disperse Stagnations of all kinds. The South facing side is Warming and strengthening. It tends to coalesce the energy and should be used for tonification and for more chronic conditions.

To check which side of a magnet is North or South, place a compass within the field of the magnet. If the North pointing end of the needle turns towards the magnet, that is the North side and should be appropriately marked for facility of use.

In general, one should begin with the North side first and if results are unsatisfactory, simply reverse the polarity to South. Since there can be acute inflammatory episodes associated with chronic conditions, there are many conditions for which a combined North and South bipolar is more effective than either used alone. Further, there are conditions where one might place a North facing magnet over the acutely sensitive area of pain and inflammation and a South facing magnet over a depleted Organ, such as the lower back for the Kidneys and Adrenals.

Contraindications for Magnet Therapy:

For obvious reasons, magnets should not be used on individuals with pacemakers, metal pins or metal parts in the body. They should also be avoided during pregnancy. Strong magnets can be very dangerous when they are placed near each other. Care and proper handling is essential to prevent injury of fingers or other delicate bodily parts. Strong magnets are usually a ceramic ferrite alloy that can easily shatter, so the proper method of attaching and separating them should be to slide them together and apart when needed. Finally, magnets will demagnetize computer hard disks, other computer disks, credit cards, CD's and magnetic tapes, so care should be taken to keep these away from all magnetic products.

Nasal Wash

Nasal wash is a procedure of washing the nostrils out with water or an herbal solution. This can be done to wash just the nostrils, or to additionally wash the throat. Doing this aids sinus congestion and infections, stuffy nose, allergies, difficulty of breathing through the nose, sore throats and especially recurring sinus and throat infections. It may be done on a preventative basis once a day first thing in the morning, or several times a day in the case of an infection. This is traditionally done by yogis in India to help clear the air passages for their breathing practices, and is called *neti*. [1]

To do a nasal wash you will need a water container that has a small spout, such as some watering pots have. Alternatively, a bulb syringe, squeeze bottle, eyedropper or turkey baster work fine. Fill this with about 2 cups water or herbal solution. Place the end of the spout in the right nostril while you tilt your head to the left. Now slowly pour the solution into the nostril, making sure it comes out the left nostril, rather than the one it is going in. You may have to adjust your head or tilt it more to make sure this happens. Continue doing this for half the solution. Be sure to locate yourself over a sink for this therapy!

Now reverse sides, inserting the spout into the left nostril while tilting your head to the right and making sure the solution comes out the right nostril. Use up the rest of the solution on this side. At first it may seem difficult, if not impossible, for the solution to come out the opposite nostril. This is because of the mucus blockage in the airways at the root of the nose. With repeated attempts, however, it will come out the opposite side and create a wonderful clearing of your nasal passages. You will be amazed at how well you can breathe afterwards.

Another method involves pouring the solution alternately through the right and left nostrils and having it run down the throat and out the mouth. For this, the head needs to be tilted backwards so the solution doesn't go out either nostril but down the throat instead. This method treats the throat directly. Often recurring and chronic sore throats, tonsillitis and other throat infections occur because the bacteria that causes them stay in the passages between the nose and the throat. These bacteria cannot be reached with the traditional gargle or throat medication. Using a nasal wash so it runs down the throat is about the only (comfortable) way to reach it.

When first doing nasal wash, there may be a burning sensation in your nose, similar to that of getting water up the nose while swimming. This goes away, however, and the process gets more comfortable with time and practice.

Using a warm salt water solution with a nasal wash is effective in preventing and clearing up infections and inflammations. It kills the bacteria causing these, as many people can confirm who have experienced a warm salt water gargle heal their sore throats. Alternatively, an herbal tea may be made and used as the wash instead. Good herbs to use include antibiotic, alterative and anti-inflammatory herbs, such as echinacea, chaparral, red clover, dandelion and goldenseal (which is especially valuable since it tones the mucus membranes) and astringents such as raspberry, calendula and squawvine. A small amount of demulcent may be added, like marshmallow or licorice, to soothe inflamed and irritated tissues. Make up your own customized solution and experiment to find your favorite ones.

QI GONG

Qi Gong means to work with one's Qi. It represents a broad body of study, knowledge and discipline where, like yoga, one combines breath and specific movements to open and direct the flow of Qi to vital areas of the body. What is known as Qi Gong has, according to Bob Flaws[2], "been practiced in China since not less than 400 BC." He goes on to state that "during the Han dynasty, a scholar named Wei Bo Yan wrote a book on what has now come to be known as Qi Gong." It was entitled *Chan Tong Qi* (Three in One) and discusses the relationship between Taoism, the I-Ching and Qi Gong. This book establishes the relationship of Qi Gong to "Jing Essence, Qi and Shen-spirit."

The next most famous exponent of Qi Gong was the Taoist acupuncturist and herbalist, Hua Tuo who also lived during the Han dynasty. He developed a series of Qi Gong exercises based on the movements of various animals such as the tiger and the crane.

Down through the ages and up to the present, literally thousands of forms of Qi Gong are practiced by the Chinese to maintain health and develop specific powers and capacities. Qi Gong is similar to Tai Qi and other Chinese martial arts forms except that it has no use in fighting. Tai Qi, practiced as a series of complex movements, is regarded as a very complete and powerful Qi Gong practice in itself.

The following simple Qi Gong practice is excerpted with permission of the author from *Imperial Secrets of Health and Longevity*[3]:

The Rising Eagle

The following is a very simple Don Gong, or moving Qi Gong, exercise. It helps to circulate the Qi, store the Qi and Jing Essence in the lower Dan Tian, and rids the Lungs of stale air. It is a good exercise to do on waking in the morning as per Qian Long's suggestion.

Begin by standing erect with feet planted shoulder width apart. The head and torso should be erect. The butt and hips should be allowed to release and slide forward, thus straightening out the curve of the low back. In addition, the knees should be slightly bent and the weight should be evenly distributed over the entire foot, leaning neither on the heels nor the balls and toes. Relax the shoulders and let the arms hang to one's side with the fingers gently extended. The breath should be through the nose with the mouth gently shut. Breathe in by expanding the lower abdomen and breathe out by contracting the lower abdomen.

As one breathes, let the feeling of the mind, the feeling of consciousness, sink to the lower Dan Tian. This is a spot 3-4 inches below the navel and a third of the way into the body. One should try to keep the mind fixed in this place or space and do the following exercise from the lower Dan Tian.

As one breathes in, let the wrists float up to the level of the chest. Feel as if there were a string attached to the wrists picking up the arm from that point. As the wrists reach the level of the chest, begin exhaling and let the hands move forward until the arms are almost straight out in front of one. Then breathe in and let the hands and arms float up over one's head. Breathe out and sink slowly into the knees as the arms move out to the sides and down. Keeping the knees bent, the hands move down and across the legs, left hand passing over right. As the hands swing apart again, begin to breathe in but do not straighten the legs. One should remain with the knees bent and buttocks tucked underneath the hips. As the hands reach the level of the shoulders, one turns the palms over so that they are facing downward. Then exhaling, the hands push down as one rises from the bent position. Again the wrists are drawn up towards the level of the chest as one breathes in, and the entire exercise is repeated.

When doing this exercise there a number of things to keep in mind. First, the mind leads the breath, the breath leads the Qi, and it is the Qi that leads the motion. The Qi goes where the mind and breath lead it. That's why what we call moving Qi Gong today was simply part of what was called Dao Yin, or leading and guiding. As one moves, feel as though the air is as thick as water. Try to move very slowly with one motion blending into the next. Try to accomplish each movement with the minimal amount of physical strain or effort. Let the entire body remain relaxed yet erect as if suspended from a string tied to the crown of the head. Repeat this exercise 9 times.

Another more famous Qi Gong practice that has infinite variations is known as The Eight Silk Brocades (Ba Duan Jin) as follows:

Supporting the Sky with the Hands
Preparation Pose: Stand relaxed and erect, looking straight ahead while breathing gently through the nose:
Slowly raise the arms upwards and sideways until the fingers of the hands lock over the head as if holding up the sky. At the same time gradually lift the heels off the ground. Lower the arms and heels and return to the starting posture. Repeat several times.

Benefits: it relaxes the muscles of the arms, legs and torso and with the deep breathing benefits the Lungs, abdomen and pelvis.

Horse Riding Posture: This stance is assumed after the preparation pose in several of the Brocades. It is accomplished by spreading the feet apart, slightly wider than the shoulders, bending the knees so they are aligned over the toes, pushing the buttocks forward and keeping the spine erect.

The Archer Drawing the Bow Left and Right

Preparation pose:
Step out to the left, bending the knees to assume the horse riding posture. Cross the arms in front of the chest, right arm outside and left inside. Extend the thumb and forefinger of the left hand with the other three fingers curled while moving the left arm out to the left with the eyes following. Simultaneous with this, clench the right hand gently as if pulling back the string of a bow.
Return to the starting posture.
Repeat the first step but to the opposite side.
Return to the starting posture.
Repeat several times, breathing in with steps 1 and 3 and out with steps 2 and 4.
Benefits: Benefits the Lungs, Heart and Liver. Promotes Blood circulation and stretches the shoulders and arms.

Separating Heaven and Earth by Raising Arm Upwards

Preparation pose:
Raise the right arm over the head with the palm and fingers facing upwards and to the right. The fingers should be together. At the same time the left hand goes downward with the left hand and fingers pointing downward and straight forward.
Return to the preparation pose.
Repeat step one except to the opposite side and with the opposite hands.
Return to the preparation pose.
Repeat many times.
Benefits: Opposite stretching of the arms affects the Liver, Gall Bladder, Spleen and Stomach and helps the digestive system.

Twisting and Looking Backward
Preparation pose: Begin with the hands gently touching the thighs.
Turn head slowly to the left, rolling the eyeballs in the same direction as the turn and looking backwards as much as possible.
Return to the preparation pose.
Repeat in the opposite direction.
Repeat several times breathing out with steps 1 and 3 and in with step 2.
Benefits: Increases strength and flexibility of the neck muscles. Benefits the eyes and strengthens the nervous system.

Quelling Heart Fire Rotating the Head and Body
Assume the horse riding posture with the legs wide apart. Place the palms of the hands on the thighs, thumbs pointing outward:
Bend forward, making a circular movement from the waist toward the left. At the same time allow the buttocks to move to the right.
Return to the preparatory horse riding posture.
Repeat step one in the opposite direction.
Return to the preparatory horse riding posture.
Repeat several times, breathing in with steps 1 and 3 and out with steps 2 and 4.
Benefits: Good for relaxing the entire body and clearing the mind.

Raising the Heels Upward
Stand upright in the first preparatory posture.
1. Slowly raise both heels off the floor, keeping both legs straight.
Slowly lower them to the ground.
Repeat seven times with a regular slow breath.
Benefits: A simple but powerful exercise said to be good for "100 diseases". It helps the spine and all the internal Organs.

Punching Forward the Tiger
Preparation pose: Stand with legs shoulder width apart with fists and palms upward at waist level. Assume the horse riding posture:
With glaring eyes, slowly punch right fist forward, right fist down and left fist lightly clenched pointing upward at waist level.
Return to preparation posture.
Repeat step one with opposite arms to the opposite side.
Return to preparation posture.

Variations of this practice are to punch alternately forward, diagonally and to the sides.

Benefits: This is an active version of the yogic Lion pose and its essence is in releasing anger through the eyes. This helps clear the Liver and builds energy and vitality.

Bending Over to Hold the Feet with Both Hands

Stand in upright preparatory pose:

Keep the knees straight but slightly bent as the entire upper torso bends forward, reaching the toes or as close as possible.

Rise to upright position.

Put palms of the hands on the lower back and slowly bend backward without straining.

Return to upright position.

Repeat many times with normal breath.

Benefits: This exercise is good to increase flexibility and strengthen the Kidneys. It should be practiced with caution by those with lower back weakness.

Breathing Exercises

The Four Purifications[4]

The Four Purifications are a set of breathing exercises which are extremely beneficial to the body, mind and spirit. Consisting of four different breathing techniques, they calm the body, quiet the mind, energize and rejuvenate the entire body and mind, tone the Lungs, Blood, circulation, brain, Internal Organs, Heart and give strength to the whole body. Interestingly, in Chinese medicine the Lungs are considered responsible in part for giving the body strength. The Lungs have always been associated with air and its essential and vital life-giving properties.

These breathing exercises further purify the nerve channels in the body, clear and stimulate the digestive system and strengthen the nervous system. Thus, they aid such ailments as nervousness, insomnia, indigestion, lung and breathing problems, poor circulation, low energy and vitality, fatigue, lethargy and poor memory. As such, they are invaluable for helping the body recover from many health problems.

For those who have never done any breathing practices, these four techniques are safe to do. For those already doing their own form of breathing practices, these are a perfect adjunct and starting exercise. Sit quietly with your back straight, either in a chair with your feet on the floor or on the floor with your legs crossed. For those who desire, you may concentrate your attention on the space between the eyebrows while doing these exercises.

The four breathing techniques are: alternate nostril breathing, skull shining, fire wash and horse mudra. Do them in the order given. After practicing them for a few months, move on to the intermediate method described at the end.

Alternate Nostril Breathing (Nadishodhana)

Begin by gently exhaling all air. Then close the right nostril with the thumb of the right hand and inhale slowly and deeply through the left nostril. When finished, close the left nostril with the ring finger of the right hand, releasing the thumb, and exhale slowly and fully through the right nostril. Next, immediately inhale through the right nostril in a slow and steady manner. Finally, close the right nostril with the right thumb again, releasing the ring finger, and exhale through the left nostril. This completes one round. Begin with ten rounds and gradually increase to forty.

This exercise alone is extremely beneficial to the body. It is very quieting to the mind and strengthens the nervous system. It induces a wonderfully calm state, releases nervous tension, anxiety, agitation, anger and other disruptive emotions, and helps you sleep better. It also oxygenates the system, thus aiding in the circulation of energy and Blood in the body. This in turn stimulates the proper functioning of all the internal organs. Continued practice of alternate nostril breathing will strengthen the Lungs and breath control.

Skull Shining (Kapala Bhati)

Skull shining is a series of forced exhalations with the breath. Begin by inhaling quickly and lightly through both nostrils. Then quickly and fully exhale all the breath through both nostrils. Emphasize the exhale, letting the inhalation come as a natural reflex. Repeat this pattern for one round consisting of thirty exhalations. After each round, which should last no longer than one minute, rest and breathe naturally. Then repeat the round. Begin with three rounds of thirty exhalations each and gradually increase to ten rounds of sixty exhalations each.

This method purifies the head area, which calms the thoughts and the breath and aids the mind. As in alternate nostril breathing, skull shining helps release nervous tension, balance the emotions and circulate energy and Blood in the body. It also strengthens the Lungs and breath control.

Caution: Persons with high blood pressure or lung disease should not practice skull shining.

Fire Wash (*Agnisara Dhauti*)

This exercise is performed with all the air held out of the body. Begin by taking a normal inhalation and exhalation, letting all the air out from the body. Then lean forward, resting your hands on your knees and holding the breath out, pull the diaphragm up and toward the backbone and then release it suddenly. Repeat this in-and-out movement rapidly, as long as the breath can be held out without strain, about thirty pulls. Then inhale gently. This makes one round. Start with three rounds, gradually increasing to ten. Begin with thirty pulls per breath and work up to sixty.

This method strengthens the "navel lock" frequently used in breathing exercises and creates heat at the navel center (manipura chakra), which purifies the nerve channels, stimulates the digestive system, increases gastric fire, strengthens the Lungs and alleviates indigestion, abdominal diseases and menstrual disorders.

Horse Mudra (*Ashvini Mudra*)

This fourth exercise is an internal movement of the anal sphincter muscle. Begin by inhaling a complete and full breath and hold the breath in. Then contract and release the anal sphincter muscle rapidly and repeatedly. Hold the breath only so long as the following exhalation can be slow and controlled. Do not force your breath or length of holding. Begin with three rounds of thirty pulls each, and increase gradually to ten rounds of sixty each. The horse mudra strengthens mula bandha, the anal lock, which increases concentration, strengthens the reproductive glands and stimulates the gastric fire.

Intermediate Method

After performing the Four Purifications regularly for two to three months and when feeling comfortable with them, one may undertake the intermediate method. In the intermediate method, the Four Purifications are done in such a way that there are no "resting breaths" in between; that is, they are done consecutively without a breath or rest in between.

To do this, do ten to thirty rounds of alternate nostril breathing. After the last exhalation through the left nostril, inhale partially and immediately begin skull shining. At the end of one series of skull shining exhalations, inhale slowly and completely, then exhale all air, hold the breath out and do the fire wash. After a round of the fire wash, inhale completely, hold the breath and do the horse mudra. This entire series now completes one round.

After the horse mudra, exhale completely and immediately begin again with alternate nostril breathing, thus starting the next round. Do five rounds, gradually increasing the numbers of alternate nostril breathing and the duration of retention in each of the other three techniques.

Other Yogic Breathing Practices[5]

It is important to begin with the Four Purifications and perform them once or twice a day for at least three months, because they are safe and prepare the body for slightly more advanced practices. Pranayama, or controlled yogic breathing, can exert powerful physical and mental effects upon the body-mind-spirit. It is ideal that they be learned from an experienced teacher, for if they are not performed with a positive attitude or are done irregularly or are overly forced, they can cause brain, heart and/or lung damage. It is important that if any adverse reactions occur as a result of wrong pranayama, they are stopped and one should do a half shoulder stand or lay in a posture with the feet moderately elevated above the head. In general, individuals with ulcers or heart or lung disease should not practice pranayama. However, if cautiously undertaken, certain of these simple practices are powerfully effective, especially for cardio-pulmonary imbalances as described in the text.

All breathing practices should be done on an empty stomach. One should assume a meditative posture with the spine, neck and head in a relaxed, straight upright posture. This can be done cross-legged on the floor or sitting in a straight-backed chair. The eyes are closed and focused on the space between them on the forehead.

Just as foods and herbs are classified as Heating and Cooling, so also are various physical exercises and breathing practices. Yogic Pranayama is very similar to Chinese Qi Gong practices, except the latter are associated with specific physical postures and movements. Following are a few simple Yogic Pranayamas that can be utilized in the treatment of the various imbalances described in the text.

Ujjayi (The Victorious Breath)

Ujjayi, or the "Victorious Breath", allows one to gain control over prana. It is heating and dissolves phlegm. However, before practicing *ujjayi* it is best to first wash the mouth and gargle with warm salt water to loosen the phlegm in the throat.

It is done by closing the mouth and taking short inhaled sips through the nose with the glottis in the throat somewhat tightened. A slight sound is automatically produced like the sobbing of a child. This is done five times in one inhale sequence. The breath is then held in the chest for 2 or 3 seconds and next, blocking the right nostril with the thumb, it is gently exhaled through the left (cooling) nostril. Immediately upon exhalation the practice is repeated. Begin with 10 rounds and gradually over a period of several weeks increase to as many as forty.

Exhaling through the left nostril is cooling and counterbalancing to the heating effect of the inhaled breath. However, one can also exhale through both nostrils, which is balanced.

Shitali and Sitkari (The Cooling Breath)

Shitali and *sitkari* are both cooling practices which can cool and calm the mind. *Shitali* is performed by folding the tongue with the sides upwards like a straw or tube. This is slightly extended beyond the lips as one takes a long slow inhale while making a faint hissing sound. This air is then swallowed into the stomach and the breath is held for 4 or 5 seconds before being slowly released through both nostrils. One should begin with 10 rounds and gradually increase to 40 over a few weeks.

Sitkari is similar and is for those who are genetically unable to curl the tongue. Here the tongue is flattened and lightly touches the back of the teeth. The breath is taken through slightly parted lips. It is interesting that for many, this type of breath response is automatic whenever they experience being overheated.

Eight Kriyas (Swasa Yam)

This is a series of the simplest and safest breathing practices which are especially useful for calming the mind. As such, they are ideal to do before meditation. Begin with the head, neck and spine in a relaxed upright position. Take unforced slow, deep and gently relaxed breaths. There are essentially two types of breath: a shallow chest breath used when inhaling through the nostrils, and a stomach breath used when inhaling through the mouth. For the chest breath, the chest fully expands with the abdomen moving inward, while for the Stomach breath the abdomen pushes out so that the chest does not fully expand.

The Eight Kriyas can be done after pranayamas or prior to meditation. They can be used whenever there is a need for profound calming and centering.

Kriya 1: Inhale gently, deeply and slowly through both nostrils into the chest, pulling the abdomen slightly inwards. Exhale slowly and easily through both nostrils. Repeat five times.

Kriya 2: Repeat the above but this time exhale slowly and gently through a partial opening in the mouth. Repeat five times.

Kriya 3: Inhale gently, deeply and slowly into the stomach through the mouth with slightly pursed lips. This time allow the abdomen to expand outwards. Exhale slowly and gently through both nostrils, gently contracting the abdomen inwards slightly. Repeat five times.

Kriya 4: Close the right nostril with the thumb of the right hand and inhale through the chest through the left nostril, contracting the abdomen inwards slightly. Release the thumb and close the left nostril with the ring finger and gently exhale through the right nostril. Repeat five times.

Kriya 5: Close the left nostril with the ring finger and inhale into the chest through the right nostril, pulling the abdomen in slightly. Follow with closing the right nostril with the thumb and exhaling slowly through the left nostril. Repeat five times.

Kriya 6: Now exhale and completely empty the lungs slowly and gently through both nostrils, allowing the abdomen to suck gently inwards. The following inhalation should occur as a normal, and not a deep, breath while releasing the abdomen. Repeat five times.

Kriya 7: Inhale into the stomach slowly, gently and deeply through the mouth with slightly pursed lips, allowing the abdomen to push out. Then exhale gently through the mouth while the abdomen slightly contracts inwards. Repeat five times.

Kriya 8: Inhale deeply into the chest through both nostrils in five slow sips, while pulling the abdomen in slightly at the same time. Exhale slowly and gently through the mouth. Repeat five times.

Harimaki

A harimaki is a special type of underclothing traditionally worn as a wide band around the waist by the Japanese. It is worn under the clothes, although the outer sash (called "obi") on kimonos serves the same purpose. The harimaki protects the vital aspects of the body, the places where the Life Gate Fire resides. This includes the "hara," a place just below the navel, and the Kidneys and Adrenals, at waist level on either side of the spine.

Since this is where Yin, Yang, Essence, Source Qi, and the deeper immune powers of the body reside and emanate, such a simple undergarment can be very helpful in maintaining health. When these Organs are kept warm, they are better able to administer their functions and protect the body from stress, exhaustion and illnesses.

The harimaki can be worn continuously, over the cold winter months or occasionally as needed. It should be considered for low back pain, frequent and/or copious urination, night time urination, poor circulation, Coldness, low energy and vitality, poor appetite and digestion, gas and bloating with coldness, frequent colds and flu, frequent hair loss, bone and disc problems, lowered immunity, a general state of debility and at the first sign of susceptibility to colds or flu. It is also beneficial to wear a harimaki while pregnant. One Japanese woman was surprised to learn that American women didn't wear harimakis during pregnancy.

Harimakis can be difficult to obtain in America. They are easily made, however, and may even be substituted by a vest that covers the waist and lower abdomen, or a scarf wrapped around these areas. As all of these can be bulky, however, it is well worth the small effort to purchase or make your own.

To make your own harimaki, purchase enough stretch cotton (for summer) or stretch wool (for winter) material to fit snugly around your waist and hips without slipping. Keep in mind that it is to be worn under your clothes next to the skin. The material should be wide enough that it covers your hips, navel and waist, about 12" for most people. It is possible to use double this amount and then fold it in half for extra warmth and protection. Now sew the two ends together to form a tube, perhaps sewing it a little tighter at the waistline (for women) to conform to your figure better. This is then slipped on your body and pulled over your hips and waist for wearing.

BIBLIOGRAPHY

Herbals, Chinese

Bensky and Gamble. *Chinese Herbal Medicine Materia Medica*, Revised Edition. Seattle: Eastland Press, 1993.

Bensky and Gamble. *Formulas and Strategies*. Seattle: Eastland Press, 1993.

Chen and Chen. *A Comprehensive Guide to Chinese Herbal Medicine*. Long Beach, CA.: Oriental Healing Arts (Ohai), 1992. (Highly recommended)

Cheung, C.S. *Treatment of Traditional Chinese Medicine*. San Francisco: Traditional Chinese Medical Publisher, 1980.

Li Shih-Chen. *Chinese Medicinal Herbs*. San Francisco: Georgetown Press, 1973.

Lu Fei and Chen Song Yu, *A Clinical Guide to Chinese Herbs and Formulae*. Edinburgh: Churchill Livingstone, 1993. (Highly recommended.)

Ni, Maoshing. *Chinese Herbology Made Easy*. Los Angeles: The Shrine of the Eternal Breath of Tao and College of Tao and Traditional Chinese Healing, 1986, (117 Stonehaven Way, Los Angeles, CA. An economical and convenient reference, highly recommended.)

Olshevsky, Noy, Zwang, Burger. *The Manual of Natural Healing Therapy: A Practical Guide to Alternative Medicine*. New York: Citadel Press, 1989.

Pang, T.Y. *A Chinese Herbal: An Introduction*. Honolulu: Tai Chi School of Philosophy and Art, 1982. (PO Box 27273, Honolulu, Hawaii, 96827).

Reid, Daniel P. *Chinese Herbal Medicine*. Boston: Shambhala Publishers, Inc., 1987. (A beautiful introductory herbal with color plates.)

Teeguarden, Ron. *Chinese Tonic Herbs*. New York: Japan Publications, 1984.

The Revolutionary Health committee of Hunan Province. *A Barefoot Doctor's Manual*. Seattle: Cloudburst Press, 1977.

Yeung, Him-Che, *Handbook of Chinese Herbs and Formulas*, Vol. I and II, Los Angeles: Him-Che Yeung, 1985. (Two outstanding references, Volume 1 is a Materia Medica and Volume 2 is a clinical formulary.)

Yanchi, Liu, The Essential Book of Traditional Chinese Medicine, Vols. 1 and 2, Columbia University Press, 1988.

Traditional Chinese Medicine Theory
Flaws, Bob. *How To Write A TCM Herbal Formula.* Boulder: Blue Poppy Press, 1993.

Ou Ming. *Manual of Common-Used Prescriptions of TCM.* Joint Publishing (H.K.), 1989.

Kanpo (Japanese Chinese Medicine)
Bulletins of the Oriental Healing Arts Institute of USA and The International Journal of Oriental Medicine. Long Beach: Oriental Healing Arts Institute, 1945. (Palo Verde Ave. Suite 208, Long Beach, California 90815. An excellent quarterly journal on Chinese Herbalism.)

Hong-Yen Hsu, Chau-Shin Hsu. *Commonly Used Chinese Herb Formulas With Illustrations.* Long Beach, California: Oriental Healing Arts Institute, 1980.

Hong-Yen Hsu & Easer, Douglas. *Major Chinese Herbal Formulas.* Long Beach, California: Oriental Healing Arts Institute, 1980.

ENDNOTES

Chapter 2

1. *Chinese Herbal*, T.Y. Pang, Tai Chi School of Philosophy and Art.

Chapter 5

1. *How to Write a TCM Herbal Formula*, Bob Flaws, Blue Poppy Press, Boulder, CO, 1993.

2. A somewhat milder variation of this formula is made by substituting two parts powdered anise seed for the pippali long pepper.

Chapter 6

1 *Tao Te Ching*, Lao Tsu, translated. by Gia-Fu Feng and Jane English, Vintage Books, Division of Random House, NY, 1972.

2 This perspective goes beyond many practitioners' conception of Essence according to Chinese medical philosophy, which limits it to a purely physical conception based upon the more recent model of materialistic Chinese Communist medicine, rather than the more ancient traditional Taoist model. What can be learned from this is that as we delve into the deeper theoretical aspects of being, beyond the physical manifestion of Qi, Blood, Fluid and so forth, into the more subtler realms of Essence and Spirit (Shen), we will not be afraid to make the appropriate jump to more psychological and spiritual concerns as they most certainly affect all aspects of psycho-physiological health. Without accomplishing this, concepts of Essence and Spirit are practically devoid of any influence or meaning, since for the most part, such parameters exist beyond the realm of direct physical intervention with herbs or acupuncture alone.

Chapter 7

1. A fascinating study with photos gives deeper detail into the findings and comparisons of the Spleen between TCM and the Western understanding of mitocondria: "Traditonal Chinese Medicine Digest", Vol. II, 3 & 4, 1987, The People's Medical Publishing House, SHK International Services, Ltd., 22/F., 151 Gloucester Road, Hong Kong. While it is important to approach Chinese Medicine on its own terms, a broader understanding of it can be achieved through its correspondences to Western medicine, such as demonstrated in this article.

Chapter 9

1. Modified from: *Knowledge of Tongue Diagnosis: Analysis of 1,000 Cases*, J.TCM 1:10, 1961.

2. See Chapter Six for a detailed description of the Four Levels of Heat: Wei, Qi, Ying and Xue.

3. See Chapter Six for a detailed description of the Six Stages of Disease: Tai Yang, Shao Yang, Yang Ming, Tai Yin, Shao Yin and Jue Yin.

Chapter 11

1. This is a traditional undergarment worn around the kidney area of the back and waist by the Japanese during the Winter. It is used to prevent sickness and keep the Kidneys warm. See the chapter on Healing Therapies for a further description and directions for making it.

2. The Chinese concept of 'Wind' implies something that travels or changes. In some instances it suggests the process of infectious diseases, while at the same time it suggests the nervous system's ability to control the dilation and contraction of the pores of the skin. Internal Wind refers to the nervous system, especially the Central nervous system of the brain.

3. According to Chinese medical theory, Dampness or Phlegm comes from weak or incomplete digestion and assimilation, which refers to Spleen Qi. Since the Lungs require a significant amount of lubrication to offset their constant drying influence from air, it is reasonable that most of the residual Spleen Dampness would first go to the Lungs. If there is too much, therefore, the Lungs are often the first place to be adversely affected.

4. 'Trikatu' is a traditional Ayurvedic preparation easily made at home for Coldness and Dampness There are many variations, but all are based on the idea of combining three spices, usually powdered and taken with honey. The standard preparation is equal parts powdered black pepper, pippli pepper (Chinese "bibo") and dry ginger in a honey-based paste. Anywhere from a half to a full teaspoon is taken two or three times daily. For children, Pippali pepper can be substituted with two parts anise seed.

5. Heat of course refers to bacterial or viral pathogens.

6. The inside juice part of the orange is both Cold and Damp while the outer peel is spicy and drying. For this reason, the Brahman sect in India are taught from a young age to always eat a part of the peel of any fruit that is peeled. In this case, warming and drying citrus peel is an antidote for the Cold Dampness of the inner fruit.

Chapter 13

1. The acid-alkaline determination is not the pH of the food itself, but the residue ash which forms when that food is oxidized. The macrobiotic delineation of foods according to a Yang-Yin continuum fairly well matches the acid-alkaline differentiation. Foods categorized as Yang tend to be acid-forming and those classified as Yin tend to be alkaline-forming.rong or toxic herbs are contraindicated for children, the very weak or aged.

Appendix

1. The yogic methods of *neti* are described in the *Ashtanga Yoga Primer* by Baba Hari Dass, Sri Rama Publishing, 1981, Santa Cruz, California.

2. *Imperial Secrets of Health and Longevity* by Bob Flaws, 1994, published by Blue Poppy Press, Boulder, CO.

3. Ibid

4. The Four Purifications are thoroughly described and illustrated, along with many other valuable breathing and yogic techniques, in the *Ashtanga Yoga Primer* by Baba Hari Dass, Sri Rama Publishing, 1981, Santa Cruz, California.

5. The following yogic breathing practices and kriyas are described in the *Ashtanga Yoga Primer* by Baba Hari Dass, Sri Rama Publishing, 1981, Santa Cruz, CA.

SOURCES AND RESOURCES

Books on Chinese Medicine
Lotus Press
P O Box 325 Dept. CM
Twin Lakes, WI 53181 USA. 800 824 6396
www.lotuspress.com
Publisher of books by Michael Tierra and other alternative health subjects.

Redwing Book Company
44 Linden St. Brookline, MA 02146
Tel: 888-873-3947, 617-738-4664 Fax: 617-738-4620
Website: www.redwingbooks.com
The most complete catalog of Traditional Chinese Medicine books and books on healing.

Herbal Computer Programs
The Formulary
The best computer program to date in the English language on Chinese herbalism, based on Bensky's Formulas and Strategies.
East West Healing Arts Center
4174 Park Blvd., Ste. 201, Oakland, CA 94602
Phone/fax: 510-531-4346 email: ewhac@emf.net

IBIS-Interactive BodyMind Information System
PO Box 308, Beaverton, OR 97075
Phone 503-526-1972 Fax 503-6416541

Planetary Herbology Computer Program
based on the book by Michael Tierra.
Program available for Dos, Windows 3.1 and 95 operating systems.
Published by: Lotus Press, PO Box 325, Dept. CM,
Twin Lakes, WI 53181USA. 800 824 6396
Website: www.lotuspress.com

Chinese Herb Suppliers
Oriental Medical Supplies
1950 Washington St. Braintree, MA 02184
Phone: 800-323-1839 Fax: 781-335-5779
Website: www.omsmedical.com
A leading supplier of Oriental and Acupuncture medical supplies.

Botanical Therapy
126 Surfside Ave. Santa Cruz, CA 95060
Phone: 800-447-2066; 408-423-5491
email: westcliff@got.net
Supplies Chinese and Western based herb formulas and other herb products.

Brion Herb Company
9200 Jeronimo Rd. Irvine, CA. 92618
Phone: 800-333-4372 Fax: 714-587-1260 email: brionc@sunten.com.

Great China Herb Company
857 Washington St. San Francisco, CA, 94108.
Phone: 415-982-2195

Internatural (retail)
PO Box 489 Dept. CM, Twin Lakes, Wi 53181 USA.
Phone: 800-643-4221 www.internatural.com.
Supplier of herbs and herbal products, books, biomagnetic products, educational videos, essential oils and natural health items.

Lotus Light (wholesale)
PO Box 1008, Dept. CM, Silver Lake, WI. 53170 USA. 800-548-3824
Wholesale catalog of more than 8000 items including herbs, herbal products, essential oils, books, videos, alternative health items.

Lotus Brands, Inc.
PO Box 325, Dept. CM, Twin Lakes, WI 53181 USA. 800-824-6396
Source supplier of bulk herbs and spices, botanicals including Chinese Herbs.

Mayway Trading Corporation
1338 Cypress St. Oakland, CA. 94607
Tel: 800-262-9929; 510-208-3113 Fax: 800-909-2828

nuHerbs Co.
3820 Penniman Ave. Oakland, CA. 94619
Phone: 800-233-4307 Fax: 510-534-4384 email: herbal@nuherbs.com

Finemost Corp./QualiHerb
13839 Bentley Pl. Cerritos, CA. 90703
Phone: 800-533-5907 Fax: 562-533-0625

Spring Wind Herb Company
2325 Fourth St., Suite 6, Berkeley, CA 94710
Phone: 800-588-4883

Tai Sang Trading Chinese Herb Company
1018 Stockton, San Francisco, CA 94108
Phone: 415-981-5364 Fax: 415-981-2032
Chinese herbal extracts in granules, capsules, tablets (traditional formulas, single herbs.

Min Tong Herbs /Tashi Enterprises
5221 Central Ave. #5
Richmond, CA 94804
Phone: 800-538-1333 Fax: 800-875-0798; 510-558-2006
Concentrated dry extracts of traditional formulas, and individual herbs to compound and vary formulas.

East West Products
PO Box 1210
New York, NY 10025-1210
Phone: 212-864-1342
This is a retail distributor of Michael Tierra's Planetary Herb Formulas and products. Catalogs available.

For wholesale sales of Planetary Herb Products contact
Threshold/Planetary Enterprises
23 Janis Way, Scotts Valley, California, 95066
Phone: 800-777-5677, 408-438-1700 Fax: 408-438-7410

East West Herbal Correspondence Course
PO Box 712, Santa Cruz, Ca. 95061
Phone: 1-800-717-5010; 408-336-5010
Fax: 408-336-4548
A comprehensive 36 lesson course integrating Western, Chinese and Ayurvedic herbalism written by Dr. Michael Tierra. The course includes theoretical principles, traditional diagnosis, traditional diet and food therapy, a comprehensive East-West Materia Medica, Formulary and clinical treatment manual. Each year there are seminars for students to attend for direct study. Students can learn at their own pace and submit assignments at the end of each lesson for evaluation.

The course is also registered for herb students in the UK for information and ongoing programs of study in the UK and abroad contact

East West Herb Course UK, C/O David and Sarah Holland
Hartfield Marsh Green, East Sussex TN7 4ET. Great Britain.
Phone: 011-44-1-342822312, Fax: 011-44-342826347.

PlanetHerbs Online Supplies

www.planetherbs.com
Offers online availability of Michael Tierra's Planetary Formulas and other hard to find herbal supplies and educational materials.

American Herbalists Guild

PO Box 70, Roosevelt, UT 84066
Phone: 435-722-8434, Fax: 435-722-8452
email: ahgoffice@earthlink.net
Website: www.healthy.net/herbalists
A national organization for North American professional herbalists. Membership consists of professionals, associates, students and benefactors from all paths of herbalism. Members receive a quarterly newsletter and notification of herbal symposiums and other events around the country.

GLOSSARY

Terms of Traditional Chinese Medicine

Aromatic Stomachic: herbs which are aromatic and assist digestion by moving Dampness.

Blood: though broader in definition, it encompasses the physical blood in the body which moistens the tissues, muscles, skin and hair and nourishes cells and organs.

Blood Deficiency: a lack of Blood with signs of anemia, dizziness, scanty menses or amenorrhea, thin emaciated body, spots in the visual field, impaired vision, numb arms or legs, dry skin, hair or eyes, lusterless, pale face and lips, tiredness and poor memory.

Calmative: calms the mind and nerves; for nervous disorders.

Cold: low metabolism.

Cold, Coldness, Cold signs: lowered metabolism with symptoms of Coldness, clear to white bodily secretions, chills, body aches, poor circulation, pale complexion, lethargy, no thirst or sweating, frigidity, impotence, infertility, night time urination, frequent and copious urination, loose stools or diarrhea, undigested food in the stools, poor digestion, lack of appetite, achy pain in joints, slowness of speech, slow movements, low fever but severe chills, aversion to cold and craving for heat and hypo-conditions such as hypo-thyroidism, hypo-adrenalism and hypoglycemic.

Cools Blood: a function of herbs which clears Heat out of the Blood; symptoms include rashes, nosebleed, vomiting, spitting or coughing of blood, blood in the stool or urine, night fevers, delirium and hemorrhage.

Damp, Dampness: excessive Fluids in the body with symptoms of include feelings of heaviness, sluggishness, secretions that are turbid, sluggish, sinking, viscous, copious, slimy, cloudy or sticky, excessive leukorrhea, oozing, purulent skin eruptions, lassitude, edema, abdominal distention, chest fullness, nausea, vomiting, loss of appetite, lack of thirst and achy, heavy, stiff and sore joints.

Damp Heat: a condition of Dampness and Heat with symptoms of thick, greasy yellow secretions and phlegm, jaundice, hepatitis, dysentery, urinary difficulty or pain, furuncles and eczema.

Deficiency: a lack of something, usually Qi, Blood, Yin, Yang or Essence.

Deficiency: a condition of weakness of lack of either Qi, Blood, Fluids, Yin, Yang or Essence.

Deficient Heat: this is the same as Yin Deficiency.

Deficient Yang: see Yang Deficiency.

Deficient Yin: see Yin Deficiency.

Diuretic: eliminates Excess Fluids. Diuretics in Chinese medicine also enhance proper fluid metabolism by increasing absorption of fluids into the deep tissues of the body. Thus, contradictory symptoms of edema and dry skin can be eliminated together with diuretics.

Dryness: characterized by dehydration with symptoms of extreme thirst, dry skin, hair, mouth, lips, nose, throat, dry cough with little phlegm and constipation.

Essence: a highly refined fluid substance which provides the basis of reproduction, development, growth, sexual power, conception, pregnancy and decay in the body.

Excess: a condition of an accumulation of too much of something, either Yin, Yang, Heat, Cold or Fluids.

Excess Cold: a condition of too much Coldness in the body; see Cold.

Excess Heat: a condition of too much Heat in the body; see Heat.

Excess Yang: this is the same as excess Heat with symptoms of high fever, restlessness, red complexion, loud voice, aggressive actions, strong odors, yellow discharges, rapid pulse and hypertension.

Excess Yin: an imbalance of excessive fluids in the body with symptoms of edema, excessive fluid retention, lethargy, a plump or swollen appearance and overall signs of Dampness, and yet these people may have adequate energy.

Exterior: see external.

External: designates the location of an illness to be on the surface of the body; includes colds, flus, fevers, skin eruptions, sore throats and headaches.

False Yang: this is Deficient Heat, or Yin Deficiency, and results in emaciation and weakness with Heat symptoms; this type of Heat symptom occurs because the cooling moistening fluids (Yin) are lacking and so is termed, "false Heat."

Heat, Hot, Heat signs: hyper-metabolism with symptoms of fever with little chills, restlessness, constipation, thirst, dark yellow or scanty urine, craving for cold, aversion to heat and craving for cold, burning digestion, infections, inflammations, dryness, red face, sweating, strong appetite, hemorrhaging and blood in vomit, urine, stool, nose or mucus, strong orders, sticky or thick yellow bodily excretions, irritability, scanty dark yellow urination, swollen, red and painful eyes or gums and red skin eruptions, and hyper-conditions such as hypertension.

Hot: overly active metabolism.

Interior: see Internal.

Internal: designates the location of an illness to be inside the body; includes conditions affection the Qi, Blood,Fluids and Internal Organs.

Jing: see Essence.

Meridians: the pathways along which Qi circulates to supply energy and nourishment to the Organs and the surface of the body.

Moves Blood: see regulates Blood.

Nervine: strengthens the nerves; for conditions of nervousness, anxiety, insomnia, emotional instability, pain, cramps, spasms, tremors, stress, muscle tension and epilepsy.

Organs: the organs in TCM are different than in Western medicine: Organs have energetic rather than physical functions; they are dynamic interrelated processes which occur throughout every level of the body. Yin organs include the Heart, Lungs, Kidneys, Spleen and Liver; Yang organs include the Small Intestines, Large Intestines, Urinary Bladder, Stomach and Gallbladder.

Qi: energy, life force; Qi circulates, protects, holds, transforms and warms.

Qi Deficiency: a lack of Qi or energy with signs of low vitality, lethargy, weakness, shortness of breath, slow metabolism, frequent colds and flu with slow recovery, low soft voice, spontaneous sweating, frequent urination, palpitations.

Regulates Blood: smoothes the flow of Blood in the body; symptoms include bleeding, hemorrhaging, excessive menstruation, localized stabbing pain, abdominal masses, ulcers, abscesses and painful menstruation.

Regulates Energy: smoothes the flow of Qi in the body; symptoms include dull aching pain, abdominal distention and pain, belching, gas, acid regurgitation, nausea, vomiting, stifling sensation in chest, pain in the sides, loss of appetite, depression, hernial pain, irregular menstruation, swollen, tender breasts and wheezing.

Sedative: sedate, calm the mind and Spirit; for insomnia, anxiety, nervousness, irritability, fright and hysteria.

Seven Emotions: the Seven Emotions are a major cause of illness. They are: sadness, fright, fear, grief, anger, joy (overexcitability) and melancholy.

Shen: the overall Spirit and mental faculties of a person, including enthusiasm for life, charisma and capacity to behave appropriately, be responsive, speak coherently, think and form ideas and live a life of joy and spiritual fulfillment.

Spirit: see Shen.

Stomach Heat: a condition of too much Heat in the Stomach with signs of bad breath, gum bleeding and swelling, mouth ulcers, frontal headaches, burning sensation in the stomach region and extreme thirst.

TCM: abbreviation for Traditional Chinese Medicine.

Tonification, Tonify: nourishes, strengthens, builds and improves the condition of either Qi, Blood, Yin or Yang in the body.

Wind: Wind causes movement with symptoms of spasms, twitches, dizziness, spasms, rigidity of the muscles, deviation of the eye and mouth, stiff or rigid neck and shoulders, tremors, convulsions, vertigo and sudden onset of colds, chills, fever, stuffy nose and headache.

Yang: the body's capacity to generate and maintain warmth and circulation.

Yang Deficiency: : a condition of Coldness due to lack of the heating quality of Yang; symptoms include lethargy, coldness, edema, poor digestion, lower back pain, the type of constipation caused by weak peristaltic motion and lack of libido.

Yin: the body's substance, including Blood and all other Fluids in the body; these nurture and moisten the Organs and tissues.

Yin Deficiency: this is Deficient Heat and results in emaciation and weakness with Heat symptoms such as night sweats, insomnia, a burning sensation in the palms, soles and chest, malar flush, afternoon fever, nervous exhaustion, dry throat, dry eyes, blurred vision, dizziness and nervous tension.

Zang Fu: the theory of the Organs; the hollow Organs (Fu) which transport and the solid Organs (Zang) which store.

General Index

GENERAL INDEX

GENERAL INDEX

GENERAL INDEX

INDEX OF CHINESE HERBAL FORMULAS

INDEX OF CHINESE HERBAL FORMULAS

INDEX OF CHINESE HERBAL FORMULAS

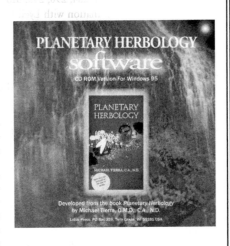

Herbs and other natural health products and information are often available at natural food stores or metaphysical bookstores. If you cannot find what you need locally, you can contact one of the following sources of supply.

Sources of Supply:

The following companies have an extensive selection of useful products and a long track-record of fulfillment. They have natural body care, aromatherapy, flower essences, crystals and tumbled stones, homeopathy, herbal products, vitamins and supplements, videos, books, audio tapes, candles, incense and bulk herbs, teas, massage tools and products and numerous alternative health items across a wide range of categories.

WHOLESALE:

Wholesale suppliers sell to stores and practitioners, not to individual consumers buying for their own personal use. Individual consumers should contact the RETAIL supplier listed below. Wholesale accounts should contact with business name, resale number or practitioner license in order to obtain a wholesale catalog and set up an account.

Lotus Light Enterprises, Inc.
PO Box 1008 CTM
Silver Lake, WI 53170 USA
262 889 8501 (phone)
262 889 8591 (fax)
800 548 3824 (toll free order line)

RETAIL:

Retail suppliers provide products by mail order direct to consumers for their personal use. Stores or practitioners should contact the wholesale supplier listed above.

Internatural
PO Box 489 CTM
Twin Lakes, WI 53181 USA
800 643 4221 (toll free order line)
262 889 8581 office phone
EMAIL: internatural@internatural.com
WEB SITE: www.internatural.com

Web site includes an extensive annotated catalog of more than 14,000 items that can be ordered "on line" for your convenience 24 hours a day, 7 days a week.

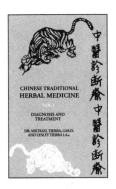
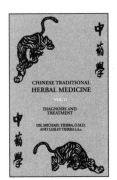

BIOMAGNETIC
and Herbal Therapy
Dr. Michael Tierra

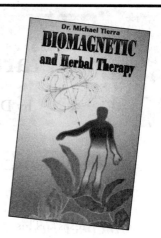

Trade Paper
ISBN 978-0-9149-5533-7
108 pp $10.95

Magnetic energy is the structural force of the universe. In this book the respected herbalist and healer, Dr. Michael Tierra, enlightens us on the healing influence of commercially available magnets for many conditions and describes the sometimes miraculous relief from such problems as joint pain, skin diseases, acidity, blood pressure, tumors, kidney, liver and thyroid problems, and more. Magnetizing herbs, teas, water and their usage in conjunction with direct placement of magnets for synergistic effectiveness is presented in a systematic, succinct and practical manner for the benefit of the professional and lay person alike. Replete with diagrams and appendices, this is a "how to do" practical handbook for augmenting health and obtaining relief from pain.

The paradigm of health in the future is based on energy flow. This paradigm reaches back to the ancient healing arts of the traditional Chinese, the Ayurvedic and the Native American cultures. It is connected to the work of Hippocrates, the "father" of Western medicine, in ancient Greek culture, and found its way through the herbal and homeopathic science that has flourished in Europe over the last few hundred years.

Dr. Tierra is the author of the all-time best selling herbal *The Way of Herbs* as well as the synthesizing work *Planetary Herbology.* He is a practicing herbalist and educator in the field with a background of studies spanning the Chinese and Ayurvedic, the Native American and the European herbal traditions.

Available at bookstores and natural food stores nationwide or order your copy directly by sending $10.95 plus $2.50 shipping/handling ($.75 s/h for each additional copy ordered at the same time) to:

Lotus Press, PO Box 325, Dept. CTM, Twin Lakes, WI 53181 USA
toll free order line: 800 824 6396   office phone: 262 889 8561
office fax: 262 889 2461   email: lotuspress@lotuspress.com
web site: www.lotuspress.com

Lotus Press is the publisher of a wide range of books and software in the field of alternative health, including Ayurveda, Chinese medicine, herbology, aromatherapy, Reiki and energetic healing modalities. Request our free book catalog.

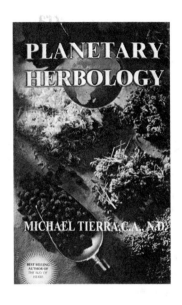

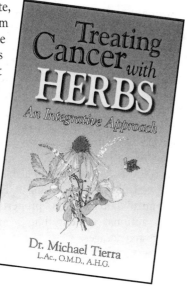